I0888329

SOCIAL JUSTICE AND MEDICAL PRACTICE

How do we understand and respond to the pressing health problems of modern society? Conventional medical practice focuses on the assessment and clinical treatment of immediate health issues presented by individual patients. In contrast, social medicine advocates an equal focus on the assessment and social treatment of underlying social conditions, such as environmental factors, structural violence, and social injustice.

Social Justice and Medical Practice examines the practice of social medicine using extensive life history interviews with a physician practicing this approach in marginalized communities. It presents a case example of social medicine in action, demonstrating how such a practice can be successfully pursued within the context of the existing structure of twenty-first-century medicine. In examining the experience of a physician on the frontlines of reforming healthcare, the book critiques the restrictive nature of the dominant clinical model of medicine and argues for a radically expanded focus for modern-day medical practice.

Social Justice and Medical Practice is a timely intervention during a period when even advanced healthcare systems are facing multiple crises. Lucidly written, it presents a striking alternative and is important reading for students and practitioners of medicine and anthropology, as well as policy makers.

Merrill Singer is a professor in the departments of anthropology and community medicine, at the University of Connecticut, USA. A medical and cultural anthropologist, his research focuses on the social determinants of health inequality, the critical biosocial nature of health, and environmental health. He is recipient of a number of prizes, including the Rudolph Virchow Professional Prize, the Society for Medical Anthropology's Career Award, and the George Foster Memorial Award for Practicing Anthropology.

Rebecca Allen completed a BA in Anthropology at the University of Connecticut, USA, where she was president of the university's chapter of Lambda Alpha, the National Collegiate Honors Society for Anthropology. She is now a medical student at George Washington University, USA.

Advances in Critical Medical Anthropology
Series Editors: Merrill Singer and Pamela Erickson

This book series advances our understanding of the complex and rapidly changing landscape of health, disease, and treatment around the world with original and innovative books in the spirit of critical medical anthropology that exemplify and extend its theoretical and empirical dimensions. Books in the series address topics across the broad range of subjects addressed by medical anthropologists and other scholars and practitioners working at the intersections of social science and medicine.

Titles in series

Drug Effects: Khat in Biocultural and Socioeconomic Perspective
Lisa L. Gezon

Syndemic Suffering: Social Distress, Depression, and Diabetes among Mexican Immigrant Women
Emily Mendenhall

Health Policy in Crisis: Access to Abortion in the Context of Austerity
Bayla Ostrach

Thinking Through Resistance: A study of public oppositions to contemporary global health practice
Nicola Bulled

Social Justice and Medical Practice: Life History of a Physician of Social Medicine
Merrill Singer and Rebecca Allen

www.routledge.com/Advances-in-Critical-Medical-Anthropology/book-series/ACMA

SOCIAL JUSTICE AND MEDICAL PRACTICE

Life History of a Physician of Social Medicine

Merrill Singer and Rebecca Allen

Routledge
Taylor & Francis Group
NEW YORK AND LONDON

First published 2018
by Routledge
605 Third Avenue, New York, NY 10017

and by Routledge
4 Park Square, Milton Park, Abingdon, Oxon OX14 4RN

Routledge is an imprint of the Taylor & Francis Group, an informa business

Library of Congress Cataloging-in-Publication Data
A catalog record for this book has been requested.

ISBN: 978-1-62958-425-6 (hbk)
ISBN: 978-1-62958-426-3 (pbk)
ISBN: 978-1-315-11227-5 (ebk)

Typeset in Bembo
by Swales & Willis Ltd, Exeter, Devon, UK

CONTENTS

ACKNOWLEDGMENTS

William Tootle, graduate student, Department of Anthropology, University of Connecticut, conducted and transcribed interviews for this project with colleagues of Bruce Gould. We thank him for his generosity and notable contributions to this book. The authors would also like to thank the colleagues of Bruce who were willing to take the time out of their busy schedules to be interviewed for this book. Life may be short, but Bruce's life has been both broad and full, and it has been a pleasure getting to learn about it.

INTRODUCTION

A Road Less Taken

The long, hard winter of 2014–15 was finally showing signs of retreating into history as Becca Allen and I drove the short distance from the campus of the University of Connecticut to the site of E. O. Smith High School in Storrs, CT. We had come to hear a talk by celebrated physician/anthropologist and author Paul Farmer, co-founder of Partners in Health and an individual who has emerged both as a very prominent public figure because of his tireless efforts on behalf of the health needs of the world's poor, but also as the best-known anthropologist of our time. Our plans were to meet up with Bruce Gould, the physician and University of Connecticut professor whose life and work is the focus of this book.

Although the school sits immediately next to and is partially surrounded by UConn, as the university is colloquially known, I had never been to E. O. Smith before. The high school is named after Edwin O. Smith, a Connecticut politician who served for almost three decades in the Connecticut House of Representatives. Previous to his lengthy political career, however, Smith had been president of Connecticut Agricultural College, which in 1939 was renamed the University of Connecticut. The relationship between the two educational institutions continues into the present. E. O. Smith students are allowed to take classes at the university free of charge, and receive credit on their academic records for both institutions. Additionally, UConn's Community School of the Arts partners with E.O. Smith to provide a non-traditional educational experience for students who need a smaller and more personalized instructional setting. Louis F. DeLoreto, a UConn graduate, is the principal of the high school. Thus there is a flow of students between the two institutions, and we joined that stream to hear Paul Farmer's talk.

To our surprise, we were actually the first to arrive at the public event, and as a result, the three of us were able to claim seats close to the auditorium stage, near the podium where Farmer would speak. Around us, a growing throng of high school and university students, teachers from the two schools, and community members gathered, several hundred strong. Students from the high school had come as part of the E.O. Smith READS program, which selected as its focus for 2014–15 Tracy Kidder's (2004) book *Mountains Beyond Mountains: The Quest of Dr. Paul Farmer, A Man Who Would Cure the World*. The program, a school-wide initiative, is modeled after UConn READS, further emphasizing relations between the now-sprawling university and the high school it partially encircles. As part of the program, students were given reading assignments and projects based on the award-winning biography in their grades 9–12 English classes, as well as opportunities to participate in conversations about the book and related issues in their other courses. The title of Kidder's book comes from a Haitian proverb: "beyond mountains there are mountains," which has been interpreted to mean that as you solve one problem, another problem looms before you, and so you move on in your life and try to solve that problem as well. In short, the challenges of life are great, but we all must do what we can while we are here on Earth by leading meaningful lives that deeply engage the often punishing social world around us, most notably, in the case of Paul Farmer, by confronting the health problems created around the world by massive social inequality and blatant injustice. Of Farmer, Kidder (2003), a Pulitzer Prize awardee, wrote in the book that he is

> A challenging person, the kind of person whose example can irritate you by making you feel you've never done anything as important, and yet, in his presence, those kinds of feelings tended to vanish. In the past, when I'd imagined a person with credentials like his, I'd imagined someone dour and self-righteous, but he was very friendly and irreverent, and quite funny. He seemed like someone I'd like to know, and I thought that if I did my job well, a reader would feel that way, too.

The goal of the E. O. Smith READS program is to promote college readiness, but more broadly, it seeks to promote life readiness. In selecting Kidder's book, the program embraced an issue that harmonizes with the goals of this book, namely raising the question: what kind of world do you want to live in and how can you help make visions of a better, fairer world a reality? Moreover, who might be a genuine exemplar for living such a life?

An important link in the extended social network connecting the globally active Farmer to a high school in the semi-rural and legally designated village of Storrs, CT was the co-sponsor of his talk, an organization known as Roots of Development that helps marginalized populations acquire the organizational skills and financial resources to achieve the level of empowerment needed to build and strengthen their impoverished communities. Roots of Development traces its origin to a trip its co-founder and executive director, Chad Bissonnette, took to Gran Sous, on the island of La Gonave, Haiti while an undergraduate student at American University in Washington, DC. Bissonnette grew up near Storrs and both of his parents were E.O. Smith teachers. Several years ago, the high school embraced the work of Roots of Development by holding fund raisers and hosting Ending

Apathy rallies among students. These events, which included speakers from various activist organizations and informational booths, were designed to inform students about the many issues facing people around the globe. Bissonnette, who spoke at an End Apathy rally in 2013, was able to link the high school with the always busy and often globe-trotting Farmer because of their respective development and health efforts in Haiti, the poorest country in the Western Hemisphere, despite its earlier history as the breadbasket of the French colonial regime. Moreover, like the individual who is the subject of this book, Bissonnette and Farmer early on in their lives made "all in" decisions, to swim against the tide of complacency, to live meaningful and engaged lives in a troubled and unjust world.

Specifically, this book addresses a fundamental question in contemporary healthcare: how do we understand and respond to the pressing health problems of society? The conventional biomedical response to this query involves the practice of a type of care that is based on careful clinical assessment of the immediate health issues presented by each individual patient and the provision of (usually) science-based medical treatment drawn from an arsenal of pharmaceutical, surgical, and other established strategies. As Paul Farmer and colleagues (2006) assert, "the holy grail of modern medicine remains the search for the molecular basis of disease." While there are benefits to the conventional approach to medicine, there are significant costs as well. Thus Farmer et al. (2006) add: "While the practical yield of . . . circumscribed inquiry has been enormous, exclusive focus on molecular-level phenomena has contributed to the increasing 'desocialization' of scientific inquiry: a tendency to ask only biological questions about what are in fact biosocial phenomena."

By contrast with the entrenched and dominant clinical model of medicine, a model that has been critiqued as contributing to a maintenance of the status quo, social medicine places an equal level of focus on the social conditions and structural inequalities that generate and exacerbate health problems, including social stigmatization and discrimination, adverse physical factors in built environments (e.g., overcrowding, impoverished neighborhoods, and inadequate diets), structural violence (a concept that has gained broad usage through the writings of Paul Farmer), and social injustice. Structural violence and related inequalities contribute to a biology of inequality, powered by the ways social disparity and deprivation get "under the skin" and are inscribed by disease on body systems. In other words, "we literally incorporate biologically the world around us," a world we must study to understand fully just "who and what is responsible for population patterns of health, disease, and well-being, as manifested in present, past and changing social inequalities in health" (Krieger 2007: 668). As summarized by the Prevention Institute (2002:3);

> The chief underlying cause of health disparities is increasingly understood to be social and economic inequality, i.e., social bias and institutional racism, limited education, poverty, and related environmental conditions that either directly produce ill health or promote unhealthy behaviors that lead to poor health.

Globally, this understanding has been supported by the findings of a growing body of reach (Mackenbach et al. 2008, Stringhini et al. 2010). Exemplary is a multi-cohort study and meta-analysis that included individual-level data on socioeconomic status drawn from seven high-income World Health Organization member countries, indexed by a set of risk factors (high alcohol intake, physical inactivity, current smoking, hypertension, diabetes, and obesity), and mortality, for a total population of 1,751,479 (Stringhini et al. 2017). The study found that low socioeconomic status was associated with a 2.1-year reduction in life expectancy between ages 40 and 85 years of age. The problem with many international programs to lower mortality, the authors argue, is that they fail to address powerful upstream structural determinants of health.

A reflection of this pattern is the disproportionate disease and mortality burden of African Americans. People of African descent in the US have a mortality rate for all causes that is 1.5 times that of Whites (adjusted by age) (Keppel et al. 2002). Cardiovascular diseases, and their precursor conditions, like hypertension and diabetes, are major contributors to Black/White differences in mortality rates. Thus, the risk of dying from heart disease is 1.3 times greater for African Americans compared to Whites (Mensah et al. 2005). In turn, African Americans are 1.8 times more likely to develop diabetes (CDC 2007) and rates of hypertension are between 1.5 and 2 times higher among African Americans (Mensah et al. 2005). There is a significant body of evidence indicating that these disparities have a social origin involving biosocial linkages that have been found to exist between social discrimination and related structural violence (including poverty), maternal stress during pregnancy, low birth weight, and adult onset of precursor diseases and heart disease (Kuzawa and Sweet 2009). These factors—and not genetic differences (as prevailing racial categories are very poor predictors of genetic patterns)—contribute to a significant lifelong deficit in the health and well-being of African Americans compared to Whites and to notably higher rates of cardiovascular disease. Indeed, it is accurate to say that

> Social inequality kills. It deprives individuals and communities of a healthy start in life, increases their burden of disability and disease, and brings early death. Poverty and discrimination, inadequate medical care, and violation of human rights all act as powerful social determinants of who lives and who dies, at what age, and with what degree of suffering. (Krieger 2005:15)

As discussed more fully in Chapter 1, social medicine traces to the work of Rudolf Virchow and his medical report emphasizing the economic, social, and cultural factors driving the 1848 typhus epidemic in Upper Silesia in Imperial Germany, Rather than recommending a narrow medical solution (e.g., sending more doctors or building more hospitals), he proposed a program of significant social reconstructions that would lead to full employment for laborers, decent wages, the organization of agricultural cooperatives, and universal education (Taylor 1985). In this vein, contemporary practitioners of social medicine seek to not only address the immediate health problems presented by patients but also the debilitating structural factors that lead to much disease and poor health.

In short, this book accentuates the fact that society as a whole must decide what type of medicine it wants. Unfortunately, given existing structural inequalities, not everyone has an equal voice in this discussion. A narrow clinical approach to health dominates because it generates an enormous amount of wealth—through the sale of treatments and insurance—for a powerful, well-heeled sector of society. While the United States has the dubious distinction of spending far more per capita on healthcare than any other nation in the world, it "ranks behind most [developed] countries on many measures of health outcomes, quality, and efficiency," with poor scores on the three established indicators of healthy lives: mortality amenable to medical care, infant mortality, and healthy life expectancy at age 60 (Davis et al. 2014:1). Problems in the quality of care and care access are especially notable among the poor and among marginalized ethnic minorities. In a recent assessment of the U.S. healthcare system, the country was found to have the worst record among industrialized nations in terms of equity. According to the report:

> Americans with below-average incomes were much more likely than their counterparts in other countries to report not visiting a physician when sick; not getting a recommended test, treatment, or follow-up care; or not filling a prescription or skipping doses when needed because of costs. On each of these indicators, one-third or more lower-income adults in the U.S. said they went without needed care because of costs in the past year. (Davis et al. 2014:1)

In such a system of massive inequality, at the personal level each individual physician must decide what type of doctor to be. Here we do not refer to medical specialty decisions but rather how to think about the source of health problems and, based on this consideration, how to practice medicine. The same is true of all healthcare workers whatever their area of focus, including nurses, dentists, and the array of other healthcare providers that populate the prevailing biomedical system. One can practice conventional biomedicine, focusing narrowly on the clinical presentation of the health complaints of patients providing the level of care allowable by for-profit insurance companies, engaging thereby in disease management rather than the promotion of health and social well-being, or one can choose to recognize and act on a understanding of health as socially constructed by the experiences and conditions of life. The latter option, leads healthcare providers to the realization that in this country

> black people pay for racist oppression with life spans ten years shorter than that of whites. Poor and oppressed minorities have 25 percent fewer successful encounters with the healthcare system than more privileged groups. Meanwhile, the rate of death or other harmful outcomes increases with the level of poverty in illnesses like coronary heart disease, cancer of all forms, obesity, growth retardation in children, unplanned pregnancies, and maternal mortality. (Levins 2000:6)

Inequalities in health grow even greater as the focus shifts from developed to developing nations, and hence we live in a world in which the wealth and unparalleled lifestyles of the upper classes of the West are paid for by the poverty and poor health of people living in developing nations. With reference to access to healthy diets, for example, as anthropologists Gewertz and Errington (2010:2) observe, "the foods on our plates are often obtained at the expense of foods not on other people's plates."

Unfortunately, while there are various personal accounts of the experience of becoming or working as a physician (e.g., Austin 2009, Colins 2006, Verghese 1994), at present, existing and prospective medical students have few alternative role models beside traditional individual patient/disease-focused practice. One such unconventional role model is exemplified by Paul Farmer. Farmer, as noted, has been described as "the man who would cure the world," in Kidder's biography. In truth, of course, very few physicians or other healthcare providers can be like Paul Farmer, as few current or prospective medical students can realistically hope to achieve his level of international recognition, media presence, and associated impact. Most physicians, instead, lead local lives and engage with homegrown healthcare challenges. And yet, as this books seeks to show, there are alternative, achievable role models at this level too—physicians who venture outside sanitized clinics into the gritty streets of real world human anguish and social suffering. And, as Bruce knows from the calls he gets from medical students, there are many who want an alternative, socially conscious and compassionate path to medical practice.

Based on extensive life-history interviews with Bruce Gould, this book presents one such alternative model of biomedical practice within the context of the existing structure of twenty-first-century medicine and in light of the consequential current unequal distribution of health, living and working conditions, and medical access. The type of social medicine that Bruce practices is informed by a keen awareness of the social origins of health and well-being. It is not a new approach, however, but dates to the early 1800s and to the launching of the Industrial Revolution. As noted, it came into being during an era in which it was difficult to ignore the extent to which capitalist production had impoverished workers, creating an entwined world of poverty, misery, and disease. The most famous early advocate of social medicine, Rudolf Virchow, is often cited by critical medical social scientists for his assertion that "politics is nothing more than medicine on a grand scale." He called for embedding social justice as a central theme in medical practice.

A commitment to this view of medical practice characterizes the approach adopted by Bruce during the challenging process of becoming a physician. Bruce received his M.D. from the State University of New York (SUNY) Upstate Medical University at Syracuse in 1979. He majored in biology as an undergraduate at Cornell University College of Agriculture. His internal medicine internship was completed at the University of Massachusetts Medical Center in 1980, followed by a two-year residency in internal medicine at the same institution, and one year as the Chief Medical Resident. He now serves as a professor and associate dean for primary care at the University of Connecticut's School of Medicine.

As this "bioblurb" description suggests, Bruce has a fairly conventional biomedical pedigree. Graduates of the SUNY Upstate Medical University—as described on the university's website—are expected to demonstrate safe, effective, timely, efficient and equitable patient-centered care that promotes health, quality of life, prevention of illness, and treatment of disease. This includes an assortment of skills, including eliciting an accurate history, performing an appropriate physical examination, constructing a comprehensive problem list and differential diagnosis, developing prioritized intervention and management plans using current scientific knowledge, and interpreting clinical, laboratory, radiologic and pathologic data, that are expected of all physicians of modern clinical biomedicine. Similarly, the University of Massachusetts Medical Center, while expressly committed to training physicians to work in the public sector and in underserved areas of Massachusetts, embraces a standard approach to individual patient-focused biomedical training. None the less, despite traversing traditional pathways to becoming a physician, over the years Bruce has earned a local reputation as a committed advocate for public health, primary care, and preventative social medicine.

Until the later months of this study, Bruce carried out his clinical work as medical director of the Burgdorf Health Center, a community clinic serving the underserved population in Hartford's north end. He had been in this position for 27 years until 2016. Then, as described in Chapter 6, an opportunity arose for him to take a new job as the medical director of the Practice Transformation Network at the Community Health Center Association of Connecticut (CHCACT), a federally funded program designed to help clinicians improve their service to patients, in which he would be able to help the Burgdorf and other community-based clinical centers that treat low-income populations. Despite this job change and his new responsibilities, he also continued to serve as director of the Connecticut Area Health Education Center Program and medical director of Hartford's Department of Health and Human Services. At the same time, he is the founder of and advisor to the Mobile Free Migrant Farm Worker Clinic, which has served Connecticut's low-income migrant farm worker population since 1998. He also helped to create the Youth Health Services Corps, an award-winning program that trains and places high school students as volunteers in healthcare provider agencies. Through this program, students are able to explore health careers while they acquire real life experience working with disadvantaged populations in community healthcare settings.

Reflecting his tireless commitment to improving health, Bruce has, in addition, long been involved in the development and delivery of the University of Connecticut Medical School's quality improvement and patient safety curriculum, as well as its nutrition curriculum. He helped establish the University of Connecticut's Urban Service Track, a special mentorship program designed to produce doctors, dentists, nurses, and pharmacists dedicated to serving Connecticut's urban underserved populations, and the Youth Health Services Corps, a nationally recognized recruitment program that trains and places high school students as volunteers in various healthcare agencies. Moreover, Bruce has not backed away from a decades-long struggle to protect health services for the poor in Hartford, despite the readiness of dominant medical institutions and prominent local players in the healthcare arena to cut costs by downsizing or shutting down programs and venues that care for marginalized sectors of the community. In short, transcending the conventional ways of being a doctor within the sanitized institutions of biomedicine, Bruce has chosen a different pathway that embraces both a sharp critique of medicine as it is usually practiced in the US and the dismal direction medicine is headed in the contemporary world, as well as an alternative vision of what medicine might be in the service of social transformation and justice.

For Bruce, the fact that he has consciously chosen to strive throughout his life and career to be a certain kind of person, and the fact he has been guided in this striving by particular values, are all metaphorically expressed in his favorite poem, "The Way It Is" by William Stafford. That this poem has such deep resonance with Bruce points to the ways he has tried long and hard to steer his life course with meaning and purpose. Despite setbacks and endless challenges, in the face of frustrating and often powerful opposition, and even in moments of self-doubt and personal uncertainty, Bruce has fought to never let go of his guiding thread, his embrace of the moral obligation to struggle for health and social equity for the poor, the underserved, and the publically maligned. Others, he knows, may not share his commitments, but his thread continues, it defines him and it leads him. It is, to again cite words of William Stafford, the hidden river at the core of his being.

Notably, Bruce's vision is shared with Paul Farmer, although the two had never met before the event at E. O. Smith High School. In the minutes prior to the program beginning, however, as people filed into the high school auditorium, Farmer spotted me—a fellow medical anthropologist—in the audience and came over to say hello. As a result, these two practitioners of social medicine were introduced, fulfilling my own imagined choreographing of the opening of this book. After Farmer's talk—which addressed the ebola epidemic in Western Africa in light of the social origins of disease—a diminutive but unintimidated high school freshman began her question by stating "Dr. Farmer you have been a great inspiration for me." While Farmer is an inspiration for many people, including many medical students around the country and beyond, it is, this book argues, actors on the local stages of social medicine, like Bruce Gould, who offer immediate and graspable models for those who choose to put people first and seek to build a social world founded on principles of collective responsibility, caring, and equity.

This model is twofold. On the one hand, it encompasses a particular kind of doctor/patient relationship. The orientation underlying this relationship, the kind that doctors like Bruce or Farmer strive to establish, is nicely captured (under the most difficult of circumstances) in the commencement address of Dr. Kent Bradley at the 2015 Indiana University School of Medicine (National Public Radio 2015). Bradley contracted ebola while working as a physician in Liberia and was the first person to receive ZMapp, an experimental drug used in the treatment of the disease:

> In the first seven weeks of treating patients with ebola, we had only one survivor; one survivor and nearly 20 deaths. Losing so many patients certainly was difficult. But it didn't make me feel like a failure as a physician because I had learned that there's a lot more to being a physician than curing illness. In fact, that isn't even the most important thing we do. The most important thing we do is to enter into the suffering of others. And in the midst of what was becoming the worst ebola epidemic in history, we were showing compassion to people during the most desperate and trying times of their lives.

Rather than a disease or diseased organ system, a patient in this model is seen as a fully human, intelligent, and emotional being, a being of meanings and feelings, while the doctor does not remain at a distance as a neutral expert engaged only in a sterile clinical diagnostic and disease treatment processes.

On the other hand, patients are not seen as isolated beings devoid of families and communities, or as people who are not at every moment being impacted by living conditions, working environments, social arrangements, and the consequences of living in an unequal social system colored by injustices, indignities, and suffering. And these wider conditions, which are examined here in some detail, are seen as every bit as important and as much medical concerns as pathogens, inflammation, genetics, fever, or failing organs.

1

ALTERNATIVES IN MEDICAL PRACTICE AND THEIR SOCIAL AND PERSONAL IMPLICATIONS

Wherever the art of medicine is loved, there is also a love of humanity.

Hippocrates

A Molecular Understanding of Disease

Many technical changes and modification of points of view notwithstanding, the central thrust of biomedicine, from research to training, to clinical practice, remains centered on the molecular understanding of disease, as it has since the mid-nineteenth century. The roots of this way of thinking about human health extend deeper in time to the fifteenth century, with the rise of the practice of anatomical dissection in Europe and the belief that opening up corpses would reveal "the causes of pathology lurking in the body" (Lock and Nguyen 2010: 29). In the eighteenth century, medical practitioners began to see the body as an integrated system that could be clinically examined using agreed-upon procedures to determine the nature and location of disease. This conception was significantly advanced with the rise of "germ theory" in the following century, including the view that specific infectious diseases were caused by specific microorganisms that invaded the body. The end result, as Candia, Banavar, and Losert (2013: 3) affirm, was that "gaining a molecular understanding of disease [became] the holy grail of current biomedical research and related interdisciplinary fields."

In clinical practice, as patients know well from personal visits to their doctors, this approach is actualized as individually focused physician review and recording of patient symptoms, physical examination, and the use of internal body data collection using various technologies (e.g., radiographic imaging, laboratory tests) to determine if a disease is present, to establish its nature, and to decide on a treatment course. Underlying conventional clinical practice is an understanding—or path for comprehending—what disease is from a biomedical perspective. This understanding is constructed within contemporary biomedicine as the product of a joint project carried out by the fields of molecular biology (which examines the components that make up cells and organisms), biochemistry (which studies the biomolecules of the body and the chemistry behind biological processes), and genetics (especially the analysis of deviance from normal gene patterning). The end result of this approach to health knowledge is a particular way of thinking about disease as a disruption, breakdown, or error at the molecular level that has adverse consequences at higher levels of complexity, especially the cellular and organismic levels.

The Patient-Centering of Healthcare?

In recent years, however, there has been much internal healthcare establishment and media discussion of a paradigm shift in biomedicine that includes a broadening of understanding about the nature of disease. This shift involves a new emphasis on what has been called patient-centered care that is delivered by a multidisciplinary provider team that incorporates concerns beyond the biological level (Anderson 2014, Beck 2015). Various factors have pushed for change. Most notable was popular dissatisfaction with rising medical costs.

In 2002, the average household was spending about $2,300, or just under 5 percent of its total income, on healthcare. This was an increase from 1999, when the average was under $2,000, or about 4.5 percent of household income. As medical costs continued to increase, employers began shifting more costs to their employees, forcing people in growing numbers to drop health insurance coverage or reduce their purchase of other goods and services. Employer healthcare premiums increased by almost 75 percent in the years 2000–05 and employee contributions for individual and family health insurance plans increased at about the same rate (Kaiser Family Foundation 2016). Smaller companies began to cancel work-based health insurance. As a result, the rate of coverage of employees at smaller companies declined from 68 percent in 2000 to 59 percent in 2005. Overall the proportion of employees who received health coverage from their employer dropped by 4 percentage points and, between 2000 and 2004, the rate of people without insurance for the entire year grew by 1.5 percentage points (Gould 2005). As Elise Gould (2005) notes "many prime-age working adults were left stranded by the drop in coverage and fell into the ranks of the uninsured. Middle-income Americans between the ages of 25 and 54 were 26.7% more likely to be uninsured in 2004 than in 2000."

The Commonwealth Fund Biennial Health Insurance Survey in 2003 showed that over 75 million Americans (or 37 percent of the adult population) were having difficulty paying their medical bills, and many people were beginning to accumulate medical debt. This led people to not seek needed care and suffer the health consequences. Specifically, the study found that almost two-thirds of people with either a medical bill or debt problem were forced to not get needed care. This was three times bigger than the rate of care avoidance in households that were not enduring health-related financial difficulties. Nearly one of every three adults in the US (approximately 61 million people) reported that they had problems paying medical bills in 2003 (Doty et al. 2005).

Suffering from medical debt also impacted other issues faced by families. A survey of low- and middle-income households found that half reported having medical debt and a quarter of those reported subsequent housing problems as a result (Seifert 2005). Himmelstein and colleagues (2005) studied individuals who filed for bankruptcy in five federal courts and found that about half reported medical factors pushed them into debt. In a follow-up national study, Himmelstein and colleagues (2009) found that over 60 percent of individual bankruptcies were of medical origin, with most people (92 percent) succumbing to debts of over $5,000. Over the period of these two studies (2001–07), the proportion of bankruptcies attributed to medical bills rose by just below 50 percent. Moreover, a telephone survey by the Access Project revealed that low- and middle-income households had to turn to credit cards to pay for medical care, raising their overall debt and increasing their economic vulnerability (Zeldin and Rukavina 2007). Although uninsured respondents had the highest levels of credit card debt, even those with health insurance were not completely exempt. Kohn and colleagues (2005) examined the scope and consequences of medical costs among people living in Kansas and found that medical bills were exhausting family savings and sending households into crushing debt. The result of these dire developments was a rising cry nationally for reform and relief from the far-reaching consequences of rising medical costs.

By 2007, the US had the highest healthcare costs relative to the size of its economy of any in the world, and yet almost 50 million citizens (approximately 16 percent of the population) lacked health insurance coverage (U.S. Census Bureau 2008). Lack of health insurance coverage can be dire. In 2009, a study by researchers at Harvard University (Wilper et al. 2009) found almost 45,000 excess deaths annually in the US among Americans lacking health insurance. Uninsured adults have been found to be at least 25 percent more likely to die prematurely than adults who have private health insurance. This is in no small part because the uninsured are six times more like to go without medical screenings that might detect significant illness in a timely manner, and they are much less likely to have received preventive care. Consequently, the uninsured are more likely to be diagnosed with a disease in an advanced stage than insured individuals. Ironically, in the end, they are forced to pay more for medical care, by as much as 2.5 times, than the insured (Families USA 2012). In his successful run for the presidency, Barack Obama emphasized the need for healthcare reform to cut costs and extend health insurance coverage. This stance was reflected in the passage of the federal Patient Protection and Affordable Care Act (ACA), or so-called "Obamacare," which was signed into law in 2010 and is discussed more fully in Chapter 2. In addition to extending coverage, the new law required that essential health benefits include mental health, preventive and wellness services, and chronic disease management, placing legal pressure on the healthcare system for further reform.

Yet, the ACA notwithstanding, current estimates do not paint a rosy picture. National health spending increases in the US for the period between 2015 and

2025 are projected to average 5.8 percent or about 1.3 percentage points faster growth than the gross domestic product. By the end of this period, healthcare will represent 20.1 percent of the total economy based on the use of actuarial and econometric modeling methods used by health economists (Keehan et al. 2016).

Unfairness

Another factor pressing for change has been the great health inequalities found in American society. As Oberlander (2006: 246) stresses, "Unfairness is arguably a cornerstone of the U.S. health care system." The 2001 report on healthcare issued by the Institute of Medicine (2000) emphasized that the healthcare delivery system in the US does not provide consistent, high-quality medical care to all people. Rather, and not surprisingly for those familiar with the healthcare system, the report noted that quality of care was found to vary by gender, ethnicity, geographic location, and socioeconomic status. The following year, based on a review of over a hundred studies, the Institute of Medicine (2002) issued a follow-up report entitled "Unequal Treatment: Confronting Racial and Ethnic Disparities in Health Care," that concluded that racial and ethnic minorities in the United States are less likely to receive routine medical procedures and more likely to experience a lower quality of health services. Healthcare inequality, the report pointed out, exists across ethnic lines even among people with similar incomes, insurance coverage, and medical conditions. Thus the report indicated African Americans and Hispanics are less likely to be given appropriate heart medication or receive bypass surgery compared to Whites with similar cardiac conditions. Further, they are less likely to receive dialysis or transplants when suffering from kidney disease. Use of cancer diagnostic tests and established treatments were also found to not be equitably used. As a result of such findings, Alan Nelson, the former president of the American Medical Association and chair of the committee that oversaw the writing of the report, stated: "The real challenge lies not in debating whether disparities exist, because the evidence is overwhelming, but in developing and implementing strategies to reduce and eliminate them" (Roach 2002: 26).

The Social Gradient

Mounting research findings on the importance of social factors in health has played a role pushing for a rethinking of the dominant biomedical paradigm. A key figure in directing attention to the social determinants of health was Michael Marmot, Professor of Epidemiology and Public Health at the University College of London. During his career, Marmot has conducted trail-breaking work on the role of social and economic inequality in health. As part of this effort, he examined the findings from the famous Whitehall studies of British civil servants. The original Whitehall Study was an investigation of cardiovascular disease prevalence and mortality rates among male civil servants between the ages of 20 and 64. A second study, the Whitehall II Study, examined the health of over 10,000 civil servants aged 35–55.

In his analysis, Marmot found that the lower the employment grade and income of a public employee the higher was his or her risk from most causes of death, a phenomenon called the "social gradient" (Marmot et al. 1978, Marmot et al. 1991a, Marmot et al. 1991b). Notably, even middle-class individuals have poorer health than those above them in the socioeconomic hierarchy, while those in the lowest ranks of employment have the worst health. Expanding on this insight, in 1998, Wilkerson and Marmot (1998), and members of the International Centre for Health and Society at University College London, published "The Solid Facts," a research-based policy statement on how social conditions—like the quality of one's neighborhood of residence—can impact health. In the Scottish city of Glasgow, for instance, research shows that people who live in poor districts have a life expectancy that is twelve years shorter than those dwelling in affluent districts (NHS Health Scotland 2004). Similarly, in the US, African American men who live in poor neighborhoods tend to live much shorter lives than wealthier White men living in more affluent neighborhoods. In Washington, DC, for example, in 1990, the life expectancy gap between White and Black men was 14.4 years and has not radically changed since then (Friedman and Jennings 2013). Among technologically developed nations, people living in the US have the second highest risk of dying from noncommunicable diseases like diabetes and the fourth highest risk of dying from communicable or infectious diseases (World Health Organization 2011). While death rates from noncommunicable diseases like those of the cardiovascular system have everywhere been in decline, it is less the case in the US. In fact, higher mortality is characteristic of the US across multiple categories of diseases, including respiratory diseases, endocrine disorders, congenital anomalies, and neuropsychiatric conditions. The US also has a dramatically higher rate of death from violence, especially gun-related violence. In 2003, the rate of homicide in the US was just under seven times higher than other wealthy countries, but the rate of gun-related homicide was almost twenty times higher (Richardson and Hemenway 2011). As a result of these cross-country differences in mortality rates, there are large differences in life expectancy at birth among wealthy nations. In 2007, men living in Switzerland and women living in Japan had the longest life expectancies by gender, respectively. The US, by contrast, ranked last among males and next to last among females. This translates into shorter lives for people in the US by approximately 3.7 years for males and 5.2 years for females compared to other rich countries (Ho and Preston 2011). Within-country mortality variances also are of note. For example, African American infants in the US are more than twice as likely as White infants to die before their first birthday (National Center for Health Statistics 2012). Among African American males who have fewer than 12 years of education, life expectancy in 2008 was 14.2 years shorter than for White males with 16 or more years of education (Olshansky et al. 2012).

Based on widespread interest in their policy statement, Wilkinson and Marmot subsequently were asked by the World Health Organization Regional Office for Europe to produce an updated edition (Wilkinson and Marmot 2003). The level of interest in the new version of "Solid Facts" is indicated by the fact that in the first year after it was posted online it received over 200,000 downloads (Marmot and Wilkinson 2005). In 2005, Marmot chaired the World Health Organization's Commission on Social Determinants of Health, which issued the impactful report *Closing the Gap in a Generation* (Commission on Social Determinants of Health 2008). Three years later, he appeared in the widely watched four-hour documentary film series *Unnatural Causes: Is Inequality Making Us Sick?* (California Newsreel 2008), which examined the social determinants of health based heavily on Marmot's work on the Whitehall Studies. In 2015, he published the book *The Health Gap: The Challenge of an Unequal World* (Marmot 2015), which assembled data from around the globe to support a call for a radical change in the conventional biomedical understanding of health by addressing the societal imbalances in power, finances, and resources that create health inequity. The work of Marmot and colleagues is but emblematic of the large body of research and theory affirming the need to address social determinants to improve health; in short, it supports the need for a new consideration of social medicine.

In light of the growing recognition of nonbiological influences on health, the Medical College Admission Test (MCAT), the gateway to qualifying for medical school admission, began to significantly increase the number of questions it asks about psychological and social factors in health. Further evidence of change in this direction is the fact that, compared to 25 years ago, the humanities now play a larger role in the medical education curriculum, as well as in the questions asked on the MCAT. Moreover, as part of accreditation, medical schools are now required to teach future doctors about core skills in patient-provider communication, the health impacts of prevailing societal inequalities, the role in the health-related behavior of patient culture(s), and the effect of provider bias on effective care delivery.

From the Trenches

Despite these changes, a question remains: how significant and deep-seated are the reforms that have occurred in biomedicine and its perspective in recent years? Has the paradigm really shifted to a new way of thinking about and responding to health issues? Or, as some maintain, have things only been changed enough in small ways to avoid changing at all in big ways? Alternatively, have things actually gotten worse?

In Bruce's view, based on his experience in the trenches at a clinic that serves poor and ethnic minority patients in the inner city, our healthcare system is now dysfunctional. In part, from his perspective, the problems are embedded in the structure of society, in expressions of structural violence like poverty, lack of food security, and unhealthy living conditions, and in part in the institutional racism that governs access to care. As he sees it, many cities across the country, including Hartford, CT, where the clinic he has worked in is located, are broken. Laying out his vision, he says: "My impulse is to say we have to fix Hartford. People [in positions of authority] get all concerned, and say it's not politically correct to call it broken. If you say it's not broken then you're living under a rock." The alternative, the way things should be headed, he asserts, is through the development with those living in the neighborhoods of an evidence-based, prioritized, intersectoral plan that addresses not only health problems in the clinic but the structural problems in those neighborhoods and the wider society that give rise to many of the health problems and health disparities he sees in his patients. What is needed is not a scattershot focus on this one problem or that isolated issue, or an approach that is superficial and only produces temporary or minor improvements—a tactic Bruce, referring to the arcade game, calls the "whack-a-mole" plan—but rather a systematic approach to creating "a healthier city in all aspects." To do this, he maintains, "we need to rebuild the health care system and have adequate resources in places that serve underserved populations so you can assure that people not only have access to health care and medications, but also to adequate housing, healthy food, quality education, jobs . . . that you're addressing social determinants, that you're looking at where they live, and that you can assure that people have the tools and resources they need" to stay healthy. What is needed, in short, is social medicine.

The Alternative of Social Medicine

While recognizing the contributions of conventional biomedicine, social medicine provides an alternative founded on a recognition of the social origins of health and illness. What precisely is this alternative, the one that Bruce, in word and deed, exemplifies? One answer to this question is found in a survey conducted with the active residents, faculty, and alumni of the Residency Program in Social Medicine (RPSM) founded in 1970 by the Montefiore Medical Center in New York City. Montefiore is noteworthy because it created the first hospital-based Department of Social Medicine in the US a few years after the end of World War II. It also established the Martin Luther King, Jr. Health Center in the Bronx as a model program for the interdisciplinary provision of community-based healthcare by integrated teams of nurses, doctors, social workers, and family health workers. The RPSM was set up to train socially minded primary care physicians who were dedicated to and trained to provide care for the underserved at the Bronx facility. The goals were to train excellent physicians who conceived of health and treatment within a biosocial understanding, were committed to community-oriented care, and served as advocates for change to improve community health and well-being. The study of the RPSM, involving 173 participants, was designed to identify the key characteristics of a social medicine doctor from an insider perspective.

The researchers identified three major themes in the textual responses of participants:

1. social medicine doctors possess a broad knowledge of the social determinants of health, and, as a result, as one study participant noted, they "limit fruitless or wasteful explorations of biological explanations for illness when social etiologies are glaringly present and often unaddressed or ignored by the rest of the health care system" (Karnik, Tschannerl, and Anderson 2015: 59);

2. they also have the ability to translate this broad perspective of health into a treatment plan for individual patients by, noted one participant, "willingness to step out of the clinic and outside of the biomedical model to have a positive impact on health" through advocacy, working in the community, and participating in care provider teams (Karnik, Tschannerl, and Anderson 2015: 59);
3. they see social medicine as an approach for promoting social justice based on a commitment to working with underserved communities and rejecting, emphasized one participant, "the use of health care for personal profit, suppression of others, or unethical scientific adventures" (Karnik, Tschannerl, and Anderson 2015: 60).

These attitudes express core tenets of social medicine, including the idea that social, socioenvironmental, and economic conditions have a profound effect on health and on medical practice; a starting point for policy should be that the health of the population is a critical government and community concern, there is a responsibility to promote health at all levels of society and through all major institutions of society, and, finally, medicine must address the issue of social and health inequality and social justice within and beyond the clinic.

The origin of social medicine traces to the early nineteenth century when the field study of the relationships between society, disease, and medicine began to emerge. One of the early key figures in the effort to examine the social origins of health was the German physician Rudolf Virchow. Well known still for his contribution to understanding the pathologic anatomy of various diseases, Virchow has been described as "a useful role model for physicians in our society" at a time when "many patients lament the fact that their doctor may be more technician and businessman than advisor and confidant" (Reese 1998).

Born in 1821 to a family of modest means in the town of Schivelbein, Prussia, Virchow began to stand out at school from an early age. He trained at the Friedrich-Wilhelm Institut, a division of the University of Berlin that produced medical officers for the Prussian Army. Even as a medical student, Virchow had broad intellectual interests in philosophy, history, and politics and exhibited a propensity toward boundless energy. After graduation in 1843 at the age of 22, he accepted a position as an intern at the Charite, one of Berlin's most renowned teaching hospitals, where he developed an interest in pathology, including the most current biomedical theories on the causes and treatment of disease. At the time, most such theories, each advocated by a different prominent physician, were primarily armchair hypotheses based on limited data. Overthrowing these frameworks and installing in their place a scientific medicine based on direct observation and experimentation became Virchow's goal (Reese 1998).

His own observations began in the autopsy room and laboratory. Within a few years after graduating from medical school, he already had made several major discoveries about the processes of thrombosis and embolism. In addition, he described leukemia as cancer of the white blood cells and differentiated it from severe blood poisoning caused by bacteria and the increase in white blood cells that occurs during an infection. He coined the now-common medical term "ischemia" to label the consequences of stopping blood flow to an organ or tissue, as occurs during heart attacks. In time, Virchow became the head pathologist at the Charite and in 1847, because his manuscripts were consistently rejected by established medical journals, he launched a still thriving journal, *The Archive of Pathological Anatomy and Physiology, and Clinical Medicine* (now called *Virchow's Archive: The European Journal of Pathology*) that reflected his scientific approach. In the first issue of the new journal, Virchow laid out his perspective: "The science of pathologic physiology will . . . gradually fulfill its promise, not as the creation of a few overheated heads, but from the cooperation of many painstaking investigators- a pathologic physiology which will be the stronghold of scientific medicine" (quoted in Nuland 1988: 313). Virchow read, was influenced by, and cited Frederick Engels' *The Condition of the Working Class in England* and used some of Engels' data to support his assessment of the relationships between poverty and disease.

Early in 1848, Virchow was sent by the Prussian Government to Upper Silesia to investigate a typhus epidemic that had begun the previous year and quickly claimed the lives of thousands of people. At the time, the reigning medical understanding of the cause of typhus was 'miasma' – foul air caused by rotting animal matter. Virchow concluded that the main cause of the epidemic was the appalling and unhygienic conditions in which most of the people were living. He was especially horrified by the extreme poverty of the peasant population and their exceptionally innutritious diet. He blamed the Catholic Church for sapping the people of ambition and local landowners for extracting any wealth generated in Upper Silesia to be spent elsewhere. He, therefore, argued that epidemics like typhus were best treated politically rather than medically. He subsequently applied a similar perspective in analyzing a cholera epidemic and an outbreak of tuberculosis in Berlin during 1848 and 1849. The social contradictions that Virchow most heavily emphasized were those of class inequality, noting that morbidity and mortality rates, and especially infant mortality rates, were markedly higher in urban working-class districts compared to wealthier areas. With undisguised dismay, he wrote:

> May the rich remember during the winter when they sit in front of their hot stoves and give Christmas apples to their little ones, that the ship hands who brought the coal and the apples died from cholera. It is so sad that thousands always must die in misery, so that a few hundred may live well. (Quoted in Waitzkin 2006: 7)

Virchow published his challenging findings during the intense revolutionary struggles of 1848–49. Virchow's political and humanistic views led him to participate, on the barricades (armed with a rusty sword and an antiquated rifle), in the widespread democratic uprisings of those years, struggles that sought German confederation, political freedoms, and radical improvements in living and working conditions. For his participation, he was removed from his position at the Charite but was able to find a position at the Würzberg University in Bavaria. Virchow's Würzburg research accomplishments included advancements in the understanding of infectious disease, cancer, liver and kidney disease, and mental retardation.

In July of 1848, Virchow founded the weekly magazine *Medical Reform* to promote social medicine and his belief that "physicians are the natural advocates of the poor." Although the magazine was only published for about a year, it was very influential in promoting both social medicine and improved public health for everyone in Germany, including the poor.

Based on this work, during the 1850s Virchow emerged as the leading physician-scientist in Europe, which led to him being offered a prestigious professorship at the University of Berlin, as Chair of Pathology at what was considered to be the world's leading school of medicine. It was there that he made his most significant contribution to medical science, the idea that cells are the fundamental building blocks comprising all tissues and organs, and that disease occurs when cells fail to perform their normal, dedicated functions. This was a revolutionary perspective at the time, although it has since been absorbed into the heart of medical understanding.

While back in Berlin, Virchow resumed his political work, beginning with being elected as a city counselor in 1859, an office which he held for over forty years, and which he used to improve the quality of life for people living in Berlin. His achievements included improving the city's water supply and sewer system and upgrading public hospitals. Berlin became one of Europe's most hygienic cities because of Virchow's tireless efforts. He also continued to support increased democracy and the development of social welfare programs (Reese 1998). Virchow died from heart failure at the age of 80 in Berlin on September 5, 1902.

One of the places Virchow's perspective on social medicine had its greatest impacts was in Latin America. A number of physicians who shared Virchow's vision for medicine immigrated to Latin America near the turn of the twentieth century. They became involved in developing departments of pathology in medical schools and in initiating courses in social medicine. Max Westenhofer, a prominent German pathologist influenced by Virchow, for example, headed the department of pathology at the medical school of the University of Chile where he was able to influence a generation of medical students, including Salvador Allende, the future president of Chile. Like Virchow, Allende's experiences as a physician and advocate of social medicine shaped much of his later career in politics up until the day he was killed in a U.S.-condoned military takeover in 1973 (Kornbluh 2003, Waitzkin 2006).

Following Virchow, modern practitioners of social medicine recognize that the health impacts of socioeconomic inequality are multifaceted, endure across the life cycle, and have multiple consequences (Barker and Osmond 1986, Dressler and Bindon 2000, Gravelee and Dressler 2005). They understand that to eliminate health disparities it is necessary to make structural changes in society. In the words of Michael Marmot, to reduce inequalities in health there is a need to take action in response to the social determinants of heath. Such action must "include relief of poverty but it will have the broader aim of improving the circumstances in which people live and work" (Marmot 2005: 1099). Such change is possible in a world that prioritizes principles of equity and health over advantage for some at the cost of the well-being of others (Whitehead 1990). To contribute to achieving this goal, as Levy (2013) argues, "Health professionals must be culturally competent to address the medical needs of poor people, and socially and politically competent to address the social contexts that keep poor people poor."

In other words, in additional to traditional clinical topics, physicians need to be taught to be culturally respectful of patient diversity across multiple issues, including class, ethnicity, gender, ableness, being deaf or hard of hearing, and sexual orientation. Most medical schools would probably say they agree with this point, but active education about the built-in, taken-for-granted, and unnoticed mechanisms of privilege and discrimination is another issue. In practice, privilege confers useful advantages to individuals based on their membership in dominant groups in society, specifically advantages involving access to desired resources and to institutionalized power. A key mechanism of the maintenance of social privilege in a nation that proclaims equality for all is to structure experience so that the privileged sectors of society remain unaware of the unlevel playing field of everyday life. In Roseblum and Travis's (1996) terms, privileged individuals possess an "unmarked status"—they experience their lives as normative for all members of society and do not fully grasp the very different life experience of marginalized groups. As Pease (2011: 69) indicates, "By simply exercising their prerogatives in everyday life, [the privileged] can easily ignore how others are denied the same opportunities." Moreover, they can engage in the exploitation of the socially marginalized without being conscious that this is occurring. As part of the system of privilege, distinctions of dress, manner of speech, skin color, health, dentition, behavior, and numerous other experiential differences among people come to serve as markers of normalness and devalued deviance from the norm. From the common privileged point of view, there is the norm (i.e., self, and others perceived to be similar to self) and there is the failure to live up to the norm (i.e., marginalized social groups). Based on these subjectively experienced differences flow the negative attitudes, moral judgments, and prejudices targeted to subordinate group members that shape their everyday lives but are not experienced as bigotry by the privileged. Rather they are perceived by them as objective assessments of failure. In the clinic, for example, issues of patient sexual orientation, weight, and disability have gained attention as reasons physicians deny medical services or provide subpar care, and rejected or undertreated patients feel discriminated against (Lynch 2013, Lagu et al. 2013). Additionally, differences in health outcomes, such as those seen in cardiovascular, kidney, and heart health, cancer detection, and pain alleviation, are intensified by ethnic disparities in disease prevention and treatment (Smedley et al. 2002).

In response to the factors described above, a core goal of social medicine is to reform the healthcare system to meet the health needs of all patients across social strata and other lines of discriminatory social division, rather than allow the existing system of notably unequal access to treatment and dramatically unequal patterns of disease to persist. This too, as described in subsequent chapters, is a goal of Bruce Gould as he labored in the trenches of an inner-city health clinic addressing the embodied impacts of systemic social inequality and a healthcare system resistant to meeting the clinical needs of the underserved.

2

THE SOCIAL CONSTRUCTION OF DISEASE CONCEPTION AND TREATMENT IN BIOMEDICINE

> Do we not always find the diseases of the populace traceable to defects in society?
>
> *Rudolph Virchow*

Biomedical Understanding of Disease as a Natural Entity

One of the core assumptions of biomedicine is that a disease exists as a discrete entity in nature (Gordon 1988). This conception of disease dates to the seventeenth century, especially to the work of Thomas Sydenham (Temkin 1963). The core conception of this understanding is that "disease is a phenomenon neither totally uniform nor totally variable concerning its form of appearance; rather, it presents itself in the form of certain definite, natural *kinds* or *classes* of disease" (Hucklenbroich 2014: 611). These entities are analogous to substances in chemistry, types of plants in botany, and species of animals in zoology. A primary task of biomedical research is to discover, define, and characterize "all disease entities that occur in empirical reality, and to build a comprehensive system reflecting all their similarities and differences" (Hucklenbroich 2014). Indeed, Foucault (1975) dates the emergence of biomedicine to the effort of practitioners to systematically classify diseases in families and species focused on the body and its parts, as opposed to focusing on the sick person as a whole being in a social context.

Today, disease entities are itemized in the accepted, if frequently amended, compendium of recognized diseases, known as the *International Classification of Diseases* (*ICD*). Managed by the World Health Organization (2016), the *ICD* is intended to be a "consensual, meaningful and useful framework which governments, providers and consumers can use as a common language" for disease. As a multispecialty nosological system, it is used for various purposes, such as the development of national morbidity and mortality statistics by World Health Organization member countries or policy decisions about healthcare financing, but also by physicians, nurses, and other healthcare providers for clinical diagnostic purposes.

In biomedicine, every case of disease, be it determined to be tuberculosis or autism, and every specific case of disease expression in an individual patient, is understood as an objective, clinically identifiable component of material reality, a thing-in-itself that can, in principle, be located in the *ICD*. It is assumed that not all diseases have as yet been discovered, and it is recognized that new human diseases continue to emerge, such as those caused by infectious agents that "jump" from other species to humans. Hence the compendium continues to grow and undergo revision. In the tenth edition of the *ICD*, a rather unwieldy collection for practical use, respiratory tuberculosis—a disease linked to 2 million deaths around the world each year—that has been confirmed by the microscopic examination of a patient's sputum samples, for example—is assigned the specific number A15.0, while tuberculosis of the lungs confirmed by culture only is assigned A15.1. Even if a disease is outside of patient awareness and consequently the patient suffers from no experiential symptoms (e.g., hypertension or early diabetes), the physical existence of the disease as an isolatable part of nature is accepted as part of material reality. The one medical specialty whose assemblage and specifications of diseases remains most in question is psychiatry, but here too there is a commitment to establishing an accepted, biologically rooted classification. Additionally, the *ICD* contains various other kinds of pathological findings and other conditions that strictly speaking are not diseases, such as some of the categorizations of aborted pregnancies. Moreover, there is a borderland of ambiguity between disease and non-disease. Grief can be both a normal response to loss or a pathological expression of depression, so too lethargy, which can be normal tiredness or a sign of infection. Similarly, while pain during childbirth usually is not a disease, it may still provoke the desire for medical attention. The same is true of dissatisfaction with one's appearance. Physicians, in short, do not only treat disease, and what they treat and define as being of medical concern varies over time and across nations.

In normal, everyday practice, whether it involves examination and diagnosis, patient care and treatment, or clinical research, biomedicine is guided by a confident conceptualization of diseases as distinct, discrete, and disjunctive entities that occur within individual human (or other) bodies. Diseases, in short, have acquired within biomedicine an "aura of factuality" (Rhodes 1996). Based on many years of work in medical settings, anthropologist Byron Good (1994: 70) reports that he has been struck repeatedly by "the enormous power of the idea within medicine that disease is fundamentally, even exclusively, biological." Further, diseases have an existence that is seen as separate from the social groups and social contexts in which they are found. Stresses Gordon (1988: 28), in biomedicine, disease "is essentially an individual problem and is systematically abstracted from social context."

Yet, the way disease is used in biomedicine does not mean that it can be read directly or automatically from empirical observation; thus while there are symptoms (patient-reported experience) and signs (physician and technologically recorded indications) of a disease like diabetes, deciding its existence is unavoidably rooted in a particular theory of what the world is like. Human judgment and decision making is always a factor in diagnosis. In the process of differential diagnosis, physicians seek to assign "every single abnormal or pathological phenomenon or finding, and every case of being ill . . . unambiguously [to] . . . only one single disease entity" and all such cases must be assigned to a disease category (or comorbid disease categories) because in biomedical theory "isolated pathological conditions outside any disease entity do not exist in reality" (Hucklenbroich 2014: 613–614).

In the *ICD*, infectious diseases occupy the slots between A00 and B99 as well as other slots based on body location (e.g., diseases of the respiratory tract). Seasonal influenza, for example, is number J100, namely influenza due to identified influenza B or C virus. Yet research on the disease outbreaks associated with these viruses suggests that they should be understood only as the immediate or proximate causes of influenza, necessary but not, by their mere presence, sufficient to cause disease, let alone a pandemic that annually takes thousands of lives (e.g., over 400,000 in the US in the years between 1972 and 1992 [Simonsen et al. 1997]). While infectious diseases have proximate causes—one or more of at least 1,400 known pathogens—the simple presence of a pathogen in or on a human body, which is actually a constant state for multiple infectious agents, does not automatically cause disease. There are mediating factors as well, such as social and environmental disruptions (e.g., poor nutrition, physical and emotional trauma, exposure to toxins, chronic distress, prior infections) that serve as stressors that weaken the body's immune functions and other functional systems of the body, that often play critical roles in infectious disease causation, severity, and outcome. The root causes of these pathways to infection—which have been labeled the "causes of the causes" (Rose 2007), such as oppressive social relationships and power—are integral to the making of infectious disease.

This is seen in the assessment of who is most likely to get influenza and to suffer the most severe consequences of the disease. As Mayoral et al. (2012) observe:

> Although . . . factors such as nutrition, and the socioeconomic or educational level are less-frequently considered when studying influenza, there is sufficient evidence of their impact on health and disease evolution to warrant study of their possible role in severe cases of influenza.

Social scientists commonly use the terms "downstream" and "upstream" to represent the relative position of a factor in the causal chain of disease development. While downstream factors would include infectious agents (or lack of good nutrition in the case of noncommunicable diseases), upstream factors are the ultimate and most fundamental determinants. In this framework, "midstream factors" are shaped by upstream determinants and, in turn, impact downstream or immediate causes. Thus, great social inequality is an ultimate determinant of neighborhood quality, which, following the causal chain, influences exposure to infectious agents or other immediate downstream factors. Causal pathways, from upstream social causes to health outcomes are often complex, often unfolding over many years, and replete with multiple opportunities for modification all along the way (Braveman et al. 2011a, Braveman et al. 2011b).

Assessing how these complex causal interactions play out in individuals or populations has not fallen within the traditional purview of biomedicine as practiced, where the primary focus is on identifying immediate causation and implementing appropriate treatment. In other words, conventional biomedicine tends to focus its efforts downstream, attending to immediate causes (e.g., individual risk factors) and bodily (or behavioral) consequences of midstream and upstream determinants of health. As a result, while biomedicine can have a dramatic and even wondrous impact on the immediate health of individual patients, the causes of the causes of their diseases continue unabated. Like others, Bruce calls this the "band aid effect" noting

> much of what we do is put band aids on the proximal or downstream sequelae of more distal or upstream social and economic issues that have resulted in or exacerbated the impact of disease on an individual patient, family or community.

Training Doctors to Understand the World

The approach to disease understanding described above has been engrained in the medical school curriculum and in the standard textbooks of clinical biomedicine since the early twentieth century. The transition point in the creation of the modern medical school was the critical assessment of the state of medical education by Abraham Flexner, who was commissioned by the Carnegie Foundation, in an influential statement that came to be known simply as the Flexner Report (Beck 2004). To prepare his report, Flexner, who was not a physician, visited all of the 155 medical schools in the US and Canada in the period between December 1908 and April 1910. The book-length document he produced held up Johns Hopkins School of Medicine as the pinnacle of medical school training, and was, no doubt, influenced by Flexner's education in Europe. As part of his assessment, Flexner offered a conceptual model of how medical education should be conducted. Schools that fared badly in Flexner's evaluation subsequently lost credibility in the eyes of medical licensing boards and tended to shut down. As a result, in the decade following the release of the Flexner Report, the number of medical schools in the US and Canada dropped from 155 to 85. Among those to disappear were all but two centers dedicated to training African American physicians. Flexner was unambiguous about the basis of his criticism of most such medical schools, noting that

> the physical well-being of the Negro is not only of moment to the Negro himself. Ten million of them live in close contact with sixty million whites. Not only does the Negro himself suffer from hookworm and tuberculosis; he communicates them to his white neighbors, precisely as the ignorant and unfortunate white contaminates him. Self-protection not less than humanity offers weighty counsel in this matter; self-interest seconds philanthropy. The Negro must be educated not only for his sake, but for ours. (Flexner 1910: 180)

Consequently, those African American institutions that did not emphasize germ theory, and train physicians accordingly, did not merit status as a modern school of medicine. In the aftermath of the Flexner Report, there was a significant drop in the availability of medical care for disadvantaged people, and loss of access to a medical school education for ethnic minorities and women, coupled with the significant elevation of the social status of physicians. Within surviving medical schools, as well as those founded after the report, medical training was thoroughly grounded in human physiology and biochemistry, and disease was unfailingly naturalized as a discrete, biochemically material entity.

Over time, medical understanding reinforced its model of disease with a molecular foundation. The introduction to biomedicine for first-year medical students at Stanford University Medical School, for example, consists of classes on the molecular foundations of medicine, applied biochemistry, the biological nature of cells and tissues, developmental biology, human genetics, human anatomy, and the practice of medicine. Similarly, at the University of Texas Southwestern Medical Center (2016), the first semester of training to become a physician consists of the study of the normal human body and its processes at the molecular and cellular levels. Included are courses on biochemistry, genetics, anatomy, and embryology. On this molecular bedrock, in the second year, students are introduced to disease, a period intended to reinforce "the pathophysiology of important diseases and the differential diagnosis of cardinal symptoms, as well as common treatment modalities" (UT Southwestern Medical Center 2016).

Exemplary of the inscribement of the biomedical model in the textbooks used in medical schools is *Harrison's Principles of Internal Medicine* (Longo et al. 2015), which is seen as one of the most authoritative sources in biomedicine (Malani 2012); first published in 1950, it is now in its nineteenth edition. Ironically, even Flexner came to be critical of the "narrow gaze of American medical education on biologic matters" (Cooke et al. 2006: 1340). Fifteen years after his report, he lamented "Scientific medicine in America—young, vigorous and positivistic—is today sadly deficient in cultural and philosophic background" (Flexner 1925). Part of the problem is that, since the Flexner Report, the first years of medical school stress that the so-called "hard sciences," including biology, chemistry, organic chemistry, and physics, are what really is important in understanding disease, while conceiving of health as a biosocial product in which social factors play a central role in disease, is considered soft science. This perspective was affirmed in the primary texts of medical school education, classroom lectures, and other faculty/student communications.

Since the Flexner Report, the biomedical self-image and the one communicated to policy makers and the general public is a field that firmly rests on a foundation of scientific research. As stated by the Association of American Medical Colleges (AAMC) (2009: 4), "The practice of medicine requires grounding in scientific principles and knowledge, as well as understanding how current medical knowledge is scientifically justified, and how the knowledge evolves." Research, however, suggests that many of the ideas and routine practices in biomedicine are not based solely on natural laws or scientifically supported research or principles (Welch 2003), and, further, that even the most frequently cited clinical research "seems to have replication problems, and this seems to be as large, if not larger, than the vast majority of other, less-cited clinical research" (Ioannidis 2005). Even the "gold standard" of scientific biomedical research, the double-blinded randomized controlled trial, has been described as being more gilded than solid because outcomes that are positive and have statistically significant findings have higher odds of being fully published than studies that are of equal importance but did not have positive findings (Dwan et al. 2008). Which study makes it to the biomedical scientific literature, how fast it gets there, and how frequently it is read and cited by other researchers is highly influenced not by the rigor of the research methods used, but by selective reporting and the appeal of the research findings. Moreover, "conflicts of interest may work in the direction of silencing or diminishing newly discovered associations that don't fit financial or other dogmatic perspectives," such as the effects of pharmaceutical industry sponsorship on research outcomes and quality (Ioannidis 2008: 644).

Ethnography has helped to clarify some of the less scientific aspects of everyday biomedical practice (Long et al. 2008). Pearl Katz (1999), for example, in her book *The Scalpel's Edge: The Culture of Surgeons*, informed by her hospital-based ethnographic research, reveals modern surgery as including an elaborate array of rituals that function not to fight disease per se, but to limit physician ambiguity and uncertainty. The well-known process of "scrubbing" for surgery, which is routinely depicted in medical movies and TV shows, for example, involves very strict regimented behaviors, within precisely designated time periods, such as washing each hand in particular ways for a specified amount of time. While it is possible to significantly reduce the presence of pathogens on one's hands and arms through careful cleaning, the precisely defined rules of scrubbing appear primarily to serve also to reduce physicians' and other surgical team members' anxiety about not being sufficiently germ-free to avoid infecting the vulnerable internal organs of the patient. By closely adhering to the prescribed rituals of surgery, the confidence doctors and nurses need to undertake a very delicate, very challenging, and potentially disastrous activity, such as cutting open and in some way changing a patient's internal environment, is heightened, Katz argues. Adds Jeffrey Brenner, a family physician and founder of the Camden Coalition of Healthcare Providers,

> what I think many people would be shocked to find out is that many of the things that we do with day-to-day care actually have very little evidence for them. They are habits that have been passed down from one generation to the next, but doesn't have literature backing it up. (Freakonomics 2015)

The ultimate problem with the biomedicine effort to rationalize all of its practices as science, as Jan Henderson (2012), a historian of medicine and writer, states is that by focusing on what can readily be quantified, it ignores what cannot, such as the social determinants of health and disease. Medicine's historical desire for the respectability that comes with being a science gets in the way of discovering what could actually make us healthier.

The New Medical School

Without question, there have been modifications in medical school training in recent years and more are in the planning. Various new approaches are being tested, like teaching physicians to work as team members with other healthcare providers, not as unquestionable leaders giving "orders". Structurally, the American Medical Association has been pushing for change. In 2013, through a program called Accelerating Change in Medical Education, it gave grants of $1 million each to eleven medical schools nationwide to stimulate innovations in the medical school curriculum. In 2015, 21 additional schools received $75,000 (American Medical Association 2016). Innovations that have been proposed are of various kinds, including new medical technologies, findings ways to better integrate medical students into interprofessional healthcare teams, improving the quality of the learning environment, giving students a better understanding of the overall healthcare system, moving the core early education model away from lectures and toward in-class problem solving. Traditional subjects, like biochemistry and anatomy, are being taught in new ways, moving them from encyclopedic textbook information to framing the ways they are useful in diagnosing a patient presenting with a specific health complaint. There is now greater emphasis, although in some place more in word than in deed, being placed on creating a more compassionate atmosphere in clinics, engaging patients more fully in their own care, and assisting poor patients in "overcoming financial and other barriers that might prevent them from taking medications and otherwise following their doctor's orders" (Wenner 2016). As this last quote—which defines the patient's social life outside of the clinic as a potential barrier to docile patient compliance—suggests, the old ways and the new ways have not been fully nor easily integrated; traditions and privileges die hard.

An example of resistance to change is seen in McKenna's (2010) study of biomedical education at Michigan State University. He examined a six-year, $6 million project called Community/University Health Partnerships, which was designed to train more community-oriented primary care physicians. Community participation was a dominant goal in all components of the project. In that the project directly challenged the engrained biomedical orientation towards curative care, professional rivalries, over-specialization, and narrow hospital-based education, it met with stiff opposition and ultimately collapsed, despite backing from a supportive dean who ultimately resigned from his position.

Another arena that reflects a change in medical education is the standardized Medical College Admission Test (MCAT), the multiple-choice exam administered by the Association of American Medical Colleges to about 80,000 applicants annually. Passage of the MCAT is a prerequisite for entry into almost all medical schools in both the US and Canada. Medical school admission committees rely on the MCAT because, on average, they only accept about 40 percent of their applicants. While would-be physicians tend to apply to multiple schools (an average of 15 schools per student in 2014), many applicants get no positive admission letters from any schools. In fact, more than half of applicants do not end up being accepted into any medical school in a given year (Association of American Medical Colleges 2015).

Since it was developed in 1928, the MCAT has undergone six revisions. There are four sections to the newest edition of the MCAT implemented in 2015, all of which must be completed in six hours and fifteen minutes of actual testing time, with the last section being of particular relevance to the changes occurring in medical schools: (1) Chemical and Physical Foundations of Biological Systems, (2) Critical Analysis and Reasoning Skills, (3) Biological and Biochemical Foundations of Living Systems, and (4) Psychological, Social, and Biological Foundations of Behavior. The new MCAT, while still emphasizing the biological and physical sciences, has added new sections on verbal reasoning, with great emphasis on comprehension in the humanities and social sciences. In a sense, the new MCAT is a reversion to the third edition implemented in 1962. It too had social science and general liberal arts knowledge content, but this was eliminated in 1977 and the hard science sections were expanded (McGaphie 2002). The MCAT, in short, like some of the content it now tests for, is very much a social product reflecting changing attitudes and values in society and in medicine. Whether its changing content spells a transformation in the practice of medicine is another question.

Beyond Medical School

One issue that has been raised with regard to the social content on the new MCAT is how seriously admissions committees will consider scores on the section that contains these questions; in the past, committees have not always given equal weight to outcomes on this information in making their admission decisions. More important, is the question of to what degree today do practicing doctors decide questions of healthcare, as opposed to insurance companies, pharmaceutical companies, medical technology companies, and hospital administrations (Morone 1990).

The Private Health Insurance Industry

What especially most distinguishes the U.S. healthcare system from the arrangements found in most other wealthy countries is the degree to which it is dominated by for-profit private insurance companies. By any measure, private U.S. health insurance is big business and it is an influential force shaping many features of healthcare. With $880 billion a year in revenues, the industry has grown over the years from a set of local, tax-exempt companies into a profit engine that is now largely controlled by globally active financial institutions. Along the way, health insurance companies have become a central force determining healthcare in the country, but their prime directive is maximizing returns on investments, not improving the public's health.

Assessment of the extent of the industry's role in biomedicine today, it has been argued, can be guided by political scientist Thomas Ferguson's (1995) version of the Golden Rule: to discover who rules, follow the gold.

Health insurance premiums have gone up 131 percent since 1999, forcing customers to pay more money for less insurance coverage and leaving them responsible for an ever-growing share of rising medical costs (Centers for Medicare & Medicaid Services 2010). Increasingly, doctors are having to deal with angry patients, especially middle- and lower-income individuals, upset about high insurance copays, increased deductions, and insurance denials. A survey of physicians by the magazine *Medical Economics* (Pofeldt 2016) found that 87 percent reported an increase in patient resentment compared to two years previously. Notably, doctors are encouraged by the magazine to implement several strategies to diminish patient anger, including speaking softly and slowly to patients, moving from behind the desk to sit in a more casual way with patients, acknowledging patient distress, and allowing patients to vent their upset (Pofeldt 2016). As this list of recommendations suggests, the focus is on making things easier for doctors rather than actually doing something about the causes of patient umbrage.

Driving patient anger, health insurance premium increases have gone up even faster than that of overall medical costs in recent years and the growth of premiums paid by consumers and employers corresponds with record revenues among health insurance companies. A study by the Kaiser Family Foundation (2015) found that U.S. health insurance achieved their third year of record-breaking profits in 2011 by hiking up premiums by 9 percent per year (Bass 2012). Because of continual increases, the cost of family insurance coverage about doubled between 2001 and 2011. In 2015, the Segal Health Plan Cost Trend Survey, an annual survey of managed care organizations, health insurers, pharmacy benefit managers and third-party administrators, found that health insurance costs "will increase for most medical plan options and increase substantially for prescription drug coverage to double-digit rates" (The Segal Group 2015). In the first half of 2011 alone, private health insurance companies took in $7 billion in profits (Health Care for America Now 2012). This massive level of profit making is justified by the health insurance industry with the argument that their profits represent less than one penny of every dollar spent in the US on healthcare. In fact, one penny out of every dollar spent on healthcare totals over $350 billion over a ten-year period (Health Care for America Now 2012). Importantly, some of these profits are put to use to influence healthcare policy and practice in ways that favor the industry. With its ever-growing stream of revenues to fund its efforts, the health insurance industry is now among the most powerful special interest groups in Washington, as well as in every state capital.

The Affordable Care Act and Dissents

One example of the ability of the industry to influence healthcare can be seen with the passage of the Affordable Care Act (ACA) or so-called "Obamacare."

As Wilper and colleagues (2009: 2289) note, the US "stands alone among industrialized nations in not providing health coverage to all of its citizens." Prior to passage of the ACA, 46 million people lacked any healthcare insurance. This is of critical importance because a survival analysis of data collected in the Third National Health and Nutrition Examination Survey with 17–64-year-olds found that not having health insurance is associated with over 44,000 deaths every year in the US, more than are caused by kidney disease (Willper 2009). Not having health insurance, quite literally, is deadly.

The insurance companies have tended to oppose national health insurance because they want insurance coverage to be private and hence profitable, and they do not want to include people with serious pre-existing diseases, or not be able to drop people who face big medical expenses. A Medicare-like national health insurance program run by the federal government, the health insurance industry well realized, could take advantage of lower administrative costs, employ government pricing power to underwrite lower premiums, and make insurance available to all applicants at a common price. The private insurers knew they could not reap huge profits if they tried to compete with a national health insurance program. In the words of one House Democratic aide, "They are very afraid of competing against a public plan that doesn't have their same priority—which is to make money for their shareholders . . . They'd rather have new tough rules they know they can circumvent" (quoted in Cohn 2009).

Consequently, while the ACA was under debate in Congress in 2009, insurance company representatives participated in the development of the legislation. The Senate Finance Committee headed by Max Baucus took the lead in drafting the ACA. Baucus worked hard to keep a single-payer, government-supported option out of healthcare reform discussions. He stated: "We are not Europe. We are not Canada. We are America. This is not a single pay country" (quoted in Tumulty 2009). This statement, which ignores the existence of the Medicare system and the Veterans Administration, both of which are government-sponsored single-payer healthcare programs that together cover about a fourth of the U.S. population, plays up an American exceptionalism that has been promoted by the insurance industry through intensive lobbying and expansive campaign donations. The idea that the people of the US reject a government-sponsored single-payer system is belied by a series of national polls. A Gallup poll conducted in 2015 found that approval of enrollees is highest in publicly financed health insurance programs (ranging from 75–78 percent), compared to 69 percent for employer-sponsored private coverage, and 65 percent for individually purchased private plans (Saluja et al. 2016b). A subsequent Gallup poll found that 58 percent of respondents supported a national health insurance program to replace the Affordable Care Act (Newport 2016). What studies show people want are lower prices, more comprehensive coverage, and a role in healthcare decision making, and it is these things they have had the hardest time acquiring because of dogged, self-interested industry efforts (Geyman 2015). As summarized by Robert Reich (2016), professor of public policy at the University of California, Berkeley:

> The real choice . . . is either a hugely expensive for-profit oligopoly with the market power to charge high prices even to healthy people and stop insuring sick people. Or else a government-run single-payer system—such as in place in almost every other advanced economy—dedicated to lower premiums and better care for everyone.

During the development of the ACA, Baucus repeatedly gave credit to Elizabeth Fowler, his chief health policy counsel, for her extensive role in the actual drafting of the document. Before joining Baucus's staff, Fowler was the Vice President for Public Policy and External Affairs (i.e. a lobbyist) at WellPoint, the largest health insurance provider in the country. Her predecessor as Baucus's chief health policy counsel, Michelle Easton, also went on to lobby for Wellpoint. Once the law was passed, Obama appointed Fowler to oversee its implementation as Special Assistant to the President for healthcare and Economic Policy at the National Economic Council. When Fowler left this position, she returned to the revolving door that connects the health insurance/lobbying industry and government to a senior policy position at pharmaceutical giant Johnson and Johnson (Greenwald 2012). In this regard, it merits mentioning that Obama received over half a million dollars in contributions from employees of pharmaceutical companies during his 2008 run for the presidency (Gibson and Smith 2016).

While the health insurance industry had a major hand in the crafting of the ACA, it also donated over $85 million to the U.S. Chamber of Commerce, a vocal opponent of healthcare reform. The Chamber used its cash windfall to promote a market-based healthcare system which contributed to the inclusion of private insurance companies as the providers of insurance under the ACA, including over 15 million newly insured individuals who were mandated to access private health insurance by the new program, and, as noted, the exclusion of a public option that would have allowed the government to compete with the health insurance industry in offering medical care.

After it was passed into law, conservative opposition to the ACA resulted in a significant weakening of its capacity to provide healthcare to the poorest people in the US. This involved a key element of the new program: the expansion of Medicaid eligibility to nearly all low-income individuals with incomes at or below 138 percent of the government-determined poverty level (i.e., $27,724 for a family of three in 2015). This component of the ACA was intended to close a significant gap in Medicaid eligibility for adults and was seen as a mechanism for extending insurance coverage to low-income individuals. These individuals were eligible to receive premium tax credits to use in gaining coverage. This initiative collapsed, however, in June 2012 when the Supreme Court ruled that states could opt out of Medicaid expansion. By January 2016, 19 states decided not to expand Medicaid. This meant that in those states Medicaid eligibility was limited to parents with a median income limit of only 44 percent of poverty, or an annual income of $8,840 a year for a family of three. Additionally, adults without children were ineligible for Obamacare. Assuming that low-income people would receive health care coverage through Medicaid, the ACA does not provide any other financial assistance to people below the poverty line. Consequently, in those states that did not expand Medicaid, many adults fall into what has been called a "coverage gap" of having incomes above Medicaid eligibility limits but below the lower limit for premium tax credits (Garfield and Damico 2016). Altogether, almost 3 million poor adults fall into the "coverage gap." These individuals tend to be concentrated in states with the largest uninsured populations. More than a quarter of people that have fallen into the coverage gap live in Texas, a state with both a large uninsured population and very restrictive Medicaid eligibility. Another 20 percent reside in Florida, while 11 percent are in Georgia, and 8 percent are located in North Carolina. Over half (10 out of 19) of the states that did not expand Medicaid are located in the South, a region of the country where almost 90 percent of people in the coverage gap are found. All of the states that opted out of Medicaid expansion have conservative governors and state legislatures that staunchly oppose the ACA and voted to reject billions of federal dollars that were offered for broadening their Medicaid programs. The result is continued lack of health insurance coverage for many poor working people in the US who do not receive healthcare benefits from their employer. The income of these individuals is too low to afford the purchase of insurance coverage which would cost, for the cheapest, least beneficial programs $246 a month, a sizeable amount for low-income individuals. Nationally, 45 percent of those who are still uninsured are White non-Hispanics, 23 percent are Hispanic, and 28 percent are African American. People who have been blocked from access to Obamacare and whose incomes make the purchase of health insurance prohibitively expensive often tend to leave their health needs untreated until they become eligible for Medicare at age 65, if they survive until then (McWilliams et al. 2007).

Power and Healthcare

The effect of the power of the healthcare industry and other for-profit industries (e.g., pharmaceutical companies, medical technology companies, hospital conglomerates) on the quality of healthcare in the US has been a significant issue of concern in public discourse. Russell Andrews, a neurosurgeon who authored the book *Too Big To Succeed*, argues that

> the morphing of American medicine from a function of a humanitarian society into a revenue stream for health care profits, drug and medical device companies, hospitals, and insurance companies . . . [has] transformed health care in the U.S. into an industry whose (real) goal is to be profitable. (Ubel 2014)

Similarly, Sachin Shah, a physician affiliated with Doctors For America, an organization of over 18,000 physicians and medical students committed to putting patients above politics, contrasts the struggles many patients face in paying their medical bills to the enormous profits of the insurance companies: "Profit in the health insurance industry is the single greatest barrier to building an efficient, sustainable system of health care in this country" (Ubel 2014).

Of note, the ACA was presented to the public as an initiative intended to offer health insurance for the uninsured. Certainly, ACA has lowered the number of people without coverage, although approximately 30 million people remain uninsured. Most people without health insurance are members of low-income working families. In 2014, over 80 percent were in a family with an employed worker with a blue-collar job, but more than half had family income that was below 200 percent of poverty. People of color are at higher risk of being uninsured than non-Hispanic Whites. So too are non-citizens, both legal and undocumented (Majerol, Newkirk, and Garfield 2015). Cost remains a major barrier to coverage, with nearly half of the uninsured in 2014 saying that the main reason they still did not have insurance was because it was too expensive for them to afford.

The Pharmaceutical Industry

In an article entitled "Pharmaceuticals, Political Money, and Public Policy" in the *Journal of Law, Medicine and Ethics*, Paul Jorgensen of the University of Texas (2013: 561) asks: "Why, when confronted with policy alternatives that could improve patient care, public health, and the economy, does Congress neglect those goals and tailor legislation to suit the interests of pharmaceutical corporations?" His answer is that the pharmaceutical industry has been successful in convincing legislators to define health policy issues in ways that protect the industry's profit margin. To achieve its goals, the pharmaceutical industry focuses on "educating" doctors, funneling its significant campaign contributions to influential legislators and their allies, selectively providing information to legislatures, and selling its ideas to the general public. Through these strategies, discussed below, the industry, "displaces the public's voice in developing pharmaceutical policy" (Jorgensen 2013: 561).

First, the pharmaceutical industry spends billions of dollars "informing doctors about its products." The key issue here is the difference between providing needed information and aggressively promoting the use of specific drugs for approved as well as unapproved purposes, or what Angell (2004) calls "marketing masquerading as education." An example of this industry practice involves the promotion of off-label uses. When a pharmaceutical company has a patent for a drug used to treat a specific disease, one way to increase profits is to extend its use in the treatment of other diseases, even if no evidence exists to suggest this would be a clinically sound decision. Indeed, pharmaceutical companies are restricted in marketing drugs for off-label uses; doctors, by contrast, are not so restrained and may prescribe any drug to treat a disease if they deem it appropriate. To get around this barrier, pharmaceutical company representatives seek to convince doctors about possible other uses for their products. As Angell (2004: 137) indicates, "They sponsor make-believe education, and often buttress it by references to flimsy research studies they sponsor." Additionally, to facilitate the educational process, they offer kickbacks in the form of gifts, ranging from the most lavish (paying for trips to conferences—possibly organized by companies with pharmaceutical ties—held sometimes at highly desirable vacation destinations, for continuing medical education) to the Lilliputian (e.g., pens, cups, letter openers). Even the annual meetings of many professional medical societies, which are attended by thousands of doctors, are handsomely funded by pharmaceutical companies. At these events, the drug companies host satellite symposia (about specific conditions treatable with pharmaceuticals) and offer attendees expensive free meals. At the conventions, pharmaceutical companies set up showy exhibits and energetic company sales representatives eagerly hand out promotional swag (e.g., thermoses, clocks, passport cases, paperweights), to attending doctors. In 2014, a federal report indicated that the pharmaceutical and medical device industries gave physicians $92.8 million for food and beverages, $74.1 million for travel and lodging, and $26.7 million for other educational costs. Another $19.2 was conveyed to doctors in the form of merchandise (Ornstein 2014). Altogether these industries spent a total of $3.5 billion in payments of various kinds to over half a million physicians and over 1,300 teaching hospitals.

The scale of the financial benefits some physicians receive from the pharmaceutical industry can be staggering. ProPublica, a non-profit news organization that produces investigative journalism in the public interest, including abuses of power and betrayals of public trust, has tracked and analyzed pharmaceutical industry payments to physicians since 2010. They have found that some doctors receive hundreds of thousands of dollars a year from the pharmaceutical industry. Taking the case of the doctor who ranked 250th among doctors who received industry payments in 2014, ProPublica reported 29 different pharmaceutical companies paid the physician a total $594,363 that year, mostly for promotional speaking and consulting, but also for travel expenses and meals as well. Such payments do not necessarily come as lump sums at the end of the year, but rather are spread across the calendar. ProPublica analysis found 768 doctors who received industry payments on more than half of the days of the year in 2014. More than 14,600 doctors received payments on at least a hundred days that year (Ornstein and Jones 2015). Of note, for doctors that are affiliated with hospitals, hospital ownership affects industry payment levels. Physicians at for-profit hospitals have been found to have the highest rate of industry payments (75 percent), followed by physicians at not-for-profit hospitals (66 percent), with doctors at federally owned hospitals having the lowest rates (29 percent) of payments (Ornstein and Jones 2016).

These practices have become deeply ingrained in the daily professional lives of many physicians. Aaron Kesselheim of Harvard Medical School, who had done research on the topic and has testified before Congress on *pharmaceutical* policy, summarized the current situation by observing that

> There are physician practices which have very deep relationships with pharmaceutical representatives, where they are a very integral part of the practice . . . Every day it's another drug company coming in for a lunch. Sometimes it may be some drug companies are bringing breakfast and some are bringing lunch and it's just part of the culture of the practice. (Quoted in Ornstein and Jones 2015)

And, indeed, shaping the culture of practice is precisely the pharmaceutical industry goal in relationship building with physicians. Drug company representatives refer to the tools of their culture influencing strategy as the three Fs: "food, friendship, and flattery" (Ornstein and Jones 2016).

The effect of the industry-influenced culture of physician practice is telling. As Schofferman (2011) stresses, "Physicians are as susceptible to marketing as anybody and cannot totally avoid the unconscious effect of receipt of a 'gift,'" and while they "tend to overestimate their ability to resist marketing efforts" physicians often "fail to appreciate that they can be subtly influenced."

In recent years, the efforts of pharmaceutical companies to get doctors to prescribe off-label uses of their drugs has resulted in several revealing lawsuits. In one case, Angela Maher, a former drug sales representative sued Ortho-McNeil Pharmaceutical, a subsidiary of Johnson & Johnson, alleging that the company pushed its anti-seizure drug Topamax for 27 off-label uses. The company settled the suit for $81 million (most of which went to the federal government and Massachusetts state Medicaid), and pleaded guilty to a misdemeanor charge of misbranding a drug; Maher was awarded $3 million (Department of Justice 2010). Similarly, Allergan, the company that makes Botox, created do-nothing advisory boards to reward doctors who prescribed their product. These physicians were treated to a stay at an oceanfront resort in Newport Beach, California, a city that is so exclusive that the median value of homes at the time exceeded a million dollars. Advisory board members were paid $1,500 to listen to presentations about the drug and its off-label uses. According to the sentencing document from the trial that resulted in a $600 million fine and a guilty plea to a misdemeanor, in addition to pushing multiple uses of Botox the gathering was intended to "build loyalty and solidify important relationships" with doctors (Ornstein 2010).

The big pharmaceutical companies begin to build ties with physicians early in their careers by infiltrating medical schools. Medical school teachers, department chairs, and deans are invited to sit on the boards of directors of drug companies, an experience that can influence medical educational content. Companies also donate money to support programs in many medical schools and teaching hospitals, and company representatives may be given access to young doctors to promote their product (Shapiro 2004). As a result, doctors in training not only receive industry-biased information but also learn a drug-intensive approach to the practice of medicine, as opposed to a prevention-first approach. Many come to believe that there is a drug for every disease and that new drugs are superior to old ones or generic brands (Kluger 2009). As a review of relevant studies concluded, the "pharmaceutical industry has a significant presence during residency training, has gained the overall acceptance of trainees, and appears to influence prescribing behavior" (Zipkin and Steinman 2005: 777).

Recognizing the ethical issues of allowing pharmaceutical representatives to have open access to students, whose understanding of medicine is in a formative stage, and to receive gifts from drug companies, medical school policies changed in recent years to limit contact on campus. But are such policies effective in restricting industry representatives from reaching medical students? A national survey of medical students and residents that examined the changing pattern of interactions between physician trainees and the pharmaceutical industry (Austad et al. 2013) found that industry gifts were still common although less prominent than in the past. Researchers reported that 33 percent of first-year students, 56.8 percent of fourth-year students, and 54 percent of medical residents reported receiving industry gifts. The conclusion drawn was, medical school and training hospital policy changes notwithstanding, that "a substantial number of trainees continue to receive gifts from pharmaceutical representatives" and that there was no relationship between the receipt of gifts and the existence of school policies concerning interactions with industry (Austad et al. 2013: 1064).

One mechanism the industry has adopted to deepen relations with physicians is called the "clinical preceptorship." In this practice, doctors are paid to allow a company sales representative to shadow them as they see patients throughout the day. This is presented to doctors as an educational experience for the representative, for which the physician receives an honorarium. These representatives often make friends with doctors and their staffs, and use these emotional connections to promote products produced by their companies. An ethical assessment of such preceptorships by Wall and Brown (2002) found them to be unjustifiable and unethical because they introduce an outside party with self-interest into the privacy of the doctor/patient relationship and the intimacies of the patient's clinical condition. As they note, "The 'honorarium' is merely a convenient fiction disguising the drug company's payment for access to the physician's patients" (Wall and Brown 2002: 598). The term "convenient fiction," in fact, applies to many of the tactics drug companies use to influence the practice of medicine in their own interest.

Even recent efforts by medical schools to dissuade doctors from developing relationships with pharmaceutical company representatives may not withstand industry persistence. Ferguson and co-workers (1999) conducted a mail survey with internal medicine staff members of a medical hospital and two affiliated community hospitals on the issue of contact with drug company representatives. They found that encounters between physicians and pharmaceutical sales representatives are common in everyday medical practice, especially in busy medical offices. Even policies that were implemented by some training hospitals in recent years that were designed to limit pharmaceutical sales representative access during residency training do not appear to have much lasting effect on the subsequent likelihood of a doctor meeting with pharmaceutical sales representatives, or accepting drug samples from them.

Free drug samples have an important effect on the practice of medicine. For one thing, they familiarize doctors and patients with newer, expensive drugs even though older, less expensive ones may still be available and have equal efficacy. This is why new drugs often come with lower prices initially. But as Angell (2004: 129) notes, "It is a form of bait and switch, although what is switched is the price, not the product." Moreover, research suggests that the more money doctors receive from drug companies, the more brand-name drugs they tend to prescribe.

The research affirming this point involved matching records on payments received from pharmaceutical companies (and medical device makers) in 2014 with data on doctors' prescriptions in Medicare's drug program. The researchers found that doctors who received industry payments were two to three times as likely to prescribe brand-name drugs at exceptionally high rates compared to those in the same medical specialty who did not receive payments (Ornstein, Jones, and Tigas 2016). Not only does the pharmaceutical industry spend vast amounts of money in a highly organized and sophisticated attempt to influence clinical practice in this way, it presents itself as merely seeking to build the knowledge base of physicians rather than as being fully intent on persuading physicians to use its products to enhance profits, sometimes to the detriment of patients and the public. While physicians at times assert that there is no conflict of interest in partaking of the industry's largesse, research suggests otherwise (Chen 1999, Lichter 2008).

Second, beyond the clinical setting, pharmaceutical companies are focused on drug-relevant health policy. To win friends in Congress to their perspective on policy issues, the pharmaceutical industry has become a big spender on U.S. elections. Joseph Stiglitz (2013: 144), in his book *The Price of Inequality*, argues that, as a result of significant campaign spending, "increasingly, and especially in the United States, it seems that the political system is more akin to 'one dollar one vote' than to 'one person one vote.'" Jorgensen calculates that, based on industry reports, the pharmaceutical manufacturers contributed $21.3 million to candidates in federal elections in 2012, about 407 percent more than their 1990 inflation-adjusted total campaign spending. Yet, even this substantial amount is probably an underestimate as the industry also makes contributions to state-level party committees that appear not to be included in the reported amounts, and various errors exist in company reports. Based on a recalculation to include state contributions and fixed errors, Jorgensen suggested that a more accurate amount for pharmaceutical company donations to U.S. elections campaigns in 2012 was closer to $30 million.

From the standpoint of industry influence, it appears to have been money well spent. The considerable financial success of the industry has been significantly assisted by a number of policies enacted by Congress, including strong patent protections and control over patient access to medicines unregulated by controls on pricing. Dating to the 1980s, several Congressional laws allowed pharmaceutical companies to acquire profitable patents on medicines developed with taxpayer funding by the National Institutes of Health. Even though the private pharmaceutical companies did not develop the NIH drugs, Congress did not attempt to stop them from raising the prices of these medicines when selling them back to the patients whose tax dollars had paid for their development in the first place (Angell 2004).

Third, Jorgensen pointed out that the pharmaceutical industry has been able to convince Congress to define health policy issues in industry-supported ways by providing select, industry-sculpted information to legislators. Access to provide this kind of information to members of Congress is enhanced through campaign spending. Studies show that campaign contributions are associated with lobbying contacts, with greater access to legislators being facilitated by higher levels of campaign donations (Hall and Deardorff 2006). Industry lobbyists are well informed about which office holders are most sympathetic to business and particularly the drug industry. These are the Congress members they contact to offer their services in helping them and their staffs to do "the hard work of research and bill writing" (Jorgensen 2013: 566). One of the core ideas the industry has sought to embed in Congressional thinking is that only by allowing them to accrue high profits by maintaining minimal controls on consumer drug prices will pharmaceutical companies have the incentive to invest in new research and development. This is actually a unique stance globally. Notes Daemmrich (2011: 35):

> Intriguingly, arguments concerning the relationship of price to industry R&D investments (and the resulting public gains) have been persuasive only to policymakers in the United States. In Europe, Japan, and elsewhere, by contrast, pharmaceutical price control by means of reference pricing or delayed entry of new drugs has become the norm.

This assertion of the industry is further undercut by the fact that it spends about twice as much money marketing its products to physicians as it does on research and development (Gagnon and Lexchin 2008).

A second idea, triggered especially by the notable differences in costs between drugs purchased in Canada and the US, is that it is unsafe to import drugs from other countries. For years, pharmaceutical companies have lobbied Congress vigorously to stop people in the US from buying drugs, often over the Internet, from licensed pharmacies in other countries. Often times, these are the same drugs that are sold in the US at higher prices or they are generic versions of domestically sold brand-name drugs. Big drug companies have tried to emphasize the risks of such purchasing through expensive media campaigns. Exemplary is the work of Sally Pipes who writes a blog for *The Hill*, a website targeted to members of Congress. Pipes is the president of the Pacific Research Institute, a conservative institute focused on free-market policy approaches to social issues, and author of three books criticizing Obamacare. In a piece called "Letting Patients Buy Canadian Drugs Will only Import Trouble" (Pipes 2015), she argues that prescription drug spending in the US "has been stable for years." She also declares that allowing prescription drug importation "would starve pharmaceutical companies of billions of dollars they'd otherwise spend on research and development" while dramatically increasing "the potential for dangerous counterfeits to enter the American supply chain." Her assertions about the stability of drug prices are fanciful and contradicted by multiple studies. Observes Langreth (2014), "Since October 2007 the cost of brand-name medicines has soared, with prices doubling for dozens of established drugs that target everything from multiple sclerosis to cancer, blood pressure, and even erectile dysfunction, according to an analysis conducted for Bloomberg." While in the past, major drug companies implemented one price increase a year, today they issue multiple price increases a year. Exemplary of the kinds of price rises now seen in the largely unregulated pharmaceutical price market was the 2015 increase in the price of the drug Daraprim by Turing Pharmaceuticals. The most effective treatment for toxoplasmosis, an infection that has plagued people living with HIV/AIDS or cancer who have impacted immune systems, the price of Daraprim was raised from $13.50 to $750 per pill overnight. Similarly, the generic drug hydroxychloroquine, used to treat rheumatoid arthritis and lupus (and also used to treat malaria) went from about $30 for 180 tablets in 2014 to $500 by the end of 2015 (Consumer Reports 2015). One of the factors feeding these huge increases is industry consolidation. As pharmaceutical companies buy up other companies, they jack up the prices on products owned by their acquisitions, medicines on which they incurred no research and development costs. Increased prices instead provide cash to fuel further acquisitions and overall company value.

At a time when millions of people cannot afford the drugs prescribed to them and hence do not take them, it is the case that rising drug prices are the most important pharmaceutical risk faced by patients. Thus studies show that as many as three out of four people do not take medications as prescribed to them by their doctor (Consumer Reports 2012) and a survey by CVS Caremark of more than 2,400 of its retail pharmacists found that 62 percent believe the high cost of drugs is the biggest reason for noncompliance (CVS Health 2016) and skyrocketing drug prices have generated an enormous level of public frustration. Notes Quiley (2016), "One in every five US cancer patients can't afford to fill their prescriptions, and many seniors on Medicare are forced to cut their pills in half to stretch their supply." The reason, in part, is because in the period between 1995 and 2013, the average initial price of new anticancer drugs, adjusted for inflation and health benefits, increased by 10 percent annually, which is an average of $8,500 per year (Howard et al. 2015).

Despite problems with the veracity of the information regularly supplied to lawmakers by manufacturers, pharmaceutical company perspectives have remained a dominant influence on policy. One result of this sway is the inclusion of Section 708 in the Food and Drug Administration Safety and Innovation Act, which was passed by Congress in 2012. This section of the law allows customs to seize and destroy medications mailed to U.S. patients from Canadian and other foreign pharmacies. Certainly, the argument could be made based on the facts that are available that it is the drug industry's profits and not public health that is protected by this federal policy.

Finally, in recent years, pharmaceutical companies have taken their messages directly to the drug-consuming public as part of a wider pattern involving the pharmaceuticalization of illness (Bell, Kravatz, and Wilkes 1999; Petryna and Kleinman 2006). Passed in 1962, the Kefauver Harris Amendments to the Food, Drug, and Cosmetic Act required pharmaceutical companies to provide detailed information about drugs' side-effects, contraindications, and efficacy in their advertisements, as well as requiring them to present a "fair balance" between the benefits and risks of use, and banning false or misleading claims. In 1985, however, the Federal Drug Administration lifted its moratorium on print media direct-to-consumer (DTC) advertisements for prescription products, signaling the beginning of a sea change in the role of the pharmaceutical industry's approach to consumers (Bradley 2010). Even before this, in 1981, the pharmaceutical company Merck, Sharp, and Dohme published a DTC ad for the prescription drug Pneumovax. At the time, this act was so novel that it was reported as news by the *New York Times* in an article that presciently stated "Physicians may suddenly find themselves assailed by a patient's demands for drugs that doctors know little about, or drugs more scientifically controversial than the advertisement implies" (Altman 1982).

The ability of the pharmaceutical industry to influence consumer behavior was even more radically accelerated in 1997 when the Food and Drug Administration (FDA), under pressure from the pharmaceutical industry lobby, issued relaxed guidelines for the DTC marketing of prescription drugs (Singer, Ostrach, and Evans 2013). Specifically, the FDA stopped requiring that drug ads provide comprehensive information about all possible side effects, although this information still had to be provided on the inserts in prescription drug packaging. Unfortunately, it has been found, these are "often inconsistent, incomplete, and difficult for patients to read and understand" (Shrank and Avorn 2007: 731). Rather than helping patients, drug inserts are "written in dense technical jargon [that] assumes the reader is a health professional" and with input from company attorneys they are intended "to limit the liability of the manufacturer in the event that an adverse drug reaction injures a consumer" (Furberg, Furberg, and Sasich 2016: 110).

Based on this federal policy change, pharmaceutical industry spending on DTC advertising rocketed to just under $5 billion by 2006. From the change in FDA policy through 2005, DTC advertising increased by 330 percent (Donahue, Cevasco, and Rosenthal 2007). For every $1 invested by the industry in DTC advertising, the market produced a gain of $4.20 in increased drug sales. Between 1998 and 1999, the 25 most advertised drugs accounted for a $7.2 billion increase in spending on pharmaceutical products. Moreover, between 2000 and 2004, U.S. healthcare costs jumped by 9.6 percent annually, much of it the result of rising spending on pharmaceutical products (Porter 2011). Notably, Merck spent almost $100 million on DTC advertising for Vioxx, a pain-relief medication, a fraction of what a study designed to test the drug's deadly side effects—heart attacks, strokes, and death—would have cost. There is evidence that Merck not only attempted to conceal the risks associated with Vioxx but was assisted in this effort by federal drug regulators to keep findings on adverse effects hidden for as long as possible (Avorn 2005; Singer and Baer 2009).

The impact of the major increase in DTC advertising is revealed by a survey conducted by the FDA which found that by 2002, 81 percent of public respondents reported seeing or hearing an ad for a prescription drug (Aikin 2003, U.S. Food and Drug Administration 2011). Today, DTC pharmaceutical advertising is the most frequent type of health communication encountered by the public (Greene and Herzberg 2010). Regular television viewers in the US see as many as 16 hours of prescription advertising a year in half to full minute doses (Frosch et al. 2007). After slowly dropping for several years, drug industry spending on DTC advertising totaled $5.4 billion in 2015 compared to $4.3 billion in 2014, a 19 percent increase and a return to 2006 levels despite the fact the majority of people in the US favor banning prescription drug advertisements on television (Mack 2016, Mangan 2016). At this point, when the issue of a ban on consumer-targeted drug advertising on television has gained a voice in public discourse, DTC advertising has spread beyond television to social media and other digital platforms.

As *Consumer Reports* (2011) emphasizes, "Consumers are besieged daily by ads for prescription drugs, all beseeching you to 'ask your doctor' for a given brand-name drug for an ailment that you might, or might not, actually have." Moreover, a survey of 2,004 adults conducted by Consumer Reports National Research Center (ConsumerReports.org 2009) found that one-fifth of survey respondents reported asking their doctor for a drug seen advertised on television or elsewhere. In most cases (70 percent), doctors comply with patient requests. As a result, demanding and receiving DTC-advertised drug prescriptions can be seen as a form of self-medication. Notably, however, the most heavily advertised drugs are often not the most effective or safest treatments. They are, however, frequently the most expensive ones (ConsumerReports.org 2009).

Moreover, a content analysis of claims made on DTC advertisements that aired in 2008–10 by Faerber and Kreling (2013) found that only 43 percent of claims were objectively true, while 55 percent were potentially misleading. The authors of the study conclude that their findings are in conflict with industry proponents who maintain that the social value of DTC advertising is their success in informing consumers about drugs.

Ultimately, in the health arena, the enactment of power can be seen in the worldwide development of a pharmaceutically centered neoliberal model of public health that stresses access to medications over disease prevention or even clinical care (Biehl 2007). Research suggests that if there was a greater focus on preventing premature death in the US, 84,000 fewer people would die every year, based on comparisons with France, Australia, and Italy, which do emphasize prevention (Nolte and McKee 2011). The ability of pharmaceutical discourse to rise to dominance and to masquerade as "truth" is rooted in the power of the global industry to frame particular social understandings, expectations, and practices. Pharmaceutical discourse, in short, seeks to shape the way that people know and act in the world (Foucault 1972). As Park and Grow (2008: 379) found in their study of direct-to-consumer antidepressant advertising, this mode of communication "may play a role in constructing [the] social reality of diseases and medicine."

Medical Technology Industry

In addition to the healthcare and pharmaceutical industries, a third force influencing the practice of biomedicine is the medical technology industry—the set of corporations engaged in the production and promotion of high-technology diagnostic and therapeutic equipment like X-ray machines, CT scanners, mechanical ventilators, ultrasound machines, robotic surgery systems, image-guided radiotherapy machines, telemedicine technology, diverse patient-worn digital monitoring devices, and much more. Increasingly, medical professionals have come to equate progress in medicine with the escalating use of expensive technologies. In their anthropological assessment of biomedicine, Lock and Nguyen (2010: 20) note that the employment of "complex, sophisticated technology is integral to biomedicine today—increasing[ly] so as molecular biological knowledge and its associated computer technologies become ever more routinized."

But the rising cost of medical technology is a significant contributor to the spiraling size of the overall healthcare bill. This trend continues because medical technology manufacturers seek to maintain a very generous profit margin for every machine or system they sell, in order to meet investor expectations, on the one hand, and to offset both research and development expenses but also marketing costs, on the other. Yet it is not uncommon for new medical technologies to be introduced to the market with only limited evaluation of their effectiveness, a gap in research on optimal patterns of use, or awareness of what impact they will have on clinical practice (Tan and Ong 2002). As a result, there are unexpected adverse consequences of the introduction of new medical technologies (Deyo 2002). For example, there is evidence that owning imaging facilities (as opposed to referring out for such services) leads to excessive use of imaging (Hillman et al. 1990). Another example involves fetal heartbeat monitoring prior to delivery (Shy, Larson, and Luthy 1987). In retrospect, it is evident that the risks and consequences of such monitoring were not fully evaluated prior to its adoption into routine obstetric care. Currently, most women who give birth in U.S. hospitals are hooked up to an electronic fetal monitor more or less continuously throughout their labor (Declercq et al. 2007). Collectively, fetal monitors have cost U.S. hospitals hundreds of millions of dollars. For these monitors to be used, the prospective mother must remain relatively inactive in bed although an unavoidable focus on monitor output may increase her level of anxiety. The combination of inactivity and anxiety may slow down labor which, in turn, triggers clinical interventions to speed up labor. When labor is accelerated, the pain of contractions rises and pain medication may be requested by the patient. Use of the medications may lower maternal blood pressure, which contributes to abnormal monitor readings. Cesarean section rates, which have skyrocketed, are 40 percent higher when electronic monitoring is used. Except for a possible small reduction in neonatal seizures, randomized clinical trials have not found that fetal monitoring improves overall fetal outcomes in terms of improvement in Apgar scores (a simple assessment of how a baby is doing at birth), cord blood gases, admission to the neonatal intensive care unit, low-oxygen brain damage, reduction in deaths, or the development of long-term problems like cerebral palsy (Alfirevic, Devane, and Gyte 2006). In the end, this medical device demonstrates only a small level of benefit, but poses significant potential risks, and yet its use is ubiquitous in the maternity wings of hospitals across the country. The story of fetal monitors is not unique but reflects, in diverse variation, problems with many of the costly new medical technologies receiving broad adoption (Deyo 2002).

New technologies are successfully promoted through a number of techniques and marketing strategies, including lobbying Congress to relax the regulation of the industry, aggressive selling to healthcare providers, media hype about the wonders of new technologies, and political pressure from trade associations. In the period between 2009 and 2011, biotechnology and medical device companies and their trade associations spent $126 million and $86 million respectively on Congressional lobbying efforts (Union of Concerned Scientists 2012). The Pharmaceutical Research and Manufacturers of America, the drug industry's chief lobbying group, spent nearly $150 million on lobbying between 2008 and 2015, putting it in sixth place among the country's biggest lobbying spenders. This association's lobbying expenditures were greater than powerful forces like defense contractors and the oil and gas industry during this period (Ludwig 2015).

Issues promoted in such lobbying include making job creation a concern of the FDA, thereby watering down public safety as the primary mission of the agency, lowering the scrutiny the FDA gives to new medical technologies, reducing conflict-of-interest standards for individuals who sit on FDA scientific advisory committees (to allow people with close ties to the industry on committees), and lowering the standard of evidence that companies can use to demonstrate product efficacy and safety. In 2012, Richard Pops, a representative of the Biotechnology Industry Organization, for example, testified before the House Energy and Commerce Subcommittee on Health that in recent years "arbitrary limits and unnecessarily restrictive interpretations of conflict of interest rules have created barriers that have prevented FDA from consistently recruiting highly qualified scientific advisors" (Union of Concerned Scientists 2012). Lost in such assertions is the question of bias among individuals on the company payroll.

Significant amounts of money also were donated during the 2009–11 period by the industry to Congressional elections, especially to incumbents who sat on two Congressional committees, the House Energy and Commerce Committee's Subcommittee on Health and the Senate Health Education Labor and Pensions Committee, that were working at the time on amendments to the Medical Device User Fee and Modernization Act. This act implemented a user fee system under which medical device companies must make payment to the U.S. Food and Drug Administration when registering with the agency or seeking to bring a new device to market in the US. These fees are used by the FDA to try to speed up the time that safe and effective devices can be put into use in the healthcare arena. By trying to shape laws, the industry seeks to have Congress work on its behalf rather than on behalf of the public.

Trade associations have come to play a big role in the lobbying efforts of the industry. Office holders who are committed to particular issues, perhaps because of constituency-voiced concerns, do not tend to like it when lobbyists try to convince them to vote against something they support or for something they do not support. This is where trade associations step in. In addition to putting on conferences for their members, setting industry standards, or publishing an industry newsletter, trade associations often are the most public voices in industry lobbying initiatives, allowing individual member companies to avoid antagonizing Congressional office holders whose help they may need in the future. In their lobbying, the trade associations have specific goals around individual bills and broader, long-term goals or ways of thinking about issues that they would like Congress to embrace. The latter include convincing Congress that: the FDA moves too slowly in approving new products, the government does not make enough venture capital available to the industry, Medicare does not adequately value new diagnostic technology (and hence does not pay for it), there is a need to have stronger policies to protect innovation, unlike the US other countries are aggressively implementing tax and other policies that lower the cost of research, development, and manufacturing of medical technology, while the US hurts the industry by taxing the profits that companies earn abroad (Advanced Medical Technology Association 2011). As this list suggests, from the trade association perspective, the government's job is to help grow the medical technology industry at taxpayer expense and at potential health risk. This viewpoint reflects a common business orientation perhaps first articulated by Henry Ford about the Food Motor Company: "What is good for Ford is good for America."

Additionally, in its effort to expand sales, medical device companies send sales representatives to medical schools and teaching hospitals to promote their products directly to physicians and hospitals. These visits may include providing training on device use, equipment calibration, and advice on implants and other sophisticated technologies (Lo and Field 2009). As with similar efforts by pharmaceutical company representatives, influencing ideas and building relationships that favor the bottom line of industry companies is the driving force in such promotion.

Media hype is another way in which new medical technologies, including those still under development, influence public expectations and hopes about technological salvation, and may influence public understanding of the value of safety regulation. News stories about exciting new medical breakthroughs, including new technologies, are now part of the standard fare of news broadcasting. Yet a review of 101 studies published in major scientific journals between 1979 and 1983 that claimed that a new therapy or new technology was promising found that only five of the products made it to market within a decade and only one of these five was still in wide use at the time of the review (Contopoulos-Ioannidis, Ntzani, and Ioannidis 2003).

Corporate Hospitals and Conglomerates

There has been a significant movement within the hospital sector over the last forty years toward the privatization of previously philanthropic not-for-profit institutions, their adoption of corporate-like component structures, and the linking of hospitals into ever-larger conglomerates. This structural transformation has had important effects on hospital policies and medical practice (Alexander, Morlock, and Gifford 1988). The corporate hospital, like all for-profit corporations, has a private agenda, which in this case involves an emphasis on perpetual growth, treatment of healthcare providers and allied health workers as employees, and handling patients as customers (Stoeckle and Reiser 1992). From the hospital perspective, as a result, "the most dangerous thing in America is an empty hospital bed," because it is not producing income, even if it means that people who are healthy enough not to need hospitalization are admitted nonetheless (Jeffrey Brenner, quoted in Freakonomics 2015).

Borrowing from President Eisenhower's farewell address upon leaving the White House, which included a stern warning about the rise of the military-industrial complex and its threat to society, Arnold Relman (1980)—influenced by the work of Barbara and John Ehrenreich (1970, also see Ehrenreich 2016)—raised a cautionary voice about the rise of what he called the "new medical-industrial complex," comprised of a large and growing network of investor-owned businesses, including hospitals, supplying health services for profit. Relman, as the editor of the *New England Journal of Medicine* at the time, was well positioned to see this trend in the corporatization of healthcare.

Analyzing data from the American Hospital Association's Annual Survey of Hospitals for the years 1988–2000, Horowitz (2005) examined over thirty medical services to test whether healthcare service offerings differed among three hospital ownership types: for-profit, not-for-profit, and government. One comparison involved services that varied by their profitability: consistently profitable services that are well-reimbursed by insurers (e.g., open heart surgery), consistently unprofitable services (e.g., psychiatric emergency room services which are disproportionately utilized by the poor and are not well reimbursed by insurance), services with variable profitable components (e.g., home health), and services with high capital costs (e.g., extracorporeal shock-wave lithotripsy [ESWL] to break stones in the kidney, gallbladder, or liver). The data indicate that for-profit hospitals were more likely to offer open heart surgery than not-for-profit hospitals, and government-owned hospitals were the least likely to do so. The magnitude of these differences was large. Conversely, hospital-based, psychiatric emergency services, which are relatively unprofitable, were most likely to be offered by government hospitals, followed by not-for-profit, and finally for-profit hospitals. The magnitude of these differences also was large. In the case of home health services, which dropped in profitability over the period of study due to changing federal policy, the probability of offering home health services fell a conspicuous 37.5 percent among for-profits, 7.7 percent among non-profits, and 1.5 percent among government-owned hospitals. Finally, the study found that all three types of hospitals were more likely to have ESWL services over time, but patterns of adoption were significantly different. Overall, 22 percent of for-profit hospitals, 17 percent of non-profit hospitals, and 13 percent of public hospitals were likely to offer ESWL. These patterns held across all of the service sectors that were examined suggested that Steinwald and Neuhauser (1970) were correct in asserting that corporatization would lead to "cream-skimming"; a practice that allows commercialized hospitals to make a profit by concentrating on the most profitable healthcare services provided to the best-paying patients and thereby skimming the cream off the market for hospital care, while leaving the remainder to non-profit and public hospitals. Additionally, in a study that used data from the California Health Facilities Commission, Patterson and Katz (1983) compared the economic performance of investor-owned and not-for-profit hospitals in California. They found that, during the period of study, both costs and charges were higher in for-profit hospitals compared to not-for-profit hospitals, whether measured in terms of patient-days or by admissions. They also found that for-profit hospital chains used aggressive marketing strategies and pricing techniques to generate profit and growth. This evidence supports the view that hospital types differ according to their interest in pursuing profits, with resulting differences in the types of services offered to patients, an issue of consequence for healthcare practice given the trend, discussed further in Chapter 4, toward hospital corporatization.

Conclusion

Despite some efforts at reform designed to make biomedical practitioners more sensitive to their patients as whole beings that are much more than the embodied sites of treatable diseases, and to contextualize patients in their communities and in light of their cultural orientations, examination of the array of forces that now shape the practice of medicine in the contemporary world affirms Relman's and the Ehrenreichs' apprehensions about the rise of the medical industrial complex. As Relman (1980) stressed, "A private health-care industry of huge proportions could be a powerful political force in the country and could exert considerable influence on national health policy." And this is precisely what has happened.

But the rise of the medical industrial complex has not solved the crisis of medicine in the US, including unparalleled expenditures on healthcare, but rather it has produced poorer results in terms of lifespan or morbidity patterns among patients, compared to the country's neighbor to the north or other highly industrialized countries; high levels of patient dissatisfaction and cost complaints; enduring health inequalities; and physician and other healthcare provider frustration with many aspects of their career experience. In fact, the medical industrial complex has intensified the crisis of medicine in the US. In the words of Michael Winship (2016), who served as senior writer of the public television series, *Moyers & Company*, "The crime, of course, is that none of this is a crime but business as usual." The reason this is so is because of a basic yet often ignored feature of free market economic systems: "if there is a profit to be made, someone will take it up, as long as it is legal and as long as there is no public protest against it" (Akerlof and Shiller 2015). By making the vital components of healthcare into commodities, sellable at a profit, and by blocking universal health insurance coverage, there is a real and measurable cost in human lives, a tragic expression of the kind of structural violence that now pervades the healthcare arena on every level. In the words of a popular health-is-a-right slogan, "in the U.S., healthcare has become wealthcare". It is within this peculiar context that doctors face tough challenges and must make difficult decisions about how they will practice medicine. In other words, they must decide if they will swim downstream with the current, doing their job with a narrow clinical focus, accepting gifts from the pharmaceutical industry, turning their heads at gross health and healthcare inequalities, and ignoring the painful yet readily available statistics on the human costs of the medical-industrial complex-generated status quo, or they can swim against the current. Political commentator and journalist Jim Hightower advocates the latter option: "swim against the current, even a dead fish can go with the flow" (Hightower and Demarco 2009).

The remainder of this book presents the case of one physician who in spite of often vexing challenges, including endless battles that had to be fought with institutionalized power structures that were not committed to the well-being of low-income and minority populations and the limitations on the ability of one physician to address the social origins of disease, persisted and was able to swim against the tide and carve out an alternative pathway that was true to his values and ethical commitments.

Commenting on the types of issues raised in this chapter, this physician noted

> the cost structure of pharmaceuticals in the United States is very different than in Canada and every other industrialized nation. Our government allows it, whether that's through collusion or just faulty reasoning. They allow the pharmaceutical and medical device companies as well as the for-profit health care companies to take advantage of the American public. There are public policy issues . . . there are health care policy issues . . . Everyone says "we can't do it all at once, choose one [thing to change]." Unfortunately, a lot of things have to be done simultaneously if you're going to be successful. If you look at the United States, versus other fully industrialized countries, we spend more by half, than any other country on earth and yet we get some of the worst health outcomes. You can either say that we're intensely stupid, or that we're not getting value for our dollar. You have to look at where those dollars are being diverted. The courts and the legislatures should, under ideal circumstances, be protecting Americans against greed and the undue influence of the powerful, but that's not what happening. So the question is how do you recapture your government and redirect it. There are public policy interventions that we know would work: taxing soft drinks and other unhealthy foods, working with the food industry and the fast food industry to decrease salt in processed food, regulating the amount of sugar, salt and chemicals in our food supply. Government's role should be as the consumer's watchdog, and assuring that industry considers, directly or indirectly, the healthfulness of its products, as it develops and markets its wares. Perhaps it's a bit cynical, but I believe it is a fact that people, generally, and corporations specifically, will do what they believe they can get away with. It's an unfortunate reality. It's also a reality that they will not go silently into the night on the strength of an incredibly logical critical argument. There really does need to be a revolution, I'm not suggesting an armed revolution, but certainly a political revolution. In view of the results of the recent [2016] presidential and congressional election, we will have to remain vigilant, strategic and work very hard, but the stakes have never been as high and worth the effort.

3

BEING A PERSON, BECOMING A DOCTOR

> The physicians are the natural attorneys of the poor, and the social problems should largely be solved by them.
>
> *Rudolph Virchow*

Formative Years, People, and Places

When Bruce was asked about his early life, he joked about his age saying, "I was born in a log cabin on the prairie," adding that Abraham Lincoln and he were once roommates. Regular joking, in fact, is part of Bruce's routine deportment. People, he explained, "respond to my humor in general. I don't think they are humoring me." His comical side is rooted in what he calls "a sense of the absurd." Because he often can see the farcicalities lurking beneath constructed formalities, rigid bureaucracies, and self-serving behaviors, he is "able in some ways to laugh off or dismiss some of the barriers, challenges, and jerks" that stand in the way of meeting the healthcare needs of patients:

> I come in contact often with a lot of folks who are difficult and obstructive in unimagined ways. I'm able . . . not to dismiss them, I'm not being dismissive, but to hear them, embrace them and move forward despite them or with them.

And forward certainly has been the primary direction in Bruce's life.

Rather than the wind-swept prairie, or at Lincoln's birthplace in a log cabin at Sinking Springs Farm, Kentucky (which at the time was part of Virginia), Bruce actually was born in Horace Harding Hospital in Queens on Long Island, New York in 1954. His parents wanted children but had trouble conceiving. They tried again and again for nine years, and even attempted artificial insemination. Nothing helped until they began filing adoption papers, after which his mother finally got pregnant with his sister Jackie. Eighteen months later, Bruce entered the world. His parents were overjoyed; it had been so difficult the first time they thought they would never have another child. The siblings grew up a few blocks from Belmont Race Track where the famous Belmont Stakes, the third leg of the thoroughbred Triple Crown, is run annually. Despite proximity to the track, Bruce did not attend a horse race until he began medical school. As he explained, "My parents were not . . . race folks." While they had a liquor cabinet in their home, they also rarely drank, mainly at funerals and special occasions." What they were, from Bruce's perspective, were two intelligent, moral, committed and loving people who had a tremendous affirming influence on his life course. "I think," he commented, "the way we were raised [was with the understanding that] a child is a blessing."

Bruce's parents were Jewish and he was raised with a Jewish identity and within the context of Eastern European Jewish culture as it blended and merged with the cultural strains of the United States. This included some folk beliefs. Even with acculturation in the US, for example, many of his relatives retained the belief in the evil eye and the ability of some people to cause harm with a malicious gaze. This notion is referenced in the Mishnah, part of the Talmud that emerged as part of the Hebrew oral tradition that developed in years after the destruction of the Second Temple in 70 CE. Because his mother was childless for so many years, some relatives did not want her near their young children for fear that jealousy would push her to curse the baby and cause it harm. As a result, at times his mother felt ostracized within her own extended family which led to occasion exchanges of harsh words. With the birth of her children, the fear that she might have an evil eye and the tensions and pain it caused evaporated, and thus she felt doubly blessed. As a result, Bruce came into a world of many caring relatives.

A great-uncle, Ben-Tzion Abelowitz, who along with his wife were killed by the Nazis in Lithuania after the German invasion, was the source of Bruce's first name. His middle name, Ephraim, was given in memory of his maternal grandmother's brother who died in Auschwitz. After the war, a man who had known Bruce's great-uncle in the concentration camp came to his grandmother's door. The two men had sworn to each other that if either survived that they would find their friend's family and tell them what happened to him. It is an enactment called "bearing witness" so that people are not erased from history. Novelist, political activist, Nobel Peace Prize awardee, and Holocaust survivor, Elie Wiesel (1993) has written, "For the dead and the living, we must bear witness." In the aftermath of the Holocaust, witnessing and the sharing of memories became a form of resisting the Nazi "final solution." The fascists tried not only to wipe out Jews but also to exterminate all memory of them in Europe, as well as the unspeakable horror of Nazi crimes against humanity. Remembering the victims of the Nazis emerged as a form of returning people to their rightful place in the human story.

Telling this piece of his family history reminded Bruce of a famous poem by prominent Protestant pastor and outspoken public foe of Adolf Hitler, Martin Niemöller (Holocaust Museum 2016):

First they came for the Socialists, and I did not speak out—
Because I was not a Socialist.
Then they came for the Trade Unionists, and I did not speak out—
Because I was not a Trade Unionist.
Then they came for the Jews, and I did not speak out—
Because I was not a Jew.
Then they came for me—and there was no one left to speak for me.

Poems have had a noticeable impact on Bruce's articulation of his view of the world, he was reminded of them often as he explained his views and values.

Bruce remembered his family as being safe and caring, but deeply affected by the jarring events that so recently had swept away so many of their relatives in Europe. His parents were both born in the US but their parents had fled Europe, his father's parents in 1905, and his mother's about 15 years later. They had come during the pogroms (from the Slavic words for "to harm"), waves of anti-Semitic persecution and periodic massacres that targeted the Jews living in Russia and Eastern Europe during the nineteenth and early twentieth centuries. His grandparents became part of a great migration of Jews from Eastern Europe, a movement that has been called a "family migration" because people did not tend to travel across the Atlantic alone but came in small family groups huddled together aboard crowded ships. Bruce's grandmother, for example, was brought to the US by her oldest sister, who raised her in their new home. He warmly remembers his mother's mother, Sarah, the youngest of ten siblings, as a "warm and fuzzy" grandmother. He would visit her while an undergraduate student at Cornell on trips home to Long Island and felt he had a real friendship with her. The way she came to the US also has been described as a "chain migration," because commonly members of an extended family would arrive, find jobs, and begin saving to bring other relatives over on the trying transoceanic voyage. Working in a sweatshop, Bruce's uncle Sam Brodsky, was able to live frugally and save the money to pay for these two of his wife's sisters to cross the sea. But as happened with many immigrant families, it took years to save enough funds to reunite the whole family in the US and by then time ran out. The other nine siblings still in Europe, and indeed hundreds of relatives that Bruce, in his self-appointed role as family historian, has collected records on and photos of all perished in the Holocaust; "they were in Poland, so when the Germans marched in, they went to the ovens."

Bruce's father's parents came from Europe together. Their meeting was part chance, part family practice, part romance, and part scandal. Their encounter began when Bruce's great-grandmother Rena Jaffe, who lived in Kovnogobernea, Lithuania, received a letter from her sister Jane, who was living in England with her husband Morris Goldstein. In the letter, Jane lamented having no children while Rena had four, and she suggested that her niece Leah be sent to live with her. Rina knew that life would be far better for Leah in England, and given the pogroms, much safer. So at the age of about 12, Leah began living with her aunt in London. Meanwhile, Morris wrote a similar letter to his brother in Warsaw,

Poland, which was under Tsarist rule at the time. Soon Jacob Goldstein arrived to live with his uncle and aunt as well. While they lived as brother and sister, Leah and Jacob were not biological relatives and they knew it. An attraction developed between them that came to fruition after Jacob returned from service in the British Army, where he fought in the Second Boer War in Southern Africa. In 1905, the young couple boarded the S.S. *Cedric*—which would later ferry soldiers during World War I—and traveled from Liverpool to New York City. In the ship's manifest, they are listed as Jacob Goldstein and Cousin Leah according to records Bruce has discovered. For his application for naturalization in the US, his grandfather had to sign a document renouncing his allegiance to Tsar Nicholas the Second of Russia, an allegiance he no doubt never felt. For a long time, the wider family was aghast at this union of "cousins" and needlessly worried that the children would suffer from the kinds of genetic defects that can occur with inbreeding.

In New York, his paternal grandfather found work as a pattern cutter in a sweatshop clothing factory, but died 13 years later when Bruce's father, Solomon Goldstein (later changed to Sheldon Gould), was just three months old. His grandmother was left with four children to raise alone during the 1920s and the Great Depression. The family was extremely poor. At the time, immigrant families could not survive on the earnings of a single head of household (Hyman 2009). Without her husband, Bruce's grandmother could not fulfill her gendered cultural role as a *baleboosteh* (an efficient home manager) and supplemental breadwinner. As a result, his father was placed in an orphanage for a period, and it was there that he celebrated his Bar Mitzvah at age 13.

Solomon faced anti-Semitism from several corners as a teenager. He could not find work and he was subject to bullying by several local street gangs. One threat came from a group of pro-Nazi hooligans affiliated with the German American Bund. Because their party uniform included brown tops, they came to be known as brown shirts. His father also was periodically beaten up by an Irish youth gang. But the Irish hated the Nazis and one day used Bruce's father as bait to draw them out and then attacked them when they began to beat up his father. After that day, he was freed of his tormentors. These kinds of experiences made his father more assertive and willing to stand up to authority. On the down side, he had a long memory and did not easily forgive an offense and move on.

Despite the hardships he endured, Bruce remarked that his father "wound up being this really wonderful, kind, caring, mentsch [human being]." His father developed a love of music, especially of opera, in part as an escape from the poverty and multiple dangers of New York's working-class streets. He discovered that

> there were standing room tickets in the back of the Metropolitan Opera house. He would go on Saturdays, and so growing up in our house [there was always music]. He had taught himself electronics and had the wherewithal to build this enormous stereo, with huge speakers and he would just blast it, both opera and big bands, [and] we would dance. My parents were ballroom dancers.

The neighbors, however, did not always appreciate his father's commitment to loud music. In fact, Bruce recalls that

> the one fight I ever saw my father almost get into was with our neighbor [over the music]. The house I grew up in was a driveway away from the [neighbor's] kitchen window and I remember [the guy] next door yelling across and saying "turn that fucking music down." And my father turned it down, but then went out and said "how dare you use foul language in front of my children." It became this face-off but never came to blows. They later reconciled.

Bruce's maternal grandfather was a painter. He worked on painting Franklyn D. Roosevelt's apartment in New York City and met Eleanor Roosevelt while he was at the apartment. One of his grandfather's jokes was that he went to Columbia University Medical School without getting a medical degree. In truth, he went there because he was hired to repaint several buildings. His grandfather would show up at Bruce's family's home whenever it was time to repaint and he taught Bruce how to mix pigments to match colors. This training had a lasting impression on Bruce who stressed

> I've done lots of painting . . . I've always never been afraid to break a sweat. So I do woodwork, and plumbing, and electrical. I've rarely hired somebody [to work on my home] . . . In the old days, I used to take the TV apart and I used to work on my car . . . Maybe some of that transfers over to the sort of the mentality [I have] of trying to fix things. So much [in the world] is just broken.

Bruce's first, most vivid memory is of getting attacked by his neighbor's boxer when he was 3 years old. The dog had just delivered a litter of puppies and all the kids in his neighborhood went to see them. The dog got nervous with so many children hovering over her puppies and bit Bruce in the face, her teeth entering his eye socket on top and his jaw on the bottom. Blood was pouring from his wound. He quickly recovered, with no permanent injuries and only some scary images to carry with him through life. He also remembers being blown across the room in his father's workshop when he stuck his hand in a high-voltage box in the back of a television. The first words out of his father's mouth once he determined that Bruce was all right was "oh my god your mother's gonna kill me." Another time, when he was about 11, he was helping his father put an antenna on the roof. His father tied a rope from himself to Bruce but not to the chimney because if Bruce fell off the roof "he just wanted me to pull him over with me so that he wouldn't have to face my mother."

Bruce's youth unfolded during the Cold War, a period of intense rivalry between two heavily armed countries, the US and the Soviet Union, that stretched through much of the latter half of the twentieth century until the formal dissolution of the

Soviet system in December 1991. It was a time of mutual suspicions, heightened political tensions, and a number of close-call incidents that raised the possibility of global nuclear war. In both countries, an atmosphere of fear prevailed, which was exploited by politicians to gain support for particular policies. Recalled Bruce:

> [When] I was 9 years old, [it was] scary, the Russian thing, the Kennedy assassination, the Cuban missile crisis, the whole juxtaposition with the Soviet Union, and the arms race. In elementary school, we had drills where you go into the hall, stand against the wall and hold your hands over your head as though that would protect you from a nuclear blast. As a joke, we would chant, "wall, wall, please don't fall." There were drills where we would crawl under our desks in case the ceilings fell. And then there were the "go home" drills where they would put a tag on you with identification information and send you home, and then sirens would sound in the town. That was pretty frightening. There was a lot of press and stories, the nuclear Armageddon scenarios like *On the Beach*, a novel and a movie about a submarine that's at sea when a nuclear war occurs and America and much of the rest of the world is wiped out and the few places that survive will slowly die from the radiation.

Although he grew up at a time when the use of spanking to punish an errant child was common, it was the rarest of events in his home. With increased public awareness and discussion of child abuse, the whole issue of the use of corporal punishment to discipline a child has shifted. Yet, even in 2014, a YouGov/Huffington Post survey of a thousand randomly selected U.S. adults interviewed about punishing children found that people tend to support hand spanking (81 percent felt it should be legal), but not if it leaves lasting injury to a child (Moore 2014). Scientific research on the issue flows in the reverse direction. Various studies show that physical punishment tends to make kids more aggressive, does not change children's behavior in the long run, and may make it worse. Moreover, physical punishment is cyclical: children who are physically punished are more likely to try solve their conflicts with their peers and sibling physically (Taylor et al. 2010, Tomoda et al. 2009, Strauss and Pachall 2009). Bruce's parents, perhaps more as an expression of their values than because of cognizance of its negative effects, did not use physical punishment with their children. However, Bruce recalls one exception to this pattern:

> my father probably hit me once, when I was a kid, gave me a spanking per se because I had scribbled in all of his books. And then he cried, I'm not sure I did. One thing that was sacred in our household were books, learning, and education. He gave me a couple [of spanks] and that was the last time, but they never really had to because it wasn't till I was a senior in high school that I started hanging out at night, and coming home at 7 in the morning, and being a little bit of a rebel, but that was normative behavior [for teens].

Growing up, Bruce had only a flirting relationship with the youth drug culture that swirled around him. At the time he was a teenager, the size of the youth population of the US had grown substantially, and, in response to the War in Vietnam and the struggles of the civil rights movement, there was a significant cultural break with the more conventional youth values of the prior generation. The era marked an important new turning point in American drug use dynamics which included: (1) a huge increase in the number of illicit drug users in the country; (2) the addition of new populations of drug users, particularly youth and young adults from the White middle and even upper classes; and (3) the popular rise of a new set of drugs, including, but not limited to, a strong emphasis on a class of drugs known as the hallucinogenics (Singer 2006). Bruce, however, never got particularly involved in illicit drug consumption:

> marijuana whatever, never did a lot for me, but I certainly tried it. It didn't really affect me, but it certainly affected [my friend]. [One day after smoking what might have been marijuana together], we walked back into my house and my mother says "Boys how are you?" and he says, "Mrs. G, how does it feel to have a drug addict for a son?" and my mother [replied] "Oh you're so funny." I mean for all I know we were smoking camel dung. Then in college, I tried smoking [marijuana again] and it just didn't do anything. I also can't hold my liquor and I don't really drink . . . pretty boring! Once in a while if I go to a nice restaurant I'll have wine [like] Zinfandel or something sweet. My friends are into bourbon and scotch. But it just doesn't taste good [to me].

The neighborhood his family lived in was composed of small, single-family, often one-story bungalows, sometimes referred to as "Roosevelt Cottages" (a mocking comparison with the 34-room Roosevelt family summer residence) or, less fancifully, as "boxy little houses." They were built as affordable housing primarily for returning GIs after World War II. In the years between 1945 and 1954, over 13 million such units were erected in a historically significant housing boom (Konczal 2009). Construction was dictated by a shortage of building materials in the aftermath of the war, coupled with a strong demand for housing among GIs with young families. Boasting little in the way of stylistic ornamentation, the bungalows generally were small (some being under 1,000 sq. ft.), with usually only two bedrooms. Bruce recalls that in his neighborhood, the houses "were postage stamps, the same house, maybe one turned sideways, two or three floorplans, block, after block, after very rectangular block." Most of the homes were built by speculative builders, by non-union workers, and purchased by White families who could take advantage of a variety of government incentive programs that often were explicitly denied to people of color. Banks used redlining to segregate residential areas and deny access to African Americans and other denigrated groups.

"Eligible" families, by contrast, were able to buy a track home with 5 percent down 30-year mortgage terms. The result was the birth of the suburbs and of private home ownership by an unparalleled number of people. They soon populated what has been called "the least exotic place" in New York City, a sprawling terrain of small homes, shopping centers, baby carriages and "paralyzing ordinariness" (Rosenthal 1999). Long Island was, in fact, the site of one of the most famous restructurings of the Eastern Seaboard environment, Levittown, the archetype of post-World War II suburbia.

In the emergent neighborhoods of post-war suburbia, hypersegregation and the unequal distribution of health and healthcare—some of the very problems Bruce seeks to tackle by embracing an alternative path in medicine—were deeply embedded in policies and practices regarding housing access. Bruce describes his childhood neighborhood as "working class, pretty much white, back in that day, Italian and Jewish." Observe Squires and Kubrin (2006), "Racial composition of neighborhoods has long been at the center of public policy and private practice in the creation and destruction of communities and in determining access to the elements of the good life, however defined." Indeed, more than just the "good life," but often life itself. The experience of fighting for the US in Europe and then returning to a country where they faced abject discrimination in housing and in other arenas of life was a powerful blow to African American GIs. Moreover, the enduring legacy of post-war social and economic discrimination contributed to the significant wealth gap that still abides between Whites and people of color. Consequently, Squires and Kubrin (2006) argue, "Place matters. Neighborhood counts." People's access to "decent housing, safe neighborhoods, good schools, useful contacts and other benefits is largely influenced by the community in which one is born, raised and resides" (Squires and Kubrin 2006: 47). Although, as Galyean (2016) stresses, "1950s suburbia conjures visions of traditional family life, idyllic domesticity and stability," the true story of the suburbanization of the US "is also one of exclusion, segregation and persecution." The very opportunity structure that is such a compelling social influence on individual life experience and well-being, cannot be understood independent of the political economy of place (Massey and Denton 1993).

The making of neighborhoods, in other words, including the very one where Bruce grew up in a congenially supportive and caring environment, reflects the less than fully overt apparatus of structural violence that drives health and other forms of inequality in the US. As Winter and Leighton (2001) underline, structural violence is embedded "in ubiquitous social structures, normalized by stable institutions and regular experiences." It is because they are routine and longstanding that "structural inequalities usually seem ordinary—the way things are and always have been" (Winter and Leighton 2001). Adds Farmer and colleagues (2006), because the mechanisms of structural violence "seem so ordinary in our ways of understanding the world, they appear to be almost invisible."

This was no doubt the case for most of the families who were able to secure loans and to move into the type of suburban community in which Bruce was born and spent his early years. Some people, of course, having lived previously in integrated urban neighborhoods, noticed the whiteness of the suburbs, and some even participated in protesting discriminatory practice. The end result of the unequal geographic distribution of privilege, however, is not unconnected to why Bruce might go on to become a physician and a child born to an African American family the same year as Bruce was much less likely to do so. And not too much has changed since Bruce was growing up. A recent re-examination of segregation in the US found a continued if shifting pattern of high residential segregation between African Americans and Whites, especially in suburbia (Lichter, Parisi, and Taquino 2015). Using the Theil Index, an analytic tool for measuring economic and other inequality, these researchers conclude that political and economic factors "play a large and typically unappreciated role in excluding Blacks and other minorities from the geographic mainstream," acting as a mechanism for the "sorting of disadvantaged minority populations into disadvantaged place-based labor markets and school districts" (Lichter, Parisi, and Taquino 2015: 870). In the jarring irony that lies behind surface appearances in U.S. society, Bruce's life is no less a product—in a far different way—than the impoverished and ailing patients he seeks to heal or for whom he tries to at least dampen the clinical results of the insults and injuries of structural violence. Importantly, Bruce has not used his privilege to focus narrowly on his own well-being and that of his family; rather, he has mobilized it in the service of those who have been disadvantaged by structural violence.

Growing up, Bruce did not feel privileged. With reference to his family's socioeconomic status, Bruce noted:

> we were not "poor poor," but we were probably poorer than my parents ever let me feel. We ate a lot of pasta. My mother was a housewife, [but] my father would get up at five in the morning, get on the train to New York City [for work].

He recalled that his family lived on what he referred to as the lower income side of town. But it was a place where

> the summer days [were] heavy, and fragrant, with nights full of fireflies. The fireflies [were] everywhere in the neighborhood, no longer the case, due to pesticides and environmental change. I remember catching fireflies in a bottle and, I know it's cliché, but I would take them under the covers at night, and try to read a book by their light. It was just a lot of fun. And then the kids in the neighborhood, we used to play ringalevio and kickball in the street till after dark . . . [There was a] richness of summer . . . a heaviness. The warm humid time just inching along. There's something just so incredibly poignant about that. In a way that's what I want to go back to someday, that ability to just live, in that moment.

It is this sentiment that influenced Bruce to identify with the novel *Dandelion Wine* by Ray Bradbury, and it became one of his favorite books. Set in the summer of 1928 in a small town in Illinois, the book employed the symbol of dandelion wine to represent pouring all the joys of a child's summer in small-town America into a single potent bottle. Bruce expressed that the book had touched him when he first read it:

> His language is so evocative, and descriptive that you can smell the flowers, you can smell the mown grass, you can feel your feet in sneakers running. That richness of that summer growing up touched a lot of chords of my growing up.

Bruce's nostalgic and optimistic sides are also revealed in his favorite movie, Frank Capra's 1946 classic *It's a Wonderful Life*, which he watches at Christmas time every year, and still cries at the end: "Not because it's sad, it's actually happy." The appeal for Bruce is that the movie highlights the fact that people can be redeemed, they can change, there can be goodness in the world.

Unfortunately, as Bruce well knows, summers end, sometimes tragically so in a single moment. One such occurrence that had a deep emotional impact on him as a child was the assassination of President Kennedy:

> My hero, if I can be honest, [was] Jack Kennedy. When Jack Kennedy got assassinated, I was 9 years old, 1963. I remember going down in the basement and sobbing, sobbing, sobbing, I was inconsolable. He was this iconic figure, and the whole family [was upset]. I still have some Kennedy cards at home. They actually came with bubble gum. They were trading cards with pictures of Camelot, of the White House, and the [Kennedy] family. It was a very different time. The press did not vilify . . . the president . . . so you could have a purist view. I remember the moment . . . I was sitting in 4th-grade class, Mrs. Casey's class, three rows back, center of the room, when she came up in tears and said "President Kennedy's been shot." So that's one news event that I remember, and the days leading up to his funeral, and it was just devastating. And Robert Kennedy also was an iconic figure, about civil rights and human rights, and doing the right thing. And Martin Luther King . . . was brilliant and incredibly courageous at a time when we needed someone to be brilliant and incredibly courageous. I was aware of what was going on, I was 10 years old, 11 years old, I was horrified [by the assassinations].

From an early age, books began to have a deep influence on Bruce:

> when I was 5, 6 years old, I wanted to be a paleontologist and study dinosaurs. My parents had bought me a "How and Why" book about dinosaurs and I was just fascinated. First and second grade, every book report was on dinosaurs. I would just read up on different dinosaurs. And then they bought me the "How and Why" book of lost cities and so archeology would become my passion. And then they got me this book on the solar system and astronomy eclipsed all my other interests . . . I became fascinated by it. All

> sort of science-based [books], and history, that sense of recreating history. A big thing for me as a kid was lying awake at night pondering that the universe was infinite, and reaching a point, and it still happens to me, where you are trying to get your arms around what going on forever means, and you just can't quite embrace it. And that's when I would fall asleep.

Precociously when he was only 5 years old, Bruce and a friend started a little company:

> We used to weed for the neighbors. I remember [one] lawn was just all weeds. And [the owner] paid us a penny a weed. I remember we pooled our resources . . . probably had netted about a dollar fifty. At one point we had a little tiff, some sort of childhood quarrel. We divided the company holdings and dissolved the corporation.

Some time later, he got into another argument with this friend: "We were playing, and got into a minor disagreement and he hit me over the head with an old rake. I was bleeding and I came home bloody and my father probably went over and talked to his parents." This same friend years later taught Bruce to play guitar:

> I remember going over to his house, he had a guitar and I didn't. I knew basic chords. He taught me to Travis pick. Travis picking [popular in ragtime] was named after a guy named [Merle] Travis [a country and western performer, best known for his ode to coal miners called "Sixteen Tons"], It allows you to play chords with your left hand while picking out the bass notes and tune with your right as backup to singing. I learned a lot of protest songs growing up. I finally bought a guitar as a med school graduation present to myself. Still have it. Still singing those protest songs.

Another friend, Neil, the boy who lived next door to Bruce growing up, began to learn to play the saxophone, and two years later, Bruce did too. This friend went on to become a musician and a musical agent. Although decades have gone by and Neil now lives in Michigan, he still signs birthday cards to Bruce BND (Boy Next Door). As a doctor, Bruce diagnosed this friend's skin cancer: "he came to visit ten years ago and we were talking and I said, 'I would have somebody look at that, I'm a little concerned,' and he had an early skin cancer." Bruce looked up to Neil:

> [he] was little bit of a hero to me, as a kid, because he was a really nice guy, and a good guy, and he mentored me. That's really what your world is about when you're a kid. And in a way you pay that forward. You realize that those seminal moments when an adult or an older kid, mentors, helps, influences a younger one, sometimes is the turning point in someone's life. And I try to give everyone a chance at that if I can, I have trouble saying no.

Arthur and Bruce met in seventh grade, immediately bonded, and stayed best friends through high school and college at Cornell. More like brothers than friends, Art later moved his family to Simsbury, CT to pursue his business career and to allow his two daughters to grow up with Bruce's children:

> Art was a big guy in body, intellect, and heart. I was always somehow finding myself in the role as his trainer, life coach, dietitian. He taught me an enormous amount about life and challenges and keeping your sense of humor.

Arthur died of leukemia at age 48 after a ten-year struggle with the disease. Although Bruce and Arthur's family all somehow survived the catastrophe of his passing, Bruce thinks of him every day and the life lessons he left behind.

Another childhood friend was Richard, the third musketeer, with Bruce and Art in high school. He got a job at age 16 and used his earnings to buy a car, which enabled Bruce and Art, his closest friends, to "go cruising." Richard went to business school after college and went on to work in the oil industry, eventually winding up in Anchorage working on the Alaska pipeline. He is now retired and sometimes visits Boston: "I'll pick him up at the train in Hartford and we will carouse around for a few days and it's like high school all over again."

Bruce's father taught at RCA Institutes in New York City. At the time, RCA was a leading center for education and development in the communications industry. Originally the school trained operators for wireless telegraphy, the messaging system that evolved into radio. As a teenager, Bruce's father became interested in Morse code and later radio, just as the new technology was becoming available to the general public. His father had planned to become an accountant and had even enrolled in City College in New York to pursue that career. It was there that he met Bruce's mother, who did so well in school that she graduated high school at age 15. When they met, his father was 20 and his mother was just 16. Their first encounter was on a four-way blind date, but neither of their respective dates actually showed up to the meeting place, so they went out with each other instead. Bruce recalled his mother once telling him that one of the first things his father said to her was "I'm never gonna get married. I'm not the marrying kind, so don't get any ideas." Further complicating the situation, Bruce's paternal grandmother opposed the soon budding relationship and tried to torpedo it, without success.

Global events, however, namely World War II, suddenly intervened. Bruce's father enlisted and was sent to fighter pilot school in the Army Air Force. But he fell out of favor with his officers because he disobeyed orders on several occasions. On the first, he refused to eject from a plane that was malfunctioning during training and instead landed it damaged in a cornfield. On the second, he was ordered to land his plane but did not because he thought he would hit another plane in his flight pattern. As a result, because of his knowledge of Morse code and radio, he was assigned to be an instructor to train radio operators on B-17 Flying Fortresses, used during the war for strategic bombing of German factories and military targets, and the B-24 Liberator, which was used especially for anti-submarine warfare and to bomb Japan. He wrote part of the manual used to train operators how to fix a broken radio. As a result, he never left the US during the war.

While his father was based in Sioux Falls, South Dakota, his mother took a train from New York to meet him, and they were married there by an army chaplain on his mother's birthday. After the war, Bruce's father worked for a time as an NBC cameraman, before taking a correspondence course in teaching electronics, which led to his job with RCA Institutes. With the salary from RCA, and a second job fixing electrical appliances in his basement shop on the side, his parents were able to buy the Long Island house where Bruce and his sister were raised. But, it was his parents' attempt to adopt a child that actually triggered the move to Long Island. Reports Bruce:

> At that time, the adoption agency said "you're living in an apartment, its windows look out over the elevated train [part of the New York subway system], there are fumes, all of this is terrible for the baby" . . . So they literally took the plunge and bought the house in the suburbs.

Because of Bruce's mother's pregnancy, the Gould family never adopted a child.

Bruce's family is one that today would be labeled a functional nuclear family, close knit but supported by a broad network of kin that included in Bruce's words "lots of family gatherings." Studies suggest that functional families provide emotionally safe environments to their members, healthy respectful relationships, accountability, sufficient individual privacy, and support for individual growth and development, and a structure of routines and family rituals (Lewis et al. 1976). This is precisely what Bruce experienced in his family growing up, adding with reference to family rituals:

> My father's parents were not observant at all, but Rosh Hashanah, Yom Kippur, we did as a family. Saturday nights, I would always make pizza. You can buy these pizza crusts with a bag, a very square bag, of tomato sauce and cheese. I would cook pizza for the family. There was no cable. There were 13 channels, maybe half of them didn't work. But *Saturday Night at the Movies* was on Channel 4, I think, and it had either a classic movie, or a recent release, which meant five or ten years old. But again we didn't have a lot of money, so we didn't go out to the movies a lot. I [did] go to the movies with my father, mainly war movies. The women didn't want to go, so my dad and I would have "men's night out." My growing up was very much family oriented.

Feeling the World: Values and Ethics

Bruce describes his parents as highly ethical people with a political consciousness. His grandmother and mother, in fact, participated in street demonstrations, once chaining themselves to the U.N. building in New York in a protest in support of the Jews in the Soviet Union who were being subjected to government persecution. They also were involved in the elder rights movement and both parents helped to start a support organization called Friends of the Handicapped at a time when physically challenged people were routinely denied access or other civil rights. They would take people to parks or other recreational and entertainment activities. Even as a child, Bruce would accompany his parents in this work and recalls outings with

> all of these people in wheelchairs, and on crutches, people with cerebral palsy, and who couldn't talk, people of color. And at our house, my parent's friends, many of them were disabled. On a routine weekend, our living room . . . was filled with diverse people . . . I think that exposure to and love of diversity is something you absorb from your parents and family, as you go forward.

While at RCA, his father joined a teacher's union, and Bruce has memories of walking the picket line with his father when the RCA teachers went on strike. This too impacted his worldview and he sees it as influencing his sensitivity to the labor movement and the ongoing struggle of workers for decent wages and working conditions. He also walked the picket line with his grandfather for the painter's union.

In high school, he participated in demonstrations against the War in Vietnam:

> I started in [my] junior year going into New York City on the weekends. I went door to door canvassing against the war, getting signatures on petitions. I remember going out and lowering the flag to half-mast in high school and the jocks would come out put it back up and then we would go out and lower it back down . . . And there was something called the Peace Boat, which was a freighter that had all sorts of antennae on it and sailed off the shore of Israel to make peace broadcasts to both the Israeli and Arab populations. I used to clean and paint the boat.

Bruce describes his mother as a glass "half full" person, noting "she was always into something, raising this for the poor, doing that, even though we really didn't have a lot." His father he saw as "the founding member of my personal fan club, which I think is what all parents should be." Then he added, "my mother clearly was either the co-founder, or certainly the first member." Bruce's sister also became a social activist and a committed feminist. As a result, he mentioned, "she's had a tough time along the way because she has really felt there's the right and there's the wrong, and you must do the right, regardless of consequences." Adding, "to be honest, I very much have that same concept."

Remembering the activism of his family members, Bruce suddenly mentioned again the assassination of John F. Kennedy, someone who had inspired him with his famous 1961 inaugural address statement: "My fellow Americans, ask not what your country can do for you, ask what you can do for your country." To Bruce, this meant "you have to step up, you have to do the right thing." This value is a core element of Bruce's ethical compass. He explained

> As a kid, you start forming that image of who you would like to wind up being, and that can go either way. And it's really tough, I tell my students this all the time, that the acculturation [process in] the medical profession . . . will attempt to beat the humanity and ethical constructs out of you. It shouldn't, but it tries to.

He sees some students watch their peers changing, losing their humanist values and it makes them want to quit medical school. He admits to having the same experience himself as a medical student. He found he needed periodic moments to reflect on issues like what was most important to him, what he wanted to do with his life, and how to be a moral person in an often immoral world.

Bruce's ethical perspective was significantly influenced by his experience with Jewish belief and practice. As a youth, he was involved in synagogue activities, serving as president of the Long Island Federation of Temple Youth. LIFTY, he explained, "was part of the national federation, so I ran Long Island in . . . my senior year of high school." This involvement, which included giving talks and organizing activities at local synagogues, helped him to develop as a community leader, a capacity also promoted by his participation in high school student

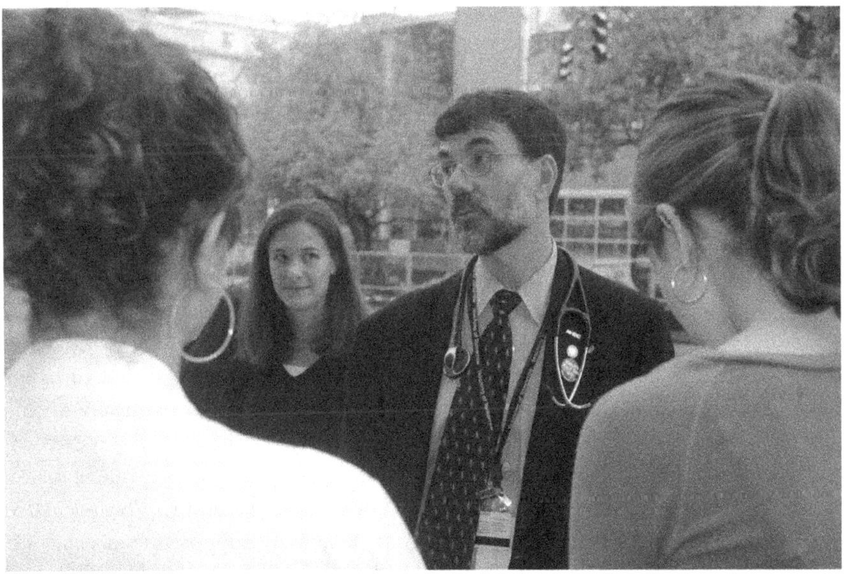

FIGURE 3.1 Bruce working with medical students

government, Key Club, as well as his membership in the boy scouts, where he became an eagle scout and senior patrol leader. He explained

> I was valedictorian of my high school class, I was valedictorian of my elementary school class, I was president of the student council in junior high school, and I was president of the Key Club, and I was treasurer. I was a senior patrol leader for the boy scouts, and I [hung out with] the "studious group" at high school.

His immersion in LIFTY also deepened his thinking about Jewish beliefs as they were relevant to his life as well. Thus he commented:

> between [the Jewish holiday of] Rosh Hashanah, which means the head of the year, the beginning of the year, and Yom Kippur there are ten days [known in Judaism as the Days of Awe]. And those are supposed to be days of introspection, and a time to review what you've done in the past year. And you can ask God for forgiveness . . . for sins against God, God can forgive you. But for sins against man, God can't forgive you, you have to actually go [to the person you offended to] ask forgiveness, and that's what you're supposed to be doing in those "days of awe."

Moreover, he mentions the

> imagery of the Book of Life, *Sefer HaChaim* [which is mentioned several times in the Bible]. It is opened on Rosh Hashanah and it is closed (claps his hands as if closing a book) on Yom Kippur. And it is in those ten days . . . that you're trying to get your name written, both figuratively and perhaps literally, in the Book of Life for the coming year [because only those whose names are written there will survive the year]. And if you look at the Rosh Hashanah service and the Yom Kippur service, it's all about that uncertainty of who will be here next year.

For Bruce, a reformed Jew, addressing transgressions—not just small interpersonal insults but the major crimes of oppression enacted through structural violence every day against subordinate groups—is central to his life values.

This attitude is expressed as well in his view of the Jewish concept of *tikkun olam*. This term literally means repairing the world, or more exotically within Jewish mysticism, repairing God (in the sense that by following the 613 commandments found in the Bible Jews help return to the Godhead the sparks of divinity that were scattered in the material world during creation). This expanded list of commandments, including 248 things people are supposed to do and 365 things they are banned from doing is mentioned in the Talmud, but a precise list is not actually provided. Notably, in the Talmud, *tikkun olam* refers specifically to social practices implemented in society to protect those who are disadvantaged (e.g., rules for freeing slaves in their seventh year of servitude). For Bruce, the concept has come to mean "while you're here, your commandment is to heal the world, to make the world a better place. This life is not a dress rehearsal!" This understanding of personal responsibility was a key value in the Gould family and was inscribed on his mother's gravestone when she died. In her last year of life, she told Bruce that it was "her hope was that the world was a little better for her having been here." Thinking about this, Bruce is reminded of the prize-winning novel *Schindler's Ark* by Australian writer Thomas Keneally, which he read several times. The book, and the epic movie it inspired, *Schindler's List*, is based on the life of Oskar Schindler, a German businessman credited with saving the lives of over a thousand Jews during the Holocaust by employing them in his factories. Bruce recalls the last scene in the movie:

> the Schindler Jews, that was what they were called, were preparing him to escape, because the Russians were going to come, and he would be [killed], he was a Nazi Party member. He starts [to cry and] . . . says "I should've done more" (or more precisely, "I should have got more," meaning more Jews working for him so they too could have been saved).

This sense of responsibility to always do more to make the world a better place, a more just and dignified place, is at the core of Bruce's understanding of who he is and who he strives to be.

An early expression of his sense of responsibility led to his first encounter with anti-Semitism:

> I remember coming out of school [one day] when I was probably in the fourth grade. These guys in leather . . . were beating up Jay. The "guys" were actually a girl and a couple of boys. They were calling him a dirty bagel, a Jewish thing. It was an anti-Semitic slur. I went over and said "you can't do that!" and they started beating me up and Jay ran home. It was one of those things. What do you do? Do you do the right thing or do you pass by and turn your head away, and let carnage, injustice, whatever you want to call it [prevail]. So I stood up, but I took a beating.

Growing up, Bruce believes he was "a nice kid," saying:

> I was polite and knew how to talk to adults and to other people, I think I was always worried about hurting people's feelings, or being kind to people. Part of that . . . was just how I was raised . . . I was taught to respect my elders and to be sensitive to my peers.

Still, Bruce readily admitted to having the usual contradictions, noting that in elementary school he suffered a "lapse of conscientiousness" involving raiding his father's change can:

> He used to come home from work each day and throw his change [in it], and he had cans of quarters, and dimes, and nickels. I was pretty strategic in that I would not take all the quarters, or all the dimes, because then he might notice. I actually looked at the distribution of coin types across "the population" and took a random sampling. I would go to the candy store after school sometimes and treat myself, [which conferred] a sense of freedom . . . sorry Dad!

Early on, Bruce faced various challenges to his budding consciousness and moral orientation. A particularly impactful one involved his friend Arthur who he met in the seventh grade. Arthur was Bruce's closest friend growing up and one of the musketeers, the triumvirate of Bruce's high school experience. While Bruce was physically fit, and fairly popular, Arthur was always the, "overweight kid." The differences in their social standing among peer networks came to a head in junior high school when Bruce would be invited to parties and Arthur would sometimes be excluded. Bruce was torn between his close friendship with Arthur and his desire to go to co-ed parties with kids who seemed "way cooler" than himself. He asked his mother what he should do. She told him, "Bruce you know what you should do." So he did not go to some of the parties and "stuck with Arthur," quite literally for the rest of Arthur's life:

> I was there at his bedside when he died, many years later. For my parents, it was doing the right thing and making sure that whatever you're doing is something a) that you can live with, and b) that you can be proud of. We all have our lapses, but I think the infractions have been relatively minor, and sometimes just my own perception, I should have called so and so, I was not attentive enough to [so and so]. But the universe of need is just so enormous that it boggles the imagination. And how do you survive it? That's [an] art form.

One of the lessons Bruce learned from Art involved stigmatization:

> Art used tell me that the only thing you can discriminate against legally anymore is obesity and the obese . . . sad! I think, growing up in a high school that was for all intents and purposes white, watching the overt discrimination, harassment, etc. that Art suffered, brought me to understand bias, made me angry and forced me to take a stand for him as a friend or abandon him, as I navigated the gauntlet of high school cliques and social groups . . . wanting to belong.

Bruce never regretted his decision regarding Arthur, who he found to be: "brilliant, funny, engaging and loving. He had a gift in nurturing his friendships and making everyone he knew feel they were special in some way. He was an amazing human being. He was trustworthy, loyal, helpful, [and] friendly."

Besides his immediate family, there were other formative influences on Bruce's direction in life. He recalled that one of his earliest memories was

> sitting in the front row pew of the synagogue on a Friday night and the rabbi, Alan Sokobin, who was intense and articulate, and kind and moral, and all of those good things, which seem to be more difficult to find [in] clergy these days, was holding an article from the *New York Times*.

The article was about Catherine Susan "Kitty" Genovese, a 28-year-old New York City woman who was stabbed to death outside her apartment building in Queens on March 13, 1964. Her murder attracted considerable attention when the *Times* reported that over 35 witnesses saw or heard the attack but failed to call the police. The incident led to conceptualization of what came to be called the "Genovese syndrome" or bystander effect (Hudson and Bruckman 2004) that seeks to explain bystander apathy. Some researchers have questioned the *Times*'s version of what occurred, and the victim's younger brother insisted that the police were summoned twice by local residents that night but failed to respond because they believed it involved a domestic dispute (Manning, Levine, and Collins 2007). As he talked about what happened to Genovese, Bruce's rabbi, who had marched for civil rights in Birmingham, was "shaking that article, and . . . he was so incensed, spittle was raining on me . . . and the remarkable thing is that I remember! And murder was not a childhood subject." The lesson for Bruce was one more reinforcement of the concept of personal responsibility, the need to work hard every day to make the world you live in the place you want the world to be. For Bruce, this is a world of fairness, tolerance, human dignity, social solidarity, and, as befits his profession, health.

The Path to Medicine

Bruce's earliest steps on the road to becoming a physician, perhaps, were in doctoring his injured sick pets when he was young. One of his earliest pets was a blue parakeet he named Yacky Doodle. When the bird became ill, he tried to nurse it back to health, but failed and he buried it in a small grave that he dug at the side of his house under the bushes. Years later, Bruce acquired a Labrador mix that developed throat cancer:

> I remember resuscitating her on the front lawn. I happened to have a banyon kit [an emergency medical kit] in the house which had oxygen. Well it was something that some guy had given me . . . some sales person that was trying to do something or another . . . So the dog started [makes gasping noise], it was a hot day, and we gave it albuterol and whatever.

But it too died.

Also laying the groundwork for his entry into medical school was Bruce's early focus on doing well in school. Everything did not always come easily to him; he had to work hard, but he was committed to the effort:

> I was a reasonably happy kid, but with my own little inner world I suppose. I worked hard in school and even back then I was driven to study. I realized early on that to learn I had to work. I was not one of those kids that reads it once and it's in there. I studied and I worked and I did well in school. My parents never had to push me. I was self-motivated in a lot of ways. Probably more then, than now.

His favorite subject in high school was science, but he liked everything he encountered, except what he termed "busy work," assignments that seemed to have no real educational value for him. Nonetheless, he got along well with teachers because they quickly perceived that he was the type of student who loves to learn, pays attention, works hard, and completes all assignments. Then, while he was a junior in high school, he went on a trip to visit his sister who was at the time a freshman at Cornell University. She introduced him to a friend of hers and asked if he would show Bruce around the campus. Bruce followed him to his classes, and to his job in the College of Architecture, Art, and Planning, and to his studio where he did metal sculpture. The very full day ended with mischievously throwing snowballs at campus buildings. Bruce was astonished by the dramatic contrasts between the controlled structure of high school and the openness and latitude of colleges: "this was freedom, freedom! I was a kid and holy shit." In response to his brief visit to Cornell, he decided was done with the kind of unexciting busy work that he had been enduring in high school. He approached his history teacher and told her

> "I don't want to do your homework anymore." She was startled, and her face revealed her dismay: how dare a student question my authority [but] we talked about control. And whoa, [this is] Bruce saying this shit? What's going on here? And, and then all of a sudden I could see the gears turning and she said, "You know Bruce, if you maintain your A average, you don't have to do it. But it's our secret" . . . The homework was the questions at the end of the chapter, which [meant] looking through the chapter and then copying over the pertinent paragraph more or less . . . It was busy work.

Another particularly important high school experience involved participation in a school-coordinated community service program. He was assigned to work at Creedmoor State Hospital, a state mental institution in Queens:

> It was horrendous. Talk about an introduction to reality! At that point, the mentally ill were just warehoused. I was on a geriatric ward, which was filled with Alzheimer's [patients] in wheelchairs, most of whom were incontinent. And my job was to be Little Mary Sunshine. It was a rude awakening.

At Creedmoor, during the second half of his senior year of high school, he met and began assisting a researcher who ran an institute for Huntington's disease, a fatal genetic disorder that causes the progressive breakdown of nerve cells in the brain. Recalls Bruce:

> Creedmoor was this incredible campus, an ancient asylum, with a large hospital building surrounded by innumerable small foreboding bungalow buildings. I worked in one of those buildings. Each day, my mother would drive me the half hour to campus or give me the car, we only had one in the family, and be stranded at home all day. The doctor I worked with was a drug researcher who was doing tracer studies, on a grant from a drug company. We were studying a vasodilator, a class of drugs commonly used to treat hypertension, angina, and congestive heart failure to determine where in the body the medication accumulated. We would feed the drug tagged with tritium, a radioactive substance, to rats which I then had to sacrifice and take samples of each of the organs, which would then be analyzed for radiation levels reflecting drug accumulation. I had to kill the rats. This bothered me quite a bit actually, because I have a very strong feelings about family members having died in the holocaust.

In preparation for a planned career in medicine, between his junior and senior year of high school, Bruce applied for a pre-med summer internship at Franklin Hospital, on Long Island in Valley Stream, NY. He did not get the internship because all of them were awarded to the children of doctors. Instead, he found a summer job as a custodian. This seemingly humbling experience later had a special effect on his style of being a physician. He, in fact, joked that it "was a formative experience":

> I learned all sorts of things about how to clean things, like how to take gum off the bottom of chairs in a 360-seat auditorium and how to clean all the light fixtures, and clean all the classrooms. It gave me a lot of respect for the custodians, because every day I would clean all these classrooms and I would move all the chairs to one side, and I would use a mop to sweep the dirt and refuse out of the way. Then I would move them to the other side, and I'd mop [that side] up. And the next day, I would come in and it was as though I'd never been there. There was litter on the floor, dirt and I'd do it all over again. It's a very Zen, a Sisyphean task, pushing the boulder up the hill. [Now] I'm friends with all the custodians. I basically know what they do, how they do it. And I've been there. And I respect that it can be a very frustrating job, and that we should all try and clean up after ourselves. Something I've passed onto my children.

A similar pattern evolved in Bruce's relationships with nurses and other hospital staff because of an early work experience:

In medical school, the summer between my first and second year, I worked in a nursing home as a nurse's aide. That gave me enormous respect for nurse's aides and all the support staff. When I became a resident, I had already done everything. At the nursing home, I had ten patients of my own each night, changing diapers and beds, undressing, bathing, dressing, feeding patients, plus I did all the toilet transfers, plus I was the night watchman too. So all night long I'd have to patrol the facility with a clock. At each corner of the building, there was a unique key that when you put it into the clock and turned it, it logged that you had been in that part of the building so they could check to make sure that I had checked the whole building. One old man that I remember vividly had been a construction worker and a plate-glass window had fallen from a building and had cut him in the neck and severed his spinal cord. So he was almost paraplegic. He could move his hands a little bit. I used to sit with him and he used to tell me stories of Foster's Meadow, which is what Elmont [where Bruce grew up] was called before it was called Elmont. Before they went to track housing, way long ago. He was pretty old. And he used to say that where all the stores were [in Elmont] was once just cornfields. There was another gentleman who called me Anonymous. He had Alzheimer's so he couldn't remember my name. So he used to scream "Anonymous! Anonymous!" which taught me an enormous amount about caring. Caring despite the filth, and the fatigue. I was very tired . . . I was doing graveyard shifts, night time 11 pm–7 am. I learned how to be gentle even though it might be the third time someone's wet their bed, and you just have to change their bed again. And you know you could let yourself get frustrated, or you just take a deep breath and you care with a capital C. It was a [very] maturing summer. I confronted a lot of things about medicine that I really had not thought about: the romantic side of saving lives versus the mundane side of keeping people clean and dry. The good news is that when I was a resident if a patient wasn't being cared for, and the nurse was busy, I would just do it myself because I knew how to change a patient in the bed, which is a little bit of an art form, flipping them to the wet side, changing one side of the bed then flipping them back. I had a head nurse at the nursing home that used to bounce a quarter off the bed [to see if the sheet was tightly fitted]. So I really knew what I was doing, feeding patients, toileting patients. I would just do it. You only have to do that a couple times as a resident, and your reputation spreads: "wow this guy's a team player." Then the nurses make your life easier, because they like you, and they realize that you understand the value of what they do, [that] you're also willing to help and you have their backs. If a patient came into the ER, they would let me sleep and they would put the IV in, they would put the nasogastric tube down, and they would do all the prep and then they would call me "hey we got a patient stabilized in the ER . . . why don't you come down and do a physical because we need a note for the chart." Versus my colleagues, [who] were sometimes sphincters. They would call them three hours before, and say "we think there might be a patient coming in from XYZ hospital, just wanted to let you know," and then an hour later they would say "they're on their way" and then they would make them get up and do it all themselves.

Bruce finished high school in the middle of his senior year and then enrolled in Cornell University with a major in biology and a pre-med focus. Between high school and college, he went to Israel "chasing a young woman" of interest to him. She was an exchange student who he met in the US through the Long Island Federation of Temple Youth:

we had three exchange students from Israel that stayed through New Years and one of them I dated while she was in the states. I was in "love." But my parents forbade me from going to Israel, fearing that I'd never come back to start college in the Fall. So I earned the money for a plane ticket myself valet parking cars at weddings, Bar Mitzvahs, tutoring Hebrew, babysitting . . . whatever odd jobs I could get . . . The day after graduation [from high school] I flew off to Israel and I got there, and she did meet at the airport, but she said, "We have to talk." She had run off with a French draft evader that she had met on her kibbutz. I think she wound up marrying him. So here I was, alone in Israel. And I ended up working on a kibbutz where the exchange student my family had hosted was from. I remember traveling around Israel alone, and meeting people, and sleeping wherever, having all sorts of incredible adventures, a summer of growth and expanding horizons.

At Cornell, he was enrolled in the School of Agriculture and Life Sciences. He made this decision because the school was a land grant college of New York State, so the tuition was $600 a year versus $5,000 for the School of Arts and Sciences. The Biology program at Cornell was, and still is a joint department of the College of Arts and Sciences and the College of Agriculture. So Bruce was able to concentrate on neurobiology and behavior and sit in on classes in biology taught by professors from Arts and Sciences, but pay a significantly reduced tuition. The difference:

When I took Sociology, I took Rural Sociology. When I took Economics, I took Agricultural Economics, which was a bit more focused on commodities, as well as rural electrification. The same economics but with a slightly different spin. For me, with my future work with migrant farm worker populations, perhaps a better spin.

Through a special program at Cornell, he was able to start medical school during what would have been his senior year of college and get his undergraduate degree after his first year of medical school. As a result, he never had to take the MCAT.

This came back to haunt him some years later when he served on his university's medical admissions committee:

> The over-achievers club of faculty on the admissions committee quizzed each of us, "what did you get on your MCATs?" It went around the room, asking the faculty what they had gotten on their MCATs and they got to me and, I'd never thought about it, I paused and then told them "I never had to take them." Everyone looked at me as though I'd snuck in the back door. I think they were just jealous.

Bruce found college to be quite stressful:

> I had gone from being the "wunderkind" in high school to just another undergraduate in Ithaca. At Cornell you can work very hard and do poorly; there is no gentleman's C. My first midterm grades were C's, at least in Biology, and I felt as though my life was over. But I pulled A's out by the end of the year. I guess I was able to figure out different study habits. My sister, Jackie, nurtured me. She was two years ahead of me at Cornell. She lived in a college town in an attic, in one of the student slums, and I used to crash there from time to time. I would say "Oh, my God, I'm never going to make it in this place." She would tell me she'd heard this before and somehow it always worked out . . . and it did."

Bruce initially shared a dorm room with a student who was anti-Semitic:

> When I arrived there, I chose a side of the room, made my bed, unpacked and put my things up on a shelf – one of those things a menorah with the Star of David on it. My roommate walked in, and looked at me, looked up at the shelf and saw the Star of David and said, "You're Jewish." Those were the first words he said to me. Not "hi, how are you doing?" He said, "You're Jewish. All the dentists and doctors in my town are Jewish." The third thing he said was "All the Jews took the seats in the medical school class. I'm a grad student." He couldn't get into medical school and on some level he blamed it on the Jews. Not an optimal start to a relationship but I suppose as a future Primary Care doctor, I've always been able to get beyond some of the barriers that some people raise to prevent you from getting to know them. I can get along with almost anyone. We would eat dinner together, study together and became friends. But during the semester that we lived together every once in a while he would say things, hurtful things. I bought a microscope used and I brought it back to the room. I said to him, "I got this microscope for $250 bucks," and he says, "Just like you people. You bargained the guy down." One time I was going home for the weekend and I joked that "Magical things happen. I put all my laundry in the trunk of my car and when I come back on Sunday it's all clean, and folded, what

> a deal. You should put your stuff in my trunk." He says, "I don't want any Rabbis touching my dirty laundry." One time, he asked me what a rube is. I said I didn't know. He said, "a New York Jew." A rube is actually an uncultured fellow, a bumpkin.

Seeking refuge from his roommate, Bruce got to know the guy who lived in the next room, who was Jewish. Steve Strongwater's room became Bruce's sanctuary during his first semester at Cornell:

> He was a very nice guy, very friendly and brilliant, brilliant, brilliant, brilliant. We became best friends, and remain so to this day. After finishing medical school, I went to UMass for residency training. Steve went to University of Michigan for a Rheumatology Fellowship. As he was finishing his fellowship, I called him to tell him there was a rheumatology position available at UMass. He took it and we practiced together for five years and then I moved to Connecticut and for five years we were separated. Then a job for an Associate Dean for Clinical Affairs opened up at UConn and I knew he wanted to do that so I called him. UConn fell in love with him and he moved to Connecticut. Our kids grew up together, our sons became best friends and wound up at Cornell together. Then about five or six years ago, when the dean retired, Steve decided to move on. A sad moment for me but we are still best friends and our families are family.

During his sophomore year at medical school, Bruce moved off campus into an apartment with friends from his class. He built a bed out of plywood and two by fours. That platform survived medical school and served as the frame for the bed he built using tongue and groove cabinetry with a stained wooden frame and six drawers on the sides, which would last through the first five years of his marriage. The bed, of which he is quite proud, is still used today by his sister in Vermont.

Bruce remembers Cornell as being harder than medical school:

> I was taking extra credits each semester to finish early and advanced biology courses. I also took the history courses for majors—the course, The History of American Foreign Policy was taught by Walter Lafebre, a world-class historian and story teller. It was a bit of a risk for a pre-med. Need to get A's to get into med school. But I love history, learned an enormous amount and still remember the essay questions on the final.
>
> I was never a drinker. I was a library guy. In fact, when I remember college, a lot of my memories are of the inside of Mann and Uris Libraries. I had all these little nooks where I could study. The Cornell Law Library had a rare books room that they no longer allow you to study in. It was in this enormous gothic building, absolutely stunning. You went into the back of the library and up these steps and there was this little room with its own stained-glass window which you could open looking out on a courtyard.

> That's where I often studied. Somehow no one else seemed to have discovered it. My own secret world!
>
> At Cornell, I worked incredibly hard but I also socialized and went to parties, but not a lot . . . life was focused on my studies. I did a lot of classes. I remember Genetics, and trudging through the winter snow to the Genetics Lab to do my fruit fly experiments to map genes. All hours of the day and night to sort and count fruit fly hatchlings before they could breed and confuse the results. I don't know if they require that anymore [breeding fruit flies for genetics research].

Bruce emphasized:

> College was not wild at all. College was all about learning. About getting to where you want to go . . . I was there to learn. Money was dear. Education was incredibly important in my family and I wasn't there to play. I wasn't there to do all sorts of other things . . . On Saturdays, I'd be in the library until 10:00 pm. I went to concerts where I'd often have a flashlight and my notes so I could study for a test the next day while listening to the concert . . . I got mainly A's, but some B's. I learned humility and hopefully learned [how] to learn, [and to] hope for the best. The competition was tough; there were a lot of really smart people.

His overall assessment was that Cornell was "a damaging experience; probably too harsh." Still, Cornell retains a distinct place in Bruce's memory:

> My wife and I have been back to Cornell reunions and I'm proud that I went to Cornell. Cornell, the mystique is probably greater for me than the real memory. But I enjoyed it. I enjoyed the history and I enjoyed the old libraries, and the traditions and the songs. I have regrets too. I didn't take as great advantage of my years at Cornell as I might have.

Bruce's biggest regret from his undergraduate days was never taking a course with Carl Sagan: "Carl Sagan, the God of astronomy and astronomy education, was a professor at Cornell. I love astronomy and I never took it, because I was focused on taking my core required courses." The best class Bruce took at Cornell was History of American Foreign Policy, an experience that influenced his thinking about the world:

> The professor was this national/international expert on foreign policy. Years later, during the Gulf War, CNN and other news programs would interview him about the implications of the war. And I went "Whoa, how cool is that?" He was an extraordinary teacher, a story teller. He'd come in and sit on the desk, lean forward and rock his legs back and forth, and say "where we left off yesterday was with Henry Clay." He would tell the stories of

people and personalities and their lives. Where they were born. How they lived and how they died. What influenced them to be the human beings they were, and do the things they did. Their lives all overlapped. Each day, a different life, and then our job was to read the history book and determine how all these lives fit together and how they influenced history.

Bruce also especially liked the ecology course he took:

The woods are really a love [of mine] and life as an ecologist, or a foresters or a park ranger would have been a good life. You have to be careful to step outside your reality once in a while, your deadlines, your pressures, and just take a deep breath, and look up at the stars. That's how I decompress . . . I don't drink, I don't smoke . . . I walk in the woods! I used to windsurf and I'd keep my board on top of my car the whole summer. If I saw a little daylight at the end of the day, I'd drive to Rhode Island . . . and step outside my reality.

When Bruce switched his major to biology, his new advisor, Professor Ari van Tienhoven, Chair of Poultry Science at Cornell, invited him to work in his lab. It was an important turning point in Bruce's undergraduate career:

that was the moment that made me feel at home at Cornell and the lab became my "home" at college. The Poultry Science lab was surreal. Dr. van Tienhoven had this zany lab tech who was probably in his 60s . . . he was nuts. When we had to sacrifice a chicken during our research, he would break its neck then throw it in an empty garbage pail. The pail would bounce around the room as the chicken, despite its broken neck, would flap its wings and try to run for some time . . . till it finally would die. It was macabre, and brought back memories of sacrificing rats during my research days at Creedmoor. I suppose I'm not cut out to be a henchman or a hunter . . . too much respect for life. I ended up doing research on the ovulatory cycle of *Gallus domesticus* [the domesticated chicken], looking at hormone levels. We varied the light cycle in the coops, shortened the day/night cycles so you could fit six days into five days to see if we could get them to lay extra eggs. [It worked] to a degree. Part of my job was drawing blood samples on chickens, using the wing vein. I became pretty good at it.

Routinely . . . I would awaken the chickens at three in the morning from a dead sleep. Because if you turn the lights on you reset their circadian rhythms. I would have to draw blood under green light; they don't see green. Then I'd have to run to the lab, spin the blood down, take off the serum, reconstitute it with saline, and then reinject the same blood into the same chicken. At this point, the chicken knew I was coming and it would flap and peck me, viciously. It was insane. But it was a great experience. It also gave me a sense of identity, which is very, very important to students.

> Before Dr. van Tienhoven, I was this anonymous student. I had a sense that if I disappeared, they would just look out at the Biology 101 class of 2,500 students, and they would see an "empty seat," and bring in another student. It was disheartening.

Affirming his independence, while at Cornell, Bruce purchased a 1959 Ford Thunderbird with the help of the tech in the lab where he worked:

> He knew a guy, that knew a guy, that had this car that had been in Pennsylvania so it hadn't been exposed to salt. He didn't tell me there were no valves left in the engine. Although I checked the compression on the cylinders before I bought it . . . they were all the same across the eight cylinders . . . I had no idea what normal was or that the compression I'd measured was low . . . leaky valves. I ended up with this car, which cost $500 and looked like the Batmobile, but burned oil like a smoke screen. The 6-year-old that lived in the apartment in the basement of my house on Quarry Street thought I was Batman . . . a guy named Bruce, with a shiny black car with fins, that left a smoke screen wherever he went. Six months later it blew up on me, but for those six months, I was in heaven.

The summer after freshman year at Cornell, Bruce came home to Long Island to work as a volunteer at Queen's Hospital Center on a cancer research project. As part of this job, he had to collect tissue samples from fetuses extracted during abortions. They were studying alpha-fetoprotein (AFP) and its correlation with various cancers and other health issues. AFP is a plasma protein that is produced by the yolk sac and the liver during fetal development. This biochemical is elevated in liver cancer and various cancerous tumors. A related peptide, a linked chain of amino acids known as alpha fetoprotein peptide, has been found to have anti-cancer effects (Richardson et al. 1998). Bruce explained that:

> During pregnancy, you can perform a blood test for alpha-fetoprotein, the results of which can diagnose the presence of Down's syndrome and other problems with the fetus. Every day I would go to the abortion clinic and be given the curretings from the day's procedures. Despite the ongoing controversy about the right to abortion, at the time, I was oblivious. It was part of the science we were doing. The abortion had been done. We were using the tissue to try to develop screening tests for genetic abnormalities, or cancer.

The following summer, he stayed at Cornell and worked with a biology professor who was studying orientation behavior in salamanders. The research focused on the pineal gland, an endocrine gland in the brain that produces melatonin. In some amphibians and reptiles, it is linked to the parapineal gland, or what has been called "the third eye," that can detect light in a different way than the rods found in the eyes:

> it turns out, if you remove salamanders from their nest and displace them a hundred miles, or even a thousand miles [away], in a few years they'll find their way back to that nest. Most people don't realize that salamanders live thirty years, have a new crop [of young] every year, and can regenerate [body parts]. You can pull the tail off and it will regenerate. The field experiment was quite elaborate. We built large release devices made up of concentric rings of fencing, 60 feet in diameter in the middle of the forest. Unfortunately, the site for the device was in the middle of an enormous poison ivy patch. The other lab assistant was quite allergic and spent a miserable summer scratching . . . I never broke out . . . lucky, I guess. We collected salamanders living along a number of brooks in a state forest, noted where they were collected along the streambed, and the orientation of the stream geographically to the release device. We disoriented the salamanders by driving them around in the back of a truck and then released them in the center of the device. The salamanders would strike out in some direction and fall in a can at compass directions along the concentric rings of fence. I would sleep out under the stars in the state forest so at night, at midnight, 3 am and 6 am, I could get up to identify which salamanders had fallen into which trap along the release device fence to determine what direction they were trying to head after being released. Science and great memories. I was working days, evenings, and nights, 120 hours a week for $80. During the mornings and afternoons I was working in the tiger salamander lab. These are enormous Midwestern spotted salamanders that we were training toward the shore of a pool and then testing whether they could use the plane of polarized light to orient in that same direction. I was also running a planetarium in the evening and testing orientation behavior in newts. I guess I was more of a biologist than a premed.

Bruce also became interested in photography:

> The summer after my junior year of college, and preceding my first year of med school I took a photography course to earn the last two credits I needed. I ran around campus taking pictures of architecture, animals, people, and learned how to develop film . . . now a lost art due to digital cameras.

Selecting Medicine

Bruce's decision to become a doctor began to emerge in between his junior and senior years of high school; there were multiple social influences in addition to various events along life's way that shaped this decision:

> My grandmother on my father's side was always telling me to be a doctor, but it was more a monetary thing: "Be a doctor! Be a doctor! You'll earn a good living!" Then there was my Uncle Harry who was married to my Aunt

> Ada for one year and then dropped dead. Ada had not married until she was 50 when she finally found a man that was good enough, and he was a doctor and he had a heart attack. I still have his watch. I have his medical dictionary, which, though way outdated, I still keep on my bookshelf. And then there was the camp doctor. I had gone to Jewish camp in Great Barrington, Massachusetts for one week the summer between junior and senior year of high school and there was a psychiatrist who as part vacation and part job was the doctor at this camp. He "adopted" me. I used to eat lunch with him each day and he told me how wonderful it was to be a doctor. And so all of a sudden [I considered it], although I had told my grandmother "no" a million times. My senior year of high school, she passed away. And I remember on her deathbed my telling her that I'd decided "to be a doctor." I went to college thinking biology and ultimately becoming a doctor . . . I was premed.

Then during his junior year at Cornell, Bruce saw a sign that read "Dual Registration Program, Upstate Medical Center State University of New York":

> Upstate wanted Cornell students and one of their ways of grabbing them before they got into other places was to offer them admission during their junior year. As part of the deal, Cornell gave students a semester's credit in biology toward their undergraduate degree after they completed their first year of medical school. So I graduated undergrad after my first year of medical school [was completed] and I walked with my [graduating] class in 1976. It was a risk, though, because had I flunked out of medical school or not done well I would also not have received my undergraduate diploma. I was apprehensive going off to med school early. I thought there was some magical maturation process that happened during your senior year of college, other than getting high and partying, that matured you in some way and prepared you for the rigors of medical school. But off I went, a year younger than most of my classmates. I figured it out. Cornell was probably tougher than medical school. Cornell was a pressure cooker and prepared me well for both medical school and the practice of medicine. It all worked out.

At first, as he had with college, Bruce found medical school unsettling:

> I had my insecurities. I don't have a bad self-image, but neither do I have an enormous ego, and I was a little worried that maybe I wasn't going to make it. I'm a more conceptual learner in general, not a memorizer. In medical school, you really have to memorize, and do it quickly, in addition to trying to formulate a conceptual construct of all this enormous knowledge or you're not going to keep up. So if you take the time to fully understand every detail and how it perfectly fits together, you'll be left in the dust. If you fall behind, you're cooked. Again, I developed a method and a pace, and it worked out fine.

To his chagrin, he found that some students were willing to sabotage others to get ahead:

> I remember one of the students in my dissection group was very nervous and high-strung and he would drop by my room and play with my head trying to psyche me out. One wonders what type of doctor he was going to make if, at that stage of his education, he was still playing competitive games. Med school is fast paced and full of pressure. Upstate was pass/fail/honors, to allow the students to work together and help each other, yet the drive to get honors motivated some people to try and climb over others. Sad!

Bruce learned about the shortcomings of the competitiveness found in some medical schools and used that experience to champion a different atmosphere when he was hired by the University of Connecticut:

> in the admissions process, we try to weed [self-absorbed students] out and look for humanistic team players. UConn is pass/fail and historically was one of two medical schools in the country that did not have a chapter of AOA (Alpha Omega Alpha), the medical school honor society. Harvard is the other one. The concern was that having an honor society where only 16 percent of the class is allowed to get in breeds a more competitive environment. One of the positives of UConn is that the students work together, they help each other. The end goal is producing good doctors and more of them. For better or worse, UConn is initiating an AOA Chapter in two years. We'll have to see how it affects the culture.

During medical school, Bruce faced a crisis when he almost flunked one of his classes:

> I got distracted but I learned that if I didn't study hard, bad things happen. I ended up flunking a mid-term. I thought, "Oh my God, my life is over." It was a course on endocrine. I regrouped, buckled down, focused, and I got an A on the final. So I ended up passing. It taught me a huge lesson. It confirmed that my study habits in college and early medical school were appropriate and worked. I understood that this was serious business, and that I really couldn't let myself get distracted. Fun was great and socializing was good, but "I'm in medical school to become a doctor." And that's what I focused on.

The curriculum Bruce encountered in medical school was typical of those being used at the time across the country: "It was pretty standard. The first two years was basic science, take the first part of the boards, and then go onto the clinical years. Not terribly avant-garde. There really weren't a lot of community experiences. It was hospital centric." On the weekends, Bruce would leave campus to go back to Cornell:

> When I'd stay at Upstate, it distracted me. I'd go out with my friends, or do whatever folks were doing. When I went to Cornell on weekends, my girlfriend, now wife, then a veterinary student at Cornell, and I would be in the library all weekend. But can you say that is healthy? I turned out okay. When I went from the basic sciences to the clinical years, I did pretty well. I didn't get honors in everything, but I got enough honors that I was up for AOA. But now, I was actually taking care of patients. I like people, and I especially like helping people. This was my attraction to the medical profession. I would attach myself to my patients, and listen and care. I believe I really helped a lot of folks, not because I made the brilliant diagnosis, but because my patients knew I heard them, cared, not only for them but about them, and would do all in my power to get them the best care possible. I realized why I'd come to medicine. Medical school . . . I remember experiences—some really good, some really bad. I remember being scared when you're left by yourself at night with intensely sick patients. Not scared in a paralyzed way, but aware of what you know and what you might not know and the repercussions of coming up short. That stimulates you to do more. But you have to be aware that you're not perfect and never will be perfect. It's just not possible.

Bruce's decision to focus on primary care came easily to him:

> I think that was where I was heading all along, even before medical school, even in high school and that's why I went into medicine in the first place, to be honest. Here's a profession that allows you to help people sometimes in really concrete ways, and, perhaps more often, in less concrete ways, through kindness, caring, listening and just being there in the moment. Helping people is what appealed to me. I really love medicine when I have all the time I need to spend with a patient. When I'm pressured and oversubscribed by an overabundance of patients, not enough help, "busy work," it can be very stressful, because humans are incredibly complex—more so in the inner city, being under resourced, and socioeconomically challenged. It takes time to "doctor" and more time to do it well, and time is the one commodity that administrators want to limit, these days. It's all about cranking 'em through and I'm a little concerned about where medicine is going. As the medical profession corporatizes, the practice of medicine is looking more and more like a sweatshop and less and less like a caring profession. As clinicians, we can't allow that to happen. I believe that in collaboration with our colleagues in care, nurse practitioners, PAs, nurses, medical assistants, and others, all members of the team, we will self-correct. I'm just not sure that it will be in my lifetime.

Finding Love

Bruce graduated early from college, which saved his parents financially: "even though they weren't wealthy, although I paid for part of college, they paid for most of it. I didn't take loans for college." When he graduated from Cornell, and after his Thunderbird blew up on the highway, his parents bought him a Toyota Corolla to take with him to medical school. But first, he used the car to travel across country. He was accompanied by his girlfriend from college, Lisa Hershkowitz, who would later become his wife and the mother of his three children: "we drove my little Toyota all across the country, through the badlands, South Dakota and Mount Rushmore, and Glacier, and Seattle, and down to San Francisco, and then back through the Grand Canyon."

Bruce met his future wife on September 30th, 1972 while they were both still freshmen at Cornell:

> It was her birthday and she was coming out of the dorm, I was going in, and we bumped into each other. We were in Donlon Hall, freshman year. I was on the fourth floor, she was on the fifth floor. She looked sort of forlorn and I said "What's wrong?" and she said "Well it's my birthday and I'm going to spend it in the library." I kissed her as I remember, a happy birthday kiss and that was the beginning. I was very focused on school, but I met Lisa, as a freshman in college. You get to school, you're looking around, and eventually you focus on someone. I remember talking to my roommate, Carl, who I still am friends with, and him saying "Bruce either you're going to ask her out or I'm going to ask her out." And so I said, "Oh, okay!" She lived in the Bronx, although she was originally was from Lawrence, Kansas, and I lived in Long Island, and over the Christmas break I went to her parents' apartment and picked her up. We went to the Museum of Modern Art in Manhattan. That was the first date and then we dated . . . through the rest of undergrad, and until I finished medical school and she finished veterinary school [at Cornell College of Veterinary Medicine]. Four days before I started residency, we were married. We were engaged about six months before our wedding. I was applying to residency programs, who knew where I'd land and I wanted her to go with me. We talked about it. We were a couple joined at the hip . . . time to commit . . . and so I asked her . . . and she said yes! And so off we went to Worcester, Mass. [to his internship and residency at the University of Massachusetts Medical Center].

He was attracted to Lisa because he found her to be

> bright, beautiful and very intuitive. She was, at that point in her life, a little bit of a hippie; a free spirit, very kind, and nice, and sweet. Your basic good human being. You meet someone and at first it's just chemistry. You just like someone, fall in love, and then after seven years of college and medical school, it was still working.

Thinking about his own situation, married to someone from another medical profession and what has happened to other doctors he knows, Bruce commented:

> I think the fact that Lisa had a career as demanding and intense as veterinary medicine allowed me to have a career and invest so much in my patients. In a relationship, a marriage, if one spouse is overly invested in work and the other spouse has less of a focus, less of a thread in their lives, it usually doesn't last. The times that you are very busy with work, the times that you are away from that person, are viewed as negative. Doctors often are super busy. And if their spouse, whether it's a male spouse or a female spouse, doesn't have a focus in their lives then that becomes a bone of contention, and it becomes a source of incompatibility. Because now as an individual you're torn between your responsibilities to your patients and your responsibility to your spouse, family, and so on. Veterinarians are also often super busy. We understood each other and worked around our careers.

The challenge, which he feels he met successfully, was meeting multiple responsibilities and fulfilling numerous commitments:

> I tried to make time for everything. When I'd be running off to Central America [on medical visits] or going to the migrant farm worker camps at night, doing all these types of things, I didn't get the negative feedback that I think a lot of people might get from their spouse . . . I'm just saying, I found the perfect spouse. We stuck together. When I look at some of my friends, things did not last . . . Lisa and I made it together . . . and are still going!

Thinking of his life with Lisa, Bruce added:

> I think with Lisa, together we're one human being . . . we complement each other. I don't say that in a flippant way. She's very detail orientated, I'm big picture orientated, and so we really are two sides of the same coin. Without her, my life would be chaos. She is the stable foundation and allows me the luxury of being able to dream. She also is a great mom. And a hiker and a partner, pretty much in everything we do. I don't know if I could've done what I've done without her support, and her guidance and her lending me her ear. Clearly when things happen, good or bad, she's the one who I wanna run and talk to about it. She's a good counselor. Obviously there are other life events, like raising three children together, and caring for our aging parents and dealing with their illness and deaths. Those are the moments when the going gets rough and the stability of family and home keeps your life from spinning out of control. We have our moments and we have our disagreements and fights and knock-down drag-outs. All part of being together for almost 45 years . . . perhaps the glue that has bonded us through all the challenges. Our visions of life are a little different, just different enough, to keep it interesting and that's probably healthy. No one gets where they are alone, good or bad. Whether you've attained the heights of

> your profession, or whether you've wound up in a crack house on the down side of town, you haven't gotten there on your own. No life outcome is totally self-determined.

Bruce and Lisa were married on June 24, 1979 in Elmont, New York, his hometown. He was 25 and she was 24. The wedding held at the synagogue his parents attended and where Bruce had his bar mitzvah a little over a decade earlier:

> it was your basic, standard 1979 wedding. I remember shopping with Lisa for her dress in Boston, because we had moved up to Worcester, Mass. There was a little store on Newbury Street in Boston, and she didn't get your standard big wedding dress with the veil and the whole nine yards. She got a cream-colored, beautiful dress. And I didn't get a tux, I just got a suit; shopped for it with my father-in-law to be, on the Lower East Side of Manhattan, his old stomping ground; in fact, my nephew wore my wedding suit to his senior prom. We had our friends from college there, our friends from medical and veterinary school, our family. We have a wedding album and all of the elders are now gone, a little bit sad. It reminds you how quickly time goes and how briefly you are here on earth. Makes you want to make it count!

As Bruce was finishing up his medical school program, he began to apply to and eventually interview at internal medicine residency programs: "I took a road trip and interviewed at programs starting in Virginia and went all the way up the coast to University of Massachusetts in Worcester. There were ten programs, including Bellevue," which was founded in 1736 and is the oldest public hospital in the US. A key factor in his final decision was his love of nature:

> I love the outdoors. At UMass they took me up to the ICU [intensive care unit] on the seventh floor of the hospital. It looked like any other ICU until you looked out the window. I found myself looking out on Lake Quinsigamond [a 4-mile-long lake located between Worcester and the nearby town of Shrewsbury]. The view was spectacular and in that moment I knew. The program was a relatively new training program and was focused on primary care and located in a mid-sized city. Worcester did not quite have the inner city that a Hartford has or a New York has, but it had underserved people and projects and challenges. The staff and faculty were young, progressive and in an instant, I felt home! That's what I tell my residents, my students, when they're interviewing: make a chart of the programs you visit, write down the details of the program and note your observations and take pictures, so when they are at the end of their interviews, trying to make a decision, they can review their chart and say, "Oh that place, right." By the end of ten, twenty interviews, all the programs begin looking the same. But, if there is a place they walk into and a little voice in their head says,

> "I'm home, these are nice people, I can survive here," then that's probably the place they're meant to be. And that's the way I ranked programs and wound up at UMass. I was an intern, then a second year, and then a third year resident and I didn't really have a plan. I really wasn't thinking academic medicine or anything, I was just thinking "I'm going to be a doctor!"

Again steered by his love of the outdoors, Bruce and Lisa moved together to Westborough, Mass., a twenty-minute drive from Worcester:

> We rented an old farm house. The farmer, who was in his 70s or 80s, and his wife, lived in an attached in-law apartment . . . I had an acquaintance who lived in Worcester, my cousin's best friend from high school, and when I interviewed at the University of Massachusetts I needed a place to stay. My cousin Carl said "Why don't you stay with Howie?" And so I called Howie and crashed at his apartment. We bonded and became really close friends. We're still friends, starting from those three days that I had stayed with him. Howie went with me house hunting, and I remember meeting with the farmer's wife who rented the Westborough place to us. At the end of the negotiation, I asked, "What about a contract?" She said, "Oh just a hand shake, that's all we need."

Bruce remembers the farm house as

> a clunky, funky place, on a hundred-acre farm with a faux waterfall in the living room and wood stove [we] huddled around to stay warm in the winter. It was a pig farm, but the pigs were on the other side of the property, which was a good thing since our dog enjoyed a good roll in pig s—t when it was handy.

The son of the farmer lived across the road:

> his daughter had a horse, a big Appaloosa. The daughter, 15, 16 years old was off in Europe, and his younger 9-year-old daughter wanted to ride the horse. Despite the fact that I had perhaps ridden a horse three times in my 25 years, they made a rule that unless I rode the horse with her, she couldn't ride. And so I would come home from the hospital after being up all night, saddle up and go riding off into the woods. Sometimes my charge would goad me into forgetting the saddle and riding bareback . . . a new experience for me, as was occasionally winding up on the ground, but I survived. This was not the usual internship experience, but it allowed me to step out of my reality and decompress quite a bit, taking my mind off the stresses of a medical internship . . . And then around February the farmer and his wife sold the house we lived in to their son across the road. He moved into the house and they rented or sold his house. So mid-internship, I was kicked out on the street.

> At that point, I was pretty upset and I decided I wasn't going to allow that to happen again, so I decided to buy a house. We bought a little two-bedroom house, a ranch, in West Boylston, Mass. for $40,000. Then we went off on a winter vacation, actually our honeymoon, in Guadalupe in the Caribbean and when we got back there had been a rainstorm and there were three feet of water in the basement. The seller, apparently had removed a sump pump so we wouldn't suspect that the house had a wet basement. So the fire department had to come and pump the water out and within two hours, the three feet of water was back. So I went off to the equivalent of Home Depot and bought a sump pump. Pumped it out, and stuck it in a hole through the foundation, and that was the last time we had trouble, though we had learned some valuable lessons.

It was during his internship that Bruce did a rotation with Professor Jon Kabat Zinn at the hospital's hospice unit. Zinn, a student of Zen Buddhism, is the father of mindfulness meditation and stress reduction. In 1979, he started a clinic at UMass—the Stress Reduction Clinic and later the Center for Mindfulness in Medicine, Health Care, and Society—where he taught dying cancer patients stress and anxiety-reduction meditation techniques that also helped lower their pain medication needs. His second book, published in 1994, *Wherever You Go, There You Are*, became a national bestseller. He also taught his mindfulness-based stress reduction techniques to interns, including Bruce, who has "used them my entire life, in and out of my doctoring roles . . . just for life!"

Parenthood

Three years after the wedding, shortly after starting his year as chief medical resident at UMass, and while coordinating the schedules and care delivered of 69 interns and residents, treating patients two days a week, and studying for his Internal Medicine Boards [which demonstrate a physician's expertise in a particular medical specialty] in his spare time, Bruce and Lisa had their first child:

> We had my daughter, Rachel, on July 26, 1982. We liked the name Rachel, and in Jewish circles you name children often to honor someone who has passed away, in order for their name not to disappear. You also supposedly want them to have some of the characteristics, hopefully, of that person. You know often you stretch the association and you say just an "R," so Rachel is representing Grandma Ruth, my father-in-law's mother, my wife's grandmother. She lived to like 101! Growing up, Rachel was my pal. In a way, because she was the oldest. She did not move with the fast crowd in high school. She was captain of the cross-country ski team. She did stuff, but she wasn't in the social in crowd. She used to go up with me to the Berkshires, and I'd bring the computer and we'd do study hall, go out to dinner, whatever. In college, she was an environmental sciences major, and during her last

> year or maybe it was the year before, she became teaching assistant of that class during her senior year. You know, conservation—environmental conservation. She asked me if she could bring the whole class up to our Berkshire home, she had spoken with the professor, and they did. The whole Brandeis class came up with Rachel and that was heaven. But then Rachel, after her freshman year of college, became a VISTA worker and was assigned to me, and spent the summer going out to the farm labor camps with me. There's nothing quite like being out at a tobacco farm, looking over the fields, the sun setting—you know, doing a good deed—you're taking care of people who really need your help—and I remember one time, I was standing next to Rachel and a worker comes up and just said "I want to thank you for being here for us." And to have that happen in the presence of your child is very significant. It's one of those moments—those Kodak moments. Another thing I remember is that she was out there with her friend, Emola. Emola is now actually a family physician—one of her best friends in high school. She was also a VISTA worker and the two of them did this after their freshman year of college. I'm out at Thralls Tobacco in Windsor. There were four hundred workers at least then, so it was like San Juan on a Saturday night. So, I'm seeing patients and then I hear laughing, whatever, and I see these two beautiful, young women surrounded by probably ten young Latino males, bantering and flirting. I went over, and I just took the two of them around, I sort of put my hands across their shoulders and I just said, "Me papa!" They all scattered, it was funny. She was the first child—and I remember when she first talked. She called herself Chi Chi because she couldn't say Rachel. You know, you just remember these things. Rachel lived in Australia for ten years, where she got her masters in environmental sciences, married her husband, Mark, had two kids, and worked for the New South Wales Conservation and Climate Control, their version of the EPA, for seven years. Now she lives in North Carolina. She's a great mom . . . the organized one that holds her family together.

After Rachel was born, the multiple challenges of work vs. parenthood began:

> I was supposed to be studying and I actually moved into the living room, because I had to get some sleep. Then all of a sudden the house got very small. We decided we needed something bigger and so we sold that house for $50,000 and bought a house in Princeton, Mass. I still love the Princeton house, it was amazing. Princeton was a rural town of 2,500, quiet, beautiful, and we lived there until 1988. The house was on a dirt road, on a two-acre wooded lot, backing on four hundred acres of forest. It was modern, contemporary . . . lots of windows and skylights . . . airy. My second daughter Taryn, was born on September 30, 1984. She is my artist, a freelance videographer, editor, and director for the music industry in New York City. She's done work for The Roots, Pearl Jam, Willie Nelson, Kiss,

Puff Daddy. She's always had an intuitive sense of the beauty around us . . . a real joy! She was named after my cousin Tina, who died at the age of 23 of vaginal carcinoma due to the fact that her mother took DES, diethylstilbestrol [a synthetic, non-steroidal estrogen given to woman from 1940 to 1971 to reduce the risk of pregnancy complications and losses, but withdrawn as a medicine when it was shown to be a carcinogen]. She was actually getting married and her fiancé was going to marry her anyway, but she died before that. I was friends with her, and especially since I was in medical school. It was especially sad, because her dad was a Holocaust survivor. And had lost a wife and children in Austerlitz but came to this country and married my mother's cousin, Muriem. They had a lot of trouble having babies, so she had taken DES and they only had one child, Tina. And then she died of this terrible cancer. It's sort of a double sadness. So when Taryn was born, it was a few years after my cousin's death, but I didn't really like the name Tina. My friend, Arthur said, "what about Taryn?" He had some associate that was named Taryn. So I said, "great." And that's how Taryn became Taryn. Her middle name is Ashera for my wife's Grandfather Hasha, a bootlegger. Taryn was always sort of this free-spirit that was always awed by the beauty of life, and she's still that way. She hasn't lost that totally—she's much more realistic and a businesswoman in a pretty fast-paced profession, but she still has not lost that. With Taryn, we have this great picture of her from her birthday—on one of her birthdays—and her friends had brought all sorts of dress-up clothing. And one day, she had put it all on—sort of a long, flowing dress with this funky hat, and a stole—a fur cape, and was carrying a shopping bag, and had these bizarre sunglasses on—she must have been four or five years old. And that's why we used to call her the bag lady. She looked like a bag lady on the streets of New York. She's just this individual who is so full of life. As Rachel ran off to Australia, Taryn really became the daughter and would come up to visit. One story with Taryn was after my father had died, and my mother was devastated, she was just devastated, and I was devastated. Somehow I didn't think I would be, because he had diabetes, and I knew he had inoperable coronary artery disease, but he was healthy. It wasn't like he was debilitated by it. He was fully healthy. I remember six months before he died, I was out raking leaves. He was up for October. He started raking leaves and I said, "Dad, are you nuts?" And he said, "Bruce, if I can't live, if I can't do things like this with you, then what's the point of it?" When he died, he died suddenly—even now I get a little lump in my throat. I remember it was a Sunday night and Zach, my son, was 9 months old maybe, in the crib, and the phone rings at 8:30, 9:00 o'clock at night, and their neighbor had called me—that she had gone over—she was a nurse and her husband was a psychiatrist—they had run in when they heard my mother screaming. They had done CPR on him and he was on his way to the hospital, but it didn't look good. I ended up packing everybody up with clothing, and funeral clothing, a week's worth for

> sitting Shiva. Again, we had two older kids and a baby. We had just moved to Connecticut. Rachel was 6 or 7, Taryn was 5, and Zach was 9 months old and my mother was just devastated. It was just so unexpected. I don't think my mother quite understood when the cardiologist came in and said "we're not going to do surgery." At first, my mother thought it was great. I looked at the films and realized that it was they couldn't—it was so clogged up. I remember Taryn going over to my mother and hugging her—she was 5 years old—and she said, "Grandma, Poppi's not gone. Everytime I look up at the sky, I see him." You know, she's always been that way. I loved hiking, and adventuring with Taryn. She then became my partner in crime a little bit when she was around. Rachel went off to college and Taryn was still there. So I would bring her up when I brought up the students for the retreats in the Berkshires. I remember one particular night—cold late October or November night—and everyone had left. We had hiked down to the lake. It was a full moon. We were standing at the lake and the wind was whipping across the surface of the lake, and the reflection of the moon was swirling in the ripples. I'm close to my kids, but it was just one of those moments where you don't have to have words or anything, and she still remembers that night.

Bruce and Lisa completed their family with their son Zach:

> My son, born on June 22, 1989, is a mechanical and aerospace engineer, lives in Anacostia, DC. He has worked all over the world; on aquaponic greenhouses in Germany, appliance recycling in Fortaleza, Brazil, and solar water pump development (for rice production) in Myanmar. He is now working on urban revitalization with two architects he lived with in college. He was really a mistake or a surprise. My wife and I had talked about having another kid. She wanted to have a boy. And I was actually the one who said, "If it's a girl, can you throw it back?" You don't want to start a child in life with a disappointment. So, she started looking for a job, and I was actually in Belize. I tried to call home and couldn't get her, couldn't get her because she had gone back to Worcester. We had just moved from the University of Massachusetts, and she was with friends in Worcester, because she was upset that she was pregnant. She had gotten beyond that idea, and had already been mapping out her going back to work, and her career, and everything else, then BOOM she's pregnant. I was at the Bullfrog Inn in Belmopan, Belize when she finally picked up the phone and I sort of got an earful. So Zachary got his name because my wife liked the name Zachary, but the connection would be my Aunt Rose—and you might say, "How does that work?" It's because Rose's real name was Zelda. All three of my children are trying to make the world a better place in their own way. And all three love each other and their parents . . . who could ask for more.

In Medical Training

Physician Howard Markel (2008: 227) writes, "Every physician recalls with relative clarity his or her first day of medical school." The memory stays with them because it is the commencement of an often jarring journey from which few survive unchanged, not just in terms of their ability to treat the sick, but in terms of the kind of person they have become. The nature of this journey was tellingly described by Stephen Bergman, under the *nom de plume* of Samuel Shem, in his classic novel *The House of God* (Shem 1978). The book sold millions of copies but was not well received by medical school deans and was maligned by older physicians. Although the author got many invitations to speak about his irreverent book, he at first refused them until grateful letters from doctors in training convinced him that he

> could be helpful to doctors who were going through the brutality of training. And so I began what has turned out to be a 35-year odyssey of speaking out, around the world, about resisting the inhumanity of medical training. The title of my talk is almost always the same: "Staying Human in Health Care." (Shem 2012)

Over time, Bergman came to see his book as part of the "fiction of resistance," writing novels as a means of giving voice to the struggle against the injustices of a system (Shem 2002). In Bergman's view as a physician, "Your patient is never only the patient, but the family, friends, community, history, the climate, where the water comes from and where the garbage goes. Your patient is the world" (Shem 2012). Hence it is the physician's responsibility to not just tend to the immediate health needs of individual patients but also to the pressing needs of the healthcare system and of society and to the social and socioenvironmental conditions that contributed to the patient's sickness. Especially important is being prepared to be a whistleblower on the ills of the healthcare system itself: "If you see a wrong in the medical system, speak out and up. It is not only important to call attention to the wrongs in the system, it is essential for your survival as a human being" (Shem 2012).

As structured in the US, medical education consists of movement through a number of stages. Stage one is medical school training through receipt of the Doctor of Medicine degree (or the less common but more or less equivalent Doctor of Osteopathic Medicine degree) over a four-year period. During the final year of medical school, students begin nervously applying for an internship in their desired area of focus, a highly competitive process that rewards you with a relatively modest salary. Internships are stressful as they require budding doctors to be "on call" on a rotating cycle often involving 36-hour shifts at the hospital, until reforms were implemented. The rationale for the long hours that physicians in training must put in is that, in the pressure cooker of hospital experience, doctors will gain broad knowledge and skills in treating many types of patients with diverse health problems, as they are adapting to the demanding and irregular hours of biomedical practice. Completion of the one-year internship is generally a requirement to be licensed to practice medicine in most states.

Medical training, in short, is not just for the mind, but for the emotions and body as well. In the past, when the social status of physicians was much higher, medical training was socially accepted as being capable of transforming a mere mortal into something akin to a demigod. As Barbara Holland (1999) writes in her book, *Wasn't the Grass Greener? Thirty-Three Reasons Why Life Isn't as Good as It Used to Be*:

> When I was a child [in the late 1930s and early 1940s] the doctor was God. Like God, in exchange for respect and obedience—"doctor's orders"—he guided us through the valley of the shadow, held out the hope of life eternal, and came when we summoned him, yea, even through snowstorms, to sit on the edge of our bed and lay his hand on our fevered brow. Our parents were wise by definition but he was infallible by definition; "The doctor knows best" was an incantation you could lean on.

A satirical quip about doctors during this era was that the difference between God and doctors is that God knows he is not a doctor (Shalof 2010). Adds Jeffrey Brenner, who practices family medicine in Camden, NJ one of the poorest cities in the US, "med school is really like being inducted into a priesthood of power, money and influence" (quoted in Freakonomics 2015).

Over time, in no small part because of the rising cost of healthcare, and the kinds of issues Bruce has had to contend with during his medical career, as hospitals have become more consolidated and corporate, as well as other changes like patient access to the Internet and pharmaceutical marketing directly to the public, the social standing and sense of personal power of physicians has declined. A definitive marker of their waning social power is the formation of physician unions. According to David Leffell, Section Chief of Dermatologic Surgery and Cutaneous Oncology at Yale School of Medicine:

> I think the time is fast approaching when a combination of trends will drive physicians to organize . . . Tensions between large hospital and health systems and doctors are increasing. Large health systems and hospitals are striving to de-professionalize doctors and create structures in which doctors have even less voice than they have now. (Quoted in Weiner 2014)

Already the Service Employees' International Union has formed physician locals as has the Union of American Physicians and Dentists, which is affiliated with the American Federation of State, County and Municipal Employees.

The specialty focus of Bruce's internship was internal medicine. This branch of medicine focuses on the prevention, diagnosis, and treatment of the wide array of diseases found in adult patients. Physicians who train in this specialty commonly are referred to as "internists" (not to be confused with "intern," the initial ranking of the medical profession) or "doctors of internal medicine." An internist is also sometimes also called the "doctor's doctor" because they are frequently called in as consultants to other physicians to help resolve perplexing diagnostic problems.

Following the one-year internship, and in order to be able to subsequently practice in a particular area of specialization, doctors must then complete a multi-year focused residency, lasting from three to seven or more years depending on their area of medical concentration. The objective is to provide adequate training and experience to enable successful unsupervised practice of medicine. Historically, residency has been a challenging experience. Residencies are so demanding, according to the Accreditation Council for Graduate Medical Education (Philibert and Amis 2011: 1), because beyond their training mission they are designed to be "a cultural symbol" of a profession that, as part of its self-defined identity, puts patients first. The burden on residents' stamina and alertness, however, grew to be so great in that in 2003, that what are called the "duty hour rules," were revised to limit a resident to 80 hours per week of hospital-based work. This includes overnights stays when residents who are on call are allowed to catch some needed sleep, a break referred to by doctors as "strategic napping."

While the discussion within medicine about the appropriate load for residents has been going on for some time, the intensity of the debate ratcheted up in 1984 following the death of Libby Zion in a New York City teaching hospital. At the time of her death, Libby, age 18, was a freshman in college. She had a history of depression and on the evening of October 4, was admitted to the hospital suffering from fever, being agitated, having jerking motions in her body, and appearing disoriented. Libby was evaluated by two physicians, an intern eight months out of medical school and a resident with an additional year of training. They were uncertain of her diagnosis but decided to admit her for rehydration and observation. This decision was approved over the telephone by a senior clinician who had previously treated several members of the Zion family. Based on their assessment of her condition, the two doctors on her ward prescribed both a dose of meperidine, a narcotic analgesic used as a painkiller, and a sedative, to control her shaking (Lerner 2006). By 3 am, as the intern was off dealing with some of the forty other patients she was covering and during a period when the resident had gone to an on-call room in an adjacent building to get some sleep, Libby became more highly disturbed. Several nurses responded and contacted the resident several times on his beeper. He instructed the nurses to restrain Libby to prevent her from hurting herself and prescribed an injection of haloperidol, an antipsychotic drug with sedative properties that effectively controlled her agitation. At 6:30 am, however, a nurse's aide took Libby's temperature and found that it had climbed to 107, a level that can cause brain damage. The intern was called and emergency measures were implemented to resuscitate Libby and lower her temperature, but she suffered cardiac arrest and died. Libby's father, a graduate of the Yale School of Law and a prominent journalist, investigated his daughter's tragic death and wrote an op-ed piece in the *New York Times* in which he stressed: "You don't need kindergarten to know that a resident working a 36-hour shift is in no condition to make any kind of judgment call—forget about life-and-death" (quoted in Lerner 2006). The district attorney sued the hospital as well the doctors that were involved. The case was only resolved many years later when an appellate court absolved the defendants of wrong doing. The case, however, drew widespread attention to the medical soundness of 36-hour physician shifts and led ultimately to restrictions on duty hours.

Following completion of the residency, a physician is known as an attending (or staff) physician. At this point, they must pass written and oral exams demonstrating their mastery of required knowledge and skills in their specialty in order to become a board-certified physician—one of the several framed certificate commonly seen hanging on a physician's office wall, although this credential is not required to practice medicine.

After his internship, Bruce remained at the University of Massachusetts Medical Center for three years as a resident, the final year serving as the Chief Medical Resident in internal medicine:

> When I was offered the position I was scared out of my mind. I didn't think I was smart enough, and I knew I was not their first choice. I knew there were two or three other residents in my class that they had asked before me that had been going on to fellowship, or just didn't want the position. They asked me and I went home and I said "oh my God, I'm not sure if I can do this," but I was afraid that if I start running away from challenges at 29, I might never stop running; that is not the way to live. I'm not the brightest bulb in the pack, but I'm not stupid either, I realized that. But some of my colleagues were encyclopedic, with photographic memories. I realized that I know a lot, but my gift is problem-solving, and taking the knowledge I have and utilizing it in new ways. Before I started that year as chief resident, I feared that I'd be presented with a patient with X, Y, or Z and be asked to spout the 37 things that it could be. That was terrifying especially because I would have seventy residents [under my supervision as Chief].

Bruce also was particularly concerned about taking report each morning [morning report] on the 10–20 patients that would have been admitted the evening before. The expectation would be that he would discuss each of the cases in depth off the top of his head:

> There's that sense of one-ups-manship and who's smarter, and certainly amongst my residents there were those that really were driven to make sure everyone knew that they were smarter. My goal was to make morning report interesting and informative to the residents but especially to assure that we reviewed the cases and assured patients were getting the best possible care. The way I figured out how to be successful as chief resident was to work harder than everyone else. At 11 o'clock each night, I would call the resident

> who was admitting and I'd say "Joe" or "Joanne," "how ya doin? Who came in tonight?" They'd tell me and, with some relief, we'd talk about the cases. It also gave them the opportunity to tell me, as the chief, what patients were worrying them, and for us together to figure out if there were safety issues or patient care issues, that we'd solve then and there, rather than allowing things to deteriorate in the middle of the night and have to pick up the pieces the next day. My job was to not let them kill people and to teach them that if there is a question, to ask it now, in the middle of the night if need be rather than, God forbid, allowing a preventable tragedy to occur. It made everyone happier. What it did for me was after 15–20 minutes on the phone I had a list of every patient that had come in and what their issues were. I would then go and read for an hour and the next day at morning report when the resident presented the cases, I had cheated [in the sense of being prepared]. I had actually read up on some of the issues, and maybe I had gone and gotten the microscope slide of their blood or their tissue or their urine, or had a copy of their EKG. So my year as chief resident was different than others before me. In the past, it had been a game show, stump the stars, or the chief resident. Now it was a case conference, identifying concerning cases and assisting the team caring for the patient, to tease out the answers and get better outcomes. I got the hospital to buy a microscope that I could project on to a television screen and so the residents knew to bring slides. So when we discussed a case, I threw the slide up and would say "Well here's the blood smear, tell me what you see." For the younger residents it was teaching rounds. I was able then to keep a little bit ahead, half an inch ahead. It was a really good year. By the end of the year, the chief of medicine came up to me and said: "Bruce I want to hire you. What d'ya wanna do? We'll make a position." I was flattered and told him: "I'm a primary care doctor, I want to be in primary care." That's when the primary care folks said they didn't want me without a fellowship. I tell residents [at the University of Connecticut] all the time that life is full of serendipity, "be passionate about what you're doing now, the job at hand, and other opportunities will come your way." I really believe that if you have a master plan for what you want your career to be, [say] the Surgeon General, and you're making all your decisions based on furthering that plan, rather than optimizing the job at hand, it won't work out.

One of the contradictions of contemporary medical training is that many graduating medical students are not as lucky as Bruce in quickly finding immediate placement for residency. Decisions about acceptance into programs are made on what is known as Match Day, because it is the day students learn to which training programs they have been matched based on preferences submitted both by students and training hospitals. The process of linking students and teaching hospitals is coordinated by the National Resident Matching Program, a non-profit organization founded by medical students to help standardize the selection process and establish a uniform date of appointment to available slots in graduate medical education. The day is experienced by many medical students as the most dramatic day of medical school. On Match Day in 2016, there were over 29,000 applicants for first-year residency openings, but over 8,500 of these were not placed (Bailey 2016). These students are informed of this disheartening news a few days earlier on what has come to be known as Black Monday. Some states, like Missouri, Kansas, and Arkansas, have seen this as an opportunity to get doctors into their rural and inner-city clinics, and have passed laws that enable unmatched medical school graduates to work in underserved areas. Others wait a year and apply again and spend their time doing research (sometimes for pharmaceutical companies), getting a master's degree, or otherwise trying to strengthen their appeal. Eventually, 99 percent of US, medical school graduates are placed (Sondheimer et al. 2015).

Even the residency is not the end of training for many physicians, as some then go on to fellowships, often in a highly specialized area of treatment and possibly research. Bruce remained at the same institution for a fellowship, but not because it was his first choice:

> Over my career, every few to several years my job would change. I worked for UMass for five years or so. I was a resident, and then chief resident, and then I was forced to be a fellow. They asked me to be on faculty and then they signed the note so I could buy [my] second home, [the one] in Princeton, which was predicated on the salary that I was going to earn as faculty. Then the primary care division decided that I needed a fellowship, and that they would only hire faculty in primary care who had a fellowship. It was politics with the chair of medicine. I had just been chief resident and spent four years in the division of primary care. The primary care faculty did not want the chair of medicine telling them who to hire, I get it. It was really a control issue. So I took a deep breath and I did a fellowship in general medicine and primary care at UMass. They more or less created the fellowship for me to do. I was a fellow in the division of primary care. They allowed me to do 24-hour shifts in the emergency room as the attending physician, so I could pay my mortgage. Then a year later I graduated the fellowship and became director of the fellowship. A year after that or so, the director of the primary clinic, who had been my mentor, left, and they asked me to be the director of the adult primary care clinic at UMass. So here I was two years out of residency training and I was director of the clinic, at least in part because I had fellowship training in primary care. That's what I tell students: if you do things well, and you do it with passion, opportunities present themselves. You don't always have to climb over someone, just work hard and do a good job.

Bruce remained as clinical director in Worcester for three years, but eventually the politics of the situation led him to think about other options. He was not happy to leave the University of Massachusetts, recalling:

> I had been there nine years. I was really part of the infrastructure of the institution. I loved UMass. It was a great place and I was sad to leave. I had a lot of patients that I'd been seeing for nine years. I had my best friends, my friend Steve had moved there because of me and leaving disrupted the circle of friends that I had at that point.

Bruce decided to leave UMass none the less, although he did not have to go very far to find what appeared to be an especially appealing opportunity given his orientation to medical care. He found an opening 90 minutes from Worcester at Mount Sinai Hospital in Hartford, CT as chief of community medicine and medical director at Burgdorf Clinic in the North End of the city serving low-income patients. The position was a joint position supported by the hospital and by the University of Connecticut School of Medicine.

Bruce saw patients at the Burgdorf: "When I first got here, I really was a clinic doc, so my practice was at the Burgdorf Center. We were in the old building across the street, which makes the new building look like the Taj Mahal." The original Burgdorf Clinic was founded in 1970 as the outpatient service for the UConn Health Center. It initially occupied the old McCook State Hospital, a site owned by the City of Hartford. McCook was the city hospital of Hartford from 1932 until 1967. In its original location, Bruce recalled, the Burgdorf

> had no windows, and it had asbestos. And so wherever asbestos had leaked from the ceiling, they didn't remove it, they would just build a little room to contain it. So right in the middle of the entrance lobby for the building was this 10 x 10 floor to ceiling cubicle with a little porthole to look inside, which is where the ceiling had collapsed and asbestos had [fallen]. With asbestos containment sometimes remediating it, ripping it out, is more dangerous than just covering it. You could cover it in all sorts of creative ways to keep it in place. If you're going to pull it out then it costs millions of dollars.

As the director, Bruce supervised eighty employees, including doctors, nurses, physician's assistants, and others, as well as a full-time Master's in Public Health-level administrator:

> Jay Pinsince was this great guy, incredibly bright, and profoundly committed to what we were doing. And despite the fact that that hospital was the end of the world, the day I walked in, my first hour on the job [I got a big surprise]—I had just taken my family on a vacation to Prince Edwards Island, we drove up to Maine, took the Nova Scotia Ferry, and so I was out of communication. There were no cell phones. I get back and we moved and I started work and the day I got there they said, "Bruce, we're so happy you're here but Mount Sinai Hospital went bankrupt. We are laying off 20 percent of your staff. They're in that room over there. Go tell them." And so, that

> was my first hour at the Burgdorf. And I went in, and rather than laying people off, we cut our individual hours back by about 20 percent. No one was laid off and then in six months, patient volumes were up and the crisis to a degree was over. At the point when I walked in the door at Burgdorf, Mount Sinai was talking to Hartford Hospital [another major hospital in Hartford] about taking over the hospital. Apparently the negotiations were too Machiavellian, it was down on your knees. Hartford Hospital backed out and it fell apart.

Instead, the Catholic hospital in Hartford, St. Francis, then came on board to run both Mount Sinai Hospital and the Burgdorf Clinic in the North End of the city (in the first U.S. takeover of a Jewish hospital by a Catholic hospital):

> Sister Francis Marie, who was at that point the CEO of St. Francis, more or less said, "You're an important community resource, we're in the same boat, and we should help each other," and so, in a very open - ended way said, "we're going to help you, we're going to keep you going." But she was let go, edged out, or retired and that's when things got interesting. Anything that wasn't tied down or profitable at Mount Sinai was shipped over to St. Francis. Anything related to abortion, contraception, etc. was closed or given away to Hartford Hospital, which created an access issue for the North End. We had the only *in vitro* infertility unit in the state at that point. It had to close because it was against church policy. The condom, with its dual relationship to contraception and STD prevention, was also against church policy. Tubal ligations were also disallowed. These were access issues to essential services in a high-risk population. I was concerned and so was the state Commission on Health and Hospitals! There was concern, well-founded, that the Commission might not approve the merger. So I spoke with the Dean of the Medical School and he allowed me to testify that the University of Connecticut would take responsibility for all family planning services . . . The primary care docs at the Burgdorf were full-time UConn faculty and UConn paid a portion of the St. Francis Hospital OB/Gyn attending's salary. UConn also provided an operating subsidy to the Burgdorf and rented some space at the clinic . . . so family planning services could be provided by UConn paid faculty, on UConn paid time, in UConn rented space . . . and that's what we did so that essential family planning services would continue to be accessible to the North End of Hartford.
>
> The CON [Certificate of Need] was approved and the St. Francis/UConn family planning arrangement was part of the CON document. I became the "king of condoms," walked around with pockets full of condoms and the residents and staff knew to ask a UConn faculty if a patient needed condoms or counseling. We tried to assure that the staff [employed by St. Francis] had nothing to do with it [family planning services] . . . they could lose their jobs. So that's how it shook out. Every once in a while, I'd

> get a letter or an email or a phone call from the Burgdorf OB/Gyn doc, that he'd gotten a letter from the Chief of OB at St. Francis, who'd gotten a letter from the CEO, who'd gotten a letter from the Archdiocese that some mom had found Burgdorf condoms in their kid's drawer. But I could pull out the CON and there it was, in black and white . . . all part of a system to assure our patients got the services they needed!

The UConn Health Center, which ultimately founded the Burgdorf, dates back to the mid-1940s following the release of the findings of several studies designed to assess the need for a new medical and dental school in Connecticut. Concern about this issue grew noticeably in the late 1950s because of new reports suggesting that there was growing possibility of a physician shortage in the US as the nation's population began to grow at an accelerated pace. In the influential 1959 report, *Physicians for a Growing America (Bean 1961)*, also known as the Bean Report, the U.S. Department of Health, Education and Welfare called for the creation of 21 new medical schools, and specified that one of them should be located in Connecticut. At the time, many private medical schools across the country restricted the number of religious and ethnic minorities they would accept, adding the issue of discrimination to the growing concern about the state of medical education. In 1961, the Connecticut General Assembly passed Special Act 328 which authorized funding for the University of Connecticut to establish a medical and dental school in Hartford County. In response, the university took over McCook in the North End of Hartford in 1967, a year before the first medical and dental classes were offered at the UConn Health Center and two years before construction was begun on UConn's new John Dempsey Hospital on a 106-acre hilltop site known as the O'Meara farm in the wealthy suburbs of Farmington, CT. When the UConn Health Center formally opened its doors in 1970, medical and dental outpatient services were opened in the new Burgdorf Health Center, transferring programs from the aging McCook building (Kirk 2011). In the aftermath of the move, the McCook site, following renovation, became the new home of a multiservice center operated by the Alcohol and Drug Recovery Centers Inc. as well as providing offices for the city's social services program.

Bruce arrived in Connecticut with a plan to make the Burgdorf a successful, effective, and efficient healthcare center with broad appeal to patients in the region. According to Patricia Joyce, associate professor of pediatrics at UConn and director of the Pediatric Clinic at Burgdorf:

> I don't even know if Bruce will remember this, but I interviewed him when he came to apply, and he had a vision from the very beginning that he could come in and try to transition this into a center of excellence that people would want to come [to] from all over, not just from the North End of Hartford. He [thought he] could pull in [insured] people from Simsbury and Avon and Glastonbury. But during our interview we had time, so I put him in my car and I drove him around the North End of Hartford to say, "This

> is who comes to us." And he came and he preserved his initial vision for a long time, and then I think he realized he wasn't going to change the culture in the suburbs; no matter how good you were, they were still going to be afraid of Hartford. So then he just wanted to make us a center of excellence for care and education. This happens all the time when people come from a different institution—he was so gung-ho that he just wanted to kind of bring all of his ideas forward, and people weren't ready for it and it was hard for him to hear that at first. After a while he figured that out and he moved with it. He never loses his vision.

The fear to which Joyce refers—a product of stereotyping, discrimination, and social isolation—was very familiar to city officials in Hartford. After he became City Manager in 1990, Raymond Eugene Shipman concluded that the main source of the troubled capital city's problems was its political isolation as an urban core that was kept impoverished by state tax policies and suburban attitudes (Johnson 1991). He urged the state to stop building low-income housing in Hartford and scatter housing projects among the suburban areas surrounding the Capital. If the state failed to do this, he urged that Hartford should levy a wage tax on the thousands of commuters who flock to the city's downtown insurance and banking office towers each workday morning, only to flee back to the suburbs at night. In support of Shipman's perspective, in the early 1990s, Hartford's City Council considered filing two lawsuits intended to overturn state tax and housing laws that council members said restricted the city's revenue and unfairly added to its low-income population. Shipman's ideas were not well received by the business community. Business leaders responded that his plan to tax commuters would drive more employers from the city. Already, they pointed out, Hartford was suffering from store closings, bankruptcies, and the loss of two downtown hotels. Progressive voices in the city also faulted Shipman's desire to eliminate housing projects in the city, knowing that surrounding towns would not take in people pushed out of low-income public residences by building local housing for the poor. At the time of Shipman's arrival in Hartford, of the almost 33,000 people receiving welfare benefits in the nine towns west of the Connecticut River that are overseen by the Hartford office of the State Department of Income Maintenance, 94.5 percent lived in Hartford, comprising more than 22 percent of the city's population. By contrast, the approximately 2,000 living in the eight other towns made up less than 1 percent of their populations (Johnson 1991).

Low-income public housing in Hartford dates to the 1940s, a period when there was a growing need for affordable housing for defense industry workers during wartime. Throughout this period, there was an inflow of war industry laborers, both White and African American, along with their families. They found work in local defense plants, such as the Pratt & Whitney Machine Tool plant and the Pratt & Whitney Aircraft Company. These new apartment-style homes were constructed with federal funding from the U.S. Housing Authority and administered by the Hartford Housing Association. In the early years, African Americans were blocked from living in public housing. As David Radcliffe (1998), author of the book *Charter Oak Terrace: Life, Death and Rebirth of a Public Housing Project*, pointed out in a 2002 interview,

> Hartford's understood policy of "controlled integration" was common in many public housing authorities in the 1950s and 1960s. This approach forced many black families, living in dreadful slum conditions, to wait until a unit reserved for minorities became available, even if other "white" units sat vacant. Underneath this approach was certainly some discrimination, if not downright racism on the part of many developers and bankers who sought to maintain segregated housing and schools. (Quoted in Albert 2003)

Exemplary was the effort to keep African Americans from moving into a project that was built just over the Hartford City line in West Hartford. West Hartford homeowners were reported to be "'alarmed' and 'horrified' at the idea of 'Negroes' living in their neighborhood. One woman said she and her family would move out the day after any African Americans moved in" (Meehan 2013). An article printed at the time in a local newspaper

> described the situation in harsh, racist language, calling it an "infiltration," and reported the prevailing sentiment among community homeowners as being: "We don't want them here." The consensus among West Hartford realtors and homeowners, the newspaper reported, was that real estate values would show "an immediate and sharp" drop if "Negroes" in any considerable number moved into town. (Quoted in Meehan 2013)

Eventually, as a result of legal challenges to discrimination, and White flight to the segregated suburbs surrounding the city, African Americans and Hispanics came to represent the predominant residents of public housing in Hartford, as elsewhere. At the same time, poor building design, inferior fast-track construction methods, revisions in federal housing policy, a consistent pattern of weak local management, and regional economic decline all took their toll on the city's housing projects. Hartford officials came to view the failing projects as a blight on a city that has long held the nickname the "Insurance Capital of the World." By the mid-1990s, Hartford housing authorities demolished most housing projects around the capital (the last federally subsidized project was not razed until 2011), forcing many poor people to try and find housing elsewhere in the city or beyond city boundaries. Those who found housing in the North End of Hartford, along with others already living there, became the patients Bruce would treat for the next several decades at Burgdorf. Just as Bruce's early life had been shaped by federal policies that created private housing for returning World War II soldiers, the destruction of federally subsidized housing for defense industry workers during the war shaped the demographic of the patients Bruce would try to administer to as a physician. As Martin Luther King (1977) realized, "We are not makers of history. We are made by history."

Fatherhood and Worldhood

Thinking of the issue of fatherhood, Bruce recalled a song that touched him:

> There's a song by Garnet Rogers, a Canadian singer songwriter . . . where he talks about his brother's death. His brother [Stan Rogers], also a singer songwriter, died in an airplane crash [Air Canada Flight 797 on June 2, 1983] while running back into the burning plane to get other people out. The song ["Night Drive"] tells us that at the grave you really can't tell someone you love them. It's too late so you should say it now, and with every action you take. And so I've made sure that my kids know how much I love them and how proud I am of them. That's one memory I want them to have.

Despite the pressures of medical training and working as a doctor, Bruce never wavered in his commitment to his children:

> I was not an absentee father. I was the soccer coach. I went to all the track meets. My daughter was on the cross country ski team, and I pretty much made all the ski meets on Saturdays, despite the fact they were up in New Hampshire at 9 in the morning, which meant I was leaving the house at 6 am. So looking back, I really feel that I was there for everyone, including my wife . . . My wife lets me do this work, a little less so the last few years. When the kids were home, she was home—she took off from being a veterinarian for a few years and then went back part-time, three days a week, when the kids were older. But because she understood the commitment to medicine, I wasn't told that "you're not home, bad husband, etc., etc." It just wasn't like that . . . we were partners in life. Now it's a little tougher because I think she really would like me to retire. I'm not quite there yet. I've thought about it, I'd like to experience that feeling of not having to do anything. I haven't felt that for 57 years. I did not, as many of my colleagues, take a year off, or travel, or bum around, or do any of that. I pushed right through my education and training . . . no breaks.

Now his children are grown, their relationships have changed, although the basic pattern endures:

> We're all very close though we're distributed up and down the East Coast from North Carolina to New York. I taught all three to love music. Bought each of them a decent guitar . . . don't want to learn on a crappy one . . . taught them the basics. I had the delusion of having a family band when they were young . . . wound up with a guitar chorus. Growing up we'd all sit around the campfire up in the Berkshires and play and sing . . . it's heaven! Now whenever we're all together, we sit around and play and sing . . . it doesn't get any better than that . . . love and music. Musically, they all passed me by a long time ago . . . but I got them started . . . a gift to them from their dad.

Bruce has also counseled his children as they have confronted the challenges of life:

> When my son was a freshman in college, which was probably 2007, he came home from school, [and] we were taking a walk in the woods and he said, "Dad, how do you know you've lived a good life?" And I thought about it and said, "You know by the numbers of lives you've touched." My son also went to Cornell but had a very different experience [than me]. He took greater advantage of the excitement of being there. But, similar to me, he would call me sometimes distraught over some big test and say "Oh, my God, I'm going to flunk." He was in the School of Engineering, which is even harder than biology, but he did fine. I'd ask him if he'd studied . . . and he would say yes . . . I'd ask him if he'd learned anything . . . and he'd say yes . . . and I'd tell him that that was all I expected . . . "take a deep breath and realize that you don't always have to get an 'A.' It's what you learn that's important." I would tell him "I love you whatever happens . . . you always have a place to live . . . a place to come home to . . . no conditions!" I'd hear a deep breath . . . and he'd move on.

Reflecting on his grown children, Bruce commented:

> At this point in life, I guess we're over the hump. We're looking at going back toward adventuring. The kids are out of the house. They're sort of self-sufficient. Occasional handouts, but that's okay because I'm still working. So as long as I can afford it, I don't mind my kids needing help now and again. Our parents were generous to us as well, making sure we weren't as financially stressed as we could have been. Sometimes we have to remind ourselves. I'm definitely the one that slips them money and pushes to pay for dinner. If we want them to visit us, we're just going to have to pay for their plane fare . . . You know, I have grandchildren now and I want them to know me. They're in North Carolina . . . lot closer than Booker Bay, Australia . . . but still not a quick jump in the car after work. I need to fly there if it's for a weekend or go there for a week, if I'm going to drive. It's a 12-hour drive . . . and I get tired more than I used to.

Despite not taking any breaks during his career, Bruce has been able to find ways to travel and to see the country:

> I have travelled within the United States, certainly New England. Florida, I've gone by car. I've gone cross-country north to south, east to west. When the kids were young, we did RV trips to Yellowstone, Glacier, Olympia, Arches and Grand Canyon . . . to most of the better known National Parks . . . and to some of the out-of-the-way ones. Capital Reef is in Utah. It's one of the original Mormon settlements. The National Park Service took over the settlement—it's still there in a canyon with Anasazi [Native American] ruins in its walls, and the original orchards still in production managed by the park

> system. When we were there, apricots were in season and you could pick the apricots for a quarter a bushel—some insane price—we loaded the RV. We all got diarrhea . . . eating way too many apricots. But it was an amazing family time . . . a real adventure. I've also travelled to a lot of states on business. When I served on the National Advisory Council for Migrant Health for four years [2000–04], we met in Omaha, and Indianapolis, Sacramento, and Phoenix, and in the non-convention smaller cities, like Ashville, North Carolina. Wherever I would go I'd try to do something, explore the uniqueness of the area. Hike, rent a bike or in some other way experience a "transcendent moment" . . . what I call an instant when you're living fully in that moment. In Phoenix, I couldn't find a bike rental, so I took the bus route to the end of the line right at the edge of the city and there was a park . . . turned out it was the largest desert park in the United States. I hiked up a mountain, and then looked out over Phoenix as the sun was setting. The flowers were in bloom in the high desert . . . breathtaking! I've given a talk in Hamilton, Ontario. I've been up to Quebec, the Thousand Islands. I've been to Seattle, Vancouver, and Alaska. We've been up and down the West Coast in an RV or with family. San Francisco, my sister used to live there. You know that I've slept on the rim of the Grand Canyon in a sleeping bag. I've slept in Arches National Park on top of the RV watching the moon do its circuit through the night. It was mystical. I've been to Hawaii a number of times, and then because my daughter was in Australia, I've been to Australia five times, New Zealand, and Fiji. Also Tahiti, Bora Bora, which was the most beautiful spot in the entire world. It was unbelievably gorgeous. We're going to Burma in four weeks. My son's there [at the time of the interview]. My son's doing an engineering fellowship. Creating and producing solar irrigation pumps for the Third World. You know, he likes to travel. He's been all over the world. And I've been to the Caribbean and I've spent time in Belize in the jungles with students. That was 25 years ago. It's been a while since I've done it. I have not been to Africa. My wife wants to go and we may go. I had an opportunity to help start a clinic in Nigeria just as Boko Haram was killing everyone. So I have to see if I have the strength and see how safe it is, because I'm not stupid. I don't have a death wish. I've been to the Southern Hemisphere, not really South America, but I've been to Central America extensively . . . and to Guatemala. That's what life is made up of to me . . . those transcendent moments. I try if I can to bump into them.

This occurs with patients as well:

> Sometimes you transcend with a patient, because you've just been able to fix something or help someone through a crisis; sometimes you can't cure it, but you've made a little bit of headway. But sometimes it's just someone saying "Gee, thank you, Dr. Gould for being there." My heart soars, it doesn't take much and that's the way to live.

In Guatemala, Bruce provided free medical care to local people:

> I rented a Range Rover, an old British Army vehicle, they didn't call them Range Rovers, they called them Land Rovers. My feet were getting wet, and I lifted the carpet and there was no floor. The windshield wipers didn't work and I was in the middle of the jungle on this dirt road, where the bridges crossing rivers were just planks. You had to line the tires up to go, it was intense. And I had students with me . . . We went to a town of a couple hundred people. There was no electricity. Everyone was doing subsistence farming, everyone doing their own barter, living in shacks in the rainforest . . . real shacks with kerosene refrigerators. My contact was an American marine biologist who had built a marine biology station at a bend in the river . . . it was basically shacks up on stilts . . . You slept under mosquito netting or you got eaten alive. You had to take anti-malarials . . . so you didn't die. No running water. For a couple days we were bathing in the river . . . then we saw these eyes looking back at us . . . there were alligators and crocodiles and whatever the hell else they have down there in the water. They really hadn't bothered us. Guess I was a little naïve back then. And then for a few days I worked in the village . . . they had this little clinic. I saw kids and adults and elderly . . . and then we also did some house calls in the village and surrounding rainforest. One woman with a huge ulcer on her foot was 101 years old . . . I do have a picture of her somewhere that we took. Then we went into Belmopan, which is the capitol of Belize. The capital used to be Belize City . . . it was really a tough, a tough city, so they moved the capitol to Belmopan. I met with some of the government officials, the director or minister of health, and some asked me if I could get them a green card to come to the United States. Subsequent to that I went down to Belize a few times, taking students and residents with me. What evolved, eventually there was a rotation at the district hospital in Stann Creek. They cleared out a storeroom, and students would stay there for six weeks, making rounds, and going to clinics with the district medical officer. A clinic was just a large room . . . people would show up, be given their charts and one by one they would be called to a table in the front of the room and the doctor would ask them what the problem was and, standing at the table, look down their throat or whatever else was bothering them and write a prescription and send them off. It is really very different than U.S. medicine, where everything is about physical history and documentation and documentation and documentation. It was an adventure. It sounds wrong, but that sense of helping someone, addressing their needs and then they just say "thank you for being here," makes me feel incredibly good. I'm not dependent on gratitude, because a lot of what we do as physicians—it's part of our job. We don't have to be thanked. But in those moments when you've really touched somebody, [then] you know. Martin Buber, who was a philosopher, he coined "I/Thou" . . . the concept that it's human connection that's actually God. It's actually that transcendent connection with other people. That's what gives me a buzz.

Building a Career in Connecticut

While he fully embraced his roles as a medical director, community physician, and leader of many initiatives designed to improve public health, Bruce avoided letting his professional obligations overwhelm him and crowd out other aspects of his life that have always been of great worth to him:

> It's important to put work, family, life and all these things in perspective. The day you die, they box your stuff up and put it out on the curb. Because I've seen this happen to so many colleagues; at some point they were an integral part of this complex [health care] machine and then, in an instant they're a memory or less. Charles Huntington, my friend, my colleague and partner [associate director] in starting the AHEC system in Connecticut, died five years ago. He worked with me for twelve years in AHEC and went on to serve as the associate dean for continuing education. He was a brilliant guy and the perennial volunteer . . . he'd volunteer for committees and task forces, he'd do the minutes, create the first draft of a document . . . a team player . . . a doer! He was president of the National AHEC Association, of the CT Public Health Association. When he died, there was shock and tears, but within a month, the hole closed behind him and people moved on. I think of him every day, not sure anyone else does. Never forget, that it's family where you leave your biggest mark, not at work.

As a university professor at the University of Connecticut, Bruce was hired at the entry-level rank of assistant professor in the professional category of medical educator. Promotion to the next level of professorship, associate professor, commonly is contingent upon the completion of significant work in research (e.g., sustained publication track record), teaching (e.g., developing a meaningful new curriculum), patient care, service (e.g., development or improvement of an educational program in the medical school) and other professional activities (e.g., taking leadership roles in the university). While in other tracks of professional ranking within the university, promotion to associate is expected to take about six or seven years, the medical educator professional category does not have a clear promotional requirement. In Bruce's case, however,

> when it was time for me to be promoted to associate professor, the chair of medicine said "it's time" and it happened. Promotion to associate is a lot easier jump than to full professor, and I really resigned myself to never getting promoted to full professor. In part, maybe it was insecurity, but in larger part, I don't like judging people and I'm not sure that I wanted to subject myself to being judged. I really didn't think a lot about promotion. I realized I had done some good things, started some worthwhile programs, but it was more about the work at hand than about professional rank. I didn't think it was time to go up for promotion and they forgot to tell me that it was time. The summer came and apparently my promotional packet was due at the

> end of the summer. I got a note from the Department of Medicine asking where my packet was. People spend a year putting together their promotion packet. I had two weeks. Our secretary was gone on vacation, so I threw it together as best I could. My name was already in the hopper, based on timelines in the department. I pulled together the migrant stuff [farm worker clinic], the CQI [Continuous Quality Improvement] curriculum which I started, and the nutrition curriculum.

In the end, as white hairs gained dominance in his well-groomed beard, Bruce finally was promoted to full professor of medicine, as well as continuing to serve as associate dean for primary care. Moreover, in 2009, Bruce received the Faculty Recognition Award from the UConn Health Center Board of Directors. As part of the award ceremony, the UConn School of Medicine's dean for academic affairs observed:

> Dr. Gould has made a career of giving voice to the most vulnerable populations. He's passionate about the delivery of medical care to the underserved of today and tomorrow, through his efforts to encourage medical students to consider careers in primary care and public health, and his efforts to introduce youth from disadvantaged communities to those professions. (UConn Health 2009)

The later comment was a reference to the Youth Health Services Corps, a nationally recognized recruitment program Bruce developed with AHEC that sends educators into high schools to train and places high school students as volunteers in healthcare provider agencies, homeless shelters, and food banks. A nine-module curriculum was developed to teach students the skills they need to be of help in their assigned community service site. Students who complete the full curriculum and fifty hours of community service receive the AHEC/National Health Service Corps recognition award. These awards are presented publically at the awards ceremonies of participating high schools. Bruce is especially proud of the program because "it started from nothing and its having a real impact, not only by virtue of affecting the kids that go through it, but also the communities it's serving" (quoted in Meldrum 2010: 98).

The following year, Bruce was the first recipient of the Charles G. Huntington III Award of the Connecticut Public Health Association. The Huntington Award recognizes healthcare practitioners who demonstrate public health leadership and a commitment to the health and well-being of populations. In the almost three decades that Bruce has worked in Hartford, his commitment to bring quality healthcare to the poor and underserved has been an uphill struggle, a prolonged confrontation with social inequality and institutional failure. It is a struggle that, at times, has worn him down, but it has not worn him out.

4

INSIDE THE BEAST

An Engaged Physician and Modern Medical Institutions

> Injustice anywhere is a threat to justice everywhere.
>
> *Martin Luther King, Jr.*

Social Justice and Access to Healthcare

A primary problem impacting the health of the poor in the US is that hospitals and other clinical services are withdrawing from poorer inner-city neighborhoods, places where rates of disease are greater than nearby wealthier urban and suburban areas. An analysis of data from the largest U.S. metropolitan areas by the *Pittsburgh Post-Gazette/Milwaukee Journal Sentinel* (Thomas 2014) found people in poor neighborhoods are less healthy than their more affluent neighbors, but more likely to live in areas with physician shortages and shuttered hospitals. The result of hospital closures in poor neighborhoods has left many low-income neighborhoods with no safety-net hospitals in areas that have become healthcare deserts. The analysis revealed that nearly two-thirds of the roughly 230 hospitals that have opened since 2000 are located in wealthier, usually suburban, areas. Meanwhile, the number of hospitals in 52 major cities across the country has dropped from a high of 781 in 1970, down to 426 by 2010. Most of the closed facilities were small to mid-size community hospitals that had been serving poor urban neighborhoods and public hospitals. In a locally focused study of hospital closures in the Pittsburgh, Pennsylvania region, using data for the period between 2000 and 2010 from the Pennsylvania Health Care Cost Containment Council, Hamill (2016) found that 11 of 39 hospitals shut their doors. Furthermore, all but one of the eleven shuttered hospitals had been providing higher than average levels of uncompensated care. In other words, the greater the level of care a hospital provided to the poor, the greater its chances of shutting down. Looking at the hospital systems that closed safety-net hospitals in the region, Hamill (2016) found that they were busy expanding existing or building new hospitals in wealthier towns and neighborhoods. Hamill's research showed "not only where the poor and disabled in [the Pittsburgh] region are, but where the doctors are not–and how that was often the same place."

Hospitals serving primarily African American patient populations have been particularly hard hit by closures. One expression of the impact of hospital closures is the disappearance of emergency rooms that serve patients in critical health and those without health insurance, leading to even greater health disparities between the poor and wealthier sectors of the population. A common result of the national epidemic of inner-city hospital closures is that fewer patients see physicians especially in a timely fashion, fewer children have regular checkups, patients are less likely to get preventive care, and there is a rise in preventable premature deaths (Kirsch 2007, Williams 2013).

In the words of Greg Burt, Chief Medical Officer at the non-profit Colusa Regional Medical Center in Colusa, California, when the decision was made to shut down his hospital, it was "a disaster for the community . . . There is a very significant risk for very poor patient outcomes" (quoted in Miller 2016). In that hospitals, as key service providers, often function as social anchors in communities that can help to stabilize neighborhoods and attract other services, including private practice physicians, their loss triggers a chain reaction of service losses that contributes to community disruption, which contributes to the subjective experience of anomie which itself is a threat to health.

Commonly, when inner-city hospitals close, the doctors who worked in them and practiced locally move on to more affluent areas rather than remain in the communities with the greatest healthcare needs. To assess the geographic distribution of physicians in the US, the Health Resources and Services Administration of the U.S. Department of Health and Human Services describes locales with fewer than one physician per 3,500 residents as "health professional shortage areas" (HPSAs). The *Post-Gazette/Journal Sentinel* data analysis indicates that the majority of the 6,100 primary care HPSAs are in inner cities and rural areas. This is true as well with dental and mental healthcare. Liu (2007), for example, found that HPSA residents in West Virginia are poorer, less educated, in worse physical health, and less likely over the past six months to have received primary healthcare services than residents who do not live in an HPSA.

As a general pattern, social disinvestment in neighborhoods leads to an interconnected downward spiral of decline in locally available sustainable resources, the experiential quality of communities among residents, community trust, and neighborhood social ties, and these adverse changes, in turn, get beneath the skin and have harmful impacts on health as it is produced in everyday life (Breslow 1999, Macintyre and Ellaway 2000, Singer 2016). As noted in Chapter 1, place matters in the making of health and well-being, but so does the experience of place by people in any locale. As Hiss (1991: xii) observes, "our ordinary surroundings, built and natural alike, have an immediate and a continuing effect on the way we feel and act, and on our health and intelligence." We are hardwired by our evolutionary history to perceive our environs through multiple senses, as survival depends on perceiving risks and responding to observed opportunities. But in addition to our sensual relationship to the world around us, and our cognitive understanding of the world, there is an emotional apparatus that responds internally to our perceptions. This phenomenon, labeled "affective primacy" (Zajonc 2000), involves the feelings (somewhat independent of thoughts and cognitions) that people experience in reaction to environmental sensations or perceptions (Ulrich 1983). A simple expression of this connection is people's response to the color of the room they are in. Studies have shown consistent room color-mood associations (Wexner 1954, Yildirim, Akalin-Baskaya, and Hidayetoglu 2007, Kwallek et al. 1996). Additionally, one's surroundings, a dynamic that anthropologists include in their conception of "lived experience," impact health (Desjarlais and Throop 2011). A study in Cook County, Illinois (Wen, Hawkley, and Cacioppo 2006) of the relationship among objectively assessed neighborhood socioeconomic status (SES), people's subjective perceptions of their neighborhood environment, their individual SES statuses, and self-rated health found a significant association between neighborhood SES and self-rated health. The sense of neighborhood quality perceived by study participants (i.e., their subjective ratings of neighborhood physical, social, and service status) showed a significant effect on self-rated health (after controlling for individual socio-demographic factors as well as neighborhood SES). The effects of perceived neighborhood environment on health appear to be related to experiences like loneliness, depression, hostility, and stress. Hospital closings and doctor flight from areas with poor patients and people of color, as a result, become contributing factors in the creation of the very health problems that Bruce focuses on in his clinical practice and in his activist community efforts.

Typical of hospital closings in recent decades is the loss of UPMC Braddock Hospital, a full-service facility that drew patients from 25 communities in the Monongahela Valley near Pittsburgh. The hospital, which primarily served the African American population of Braddock, had opened its doors in 1906, and 90 years later it became part of the University of Pittsburgh Medical Center (UPMC). Then in early 2010 the hospital stopped accepting patients and soon locked its doors permanently (Twedt 2009). A community-based activist group that took the name "Save Our Community Hospital" quickly formed to voice community anger and to try to stop or delay the hospital's closure. The group organized numerous protest events. All to no avail. For the people of Braddock, the UPMC slogan, "Life Changing Medicine," proved to be quite accurate, but not in the way public relations formulators of that branding label intended.

Hospital closures add to the emerging picture of the U.S. healthcare system as a wobbly and dysfunctional structure that exhibits grossly underserved poor and minority people at one end and very well-heeled and undeniably powerful sellers of healthcare for a profit at the other, with middle-income people struggling to deal with rising health costs in the middle. Fighting this behemoth at the local level, in an effort to care for the health of the poor and minority patients, is

Bruce's life mission, day in and day out. It is the reason he has fought for many years to keep the Burgdorf Clinic open, despite multiple efforts to close it or diminish its services.

Hospital Corporatization

The term "neoliberal economics" refers to fiscal policies that promote "the deregulation of corporations, and particularly of financial institutions; the rollback of public services and benefit programs; curbing labor unions; 'free trade' policies that would pry open foreign markets; and wherever possible the replacement of public programs with private markets" (Piven 2007: 13). Much of the research on the social effects of neoliberalism have focused on developing countries and the enforced shift demanded by international loaner institutions and dominant nations toward the privatization of societal institutions and loss of public employment and social safety net programs. But similar processes are unfolding within developed nations including the US. For example, there has been considerable discussion of the defunding of universities by state governments and the associated full-on shift toward the corporate university, a change in which increasingly institutions of higher education are "busily striving to profit from teaching, research and all the other activities on campus—offering corporations the right to endow professorships, sponsor courses, bring the university's scientific discoveries to market, even advertise in campus bathrooms" (Clay 2008). Adds Noam Chomsky (2014), "When universities become corporatized, as has been happening quite systematically over the last generation as part of the general neoliberal assault on the population, their business model means that what matters is the bottom line." Structural changes like these in the wider society have been reproduced within the healthcare system. Bruce laments this fact, explained: "everything went to corporatization" and the end result is

> our dysfunctional health care system . . . The political and economic structure gives way too much power to [private] companies and producers, advertisers, etc. There's relatively too little control over resources at the level of providers and clinical teams that day to day deal with population health.

While Bruce is describing his own immediate perceptions of the changes occurring in society generally but more specifically in healthcare, his experience is backed up by a body of social research that documents significant organizational alterations in healthcare institutions.

With reference to the broader society, the Institute for Policy Studies (Anderson and Cavanagh 2007) reports that just over half of the wealthiest economic entities in the world are corporations. The biggest two hundred corporations account for 25 percent of the total global economic activity. With this kind of economic muscle, corporations can exert a commanding influence on what happens in the world, economically and otherwise, including, as has been described, the nature of the U.S. healthcare system and the quality of life for all people. Some corporate actions, like the production of useful medical technologies or the development of effective, affordable drugs are beneficial to society, although more so to some sectors than others; other corporate actions do enormous harm, and, again, this too is not evenly distributed. Bruce cited a specific case making reference to the willingness of the health insurance industry to avoid providing coverage to low-income populations. The case involved a woman with diabetes who came to the Burgdorf who was septic from a urinary infection, a potentially lethal condition. He told the woman that she needed to be admitted to the hospital. She replied,

> "I'm still paying off the last admission. I'm not going to the hospital" and she went home. For every story like her, there's a whole bunch of people just dying at home or coming in so late that there's nothing we can do, or coming in so late that they end up never returning to a functional lifestyle, so the rest of us pay. (Quoted in Becker 2010)

Fortunately, in this instance, the woman recovered after Bruce put her on what turned out to be an effective oral antibiotic regime.

Corporatization also has reshaped U.S. healthcare, including hospital-based medicine, with investor-owned hospital management companies representing one of the most dramatic changes, as noted in the discussion of the emergence of the medical-industrial complex in Chapter 2. As reported there, privatized hospitals structured around profit generation tend to delimit the services they offer to those that produce the greatest profit and to provide these services to the best-paying patients, while abandoning other needed services and poorer-paying, yet sicker patients, to less-well-funded and increasingly ailing non-profit and public hospitals. The consequence has been the pattern of hospital closures in areas with concentrated low-income populations, as noted above. A surgeon and researcher, Martin Makary (2012: 3) comments:

> A hospital is no longer the community pillar I knew growing up, with its altruistic mission guiding its decisions. Hospitals have merged and transformed into giant corporations with little accountability—and they like it that way. Patients are encouraged to think that the health care system is a well-oiled machine, competent and all-wise. It's not.

The problem, Makary (2012: 5) emphasizes, is that in the US "the health care system is broken." This too is Bruce's perspective:

> in this country, unfortunately, we have not yet reached the point where optimization of the health status of the population becomes the primary mission and goal of the health system, and then, from there, we determine the most efficient and affordable way to achieve that goal. Then we would have

> to look at the environment, and housing, and education, and poverty, and social determinants and all those other things beyond simple access to care, that stand between patients and health . . . we would figure out that the most efficient and affordable way to get to health is a single-payer health care system of some type. Lots of countries have been incredibly creative in figuring out ways to get there. And almost all of them have gotten better outcomes at a fraction of the cost. I'm not an economist, but my sense is that part of the cost of this health care system is that large amounts of money are being diverted to what is an enormous business, a very profitable business. Some of it [goes] to advertising, some of it to CEO salaries, and significant dollars to dividends and profits.

Recognition of the ills of healthcare is not limited to those with a social medicine perspective who, like Bruce, embrace "a vision of medicine and public health constructed around the principles of justice rather than commodification and profitability" (Waitzkin 2011). Awareness is found as well among those with a market orientation who believe that if healthcare were run fully as a business, with the market setting the prices of services (which are treated as commodities), the listing ship of healthcare would be righted. The problem with this perspective is that it prescribes as medicine for the dysfunctional, ailing health system, the cause of the disease: treating medicine and healthcare as a profit-making commodity. Observes Anderson (2012: 2),

> Corporations are driven by the need to maximize profit regardless of health consequences. Let us not forget that the tobacco companies make a product that eventually kills their customers. This should give us pause when we hear that we need more "business thinking" in the organization of health care services.

The quasi-religious tone of the most ardent market-based solutions for healthcare reflect an almost faith-based (because it is certainly not evidence-based) view of unfettered capitalism. The Mises Institutes, an organization that follows the teachings of libertarian economists Ludwig von Mises and Murray Rothbard, for example, argues that the restoration of the healthcare system in the US requires four changes: (1) eliminate all licensing for medical schools, hospitals, pharmacies, medical doctors, and other healthcare personnel; (2) remove all government restrictions on the production and sale of pharmaceutical products and medical devices; (3) deregulate the health insurance industry; and (4) abolish all subsidies to the sick or unhealthy (e.g., Medicare and Medicaid, as well as the Supplemental Nutritional Assistance Program (SNAP) for children) (Mises Institutes 2016). With these changes, patients—as supposedly hardnosed, self-interested consumers making the best decisions for their well-being—would create an effective healthcare system, and corporations would be free to make profits in a competitive market unfettered by government regulation. One need only glimpse the adverse effects of the weak regulation of pharmaceutical and medical technology prices, as discussed in Chapter 2, to grow suspect of market-based solutions to market-caused social ills. The Congressionally approved inability of the federal government to negotiate pharmaceutical prices has contributed to the skyrocketing of pharmaceutical costs for consumers.

A harrowing consequence of full deregulation of the pharmaceutical industry is revealed by the findings of Saluja and co-workers (2016a) who studied 17 drugs that were approved by the U.S. Food and Drug Administration (FDA) between the years 1993 and 2010 but were later withdrawn from the market as unsafe. Based on various data sets, they estimate that during this 18-year period these subsequently withdrawn drugs were prescribed during 112 million physician visits, with nine of the drugs being prescribed more than a million times. In other words, even with FDA regulation millions of people unwittingly take unsafe medications, some of which only are discovered to be harmful years after they are put on the market. The prescribing physicians do not know they are unsafe, so how could patients possibly know? The sleights of hand built into anti-regulatory proposals like the one issued by the Mises Institutes include turning a blind eye to the frequently exposed corporate misinformation and misrepresentation of products, corporate manipulation of clinical trials, corporate manipulation of prices (Taibbi 2013), and further health-threatening environmental destruction (e.g., air pollution and toxic spills), and are further complicated by the already existing inequalities that ensure that consumers are anything but a homogenous group with equal access to knowledge and other resources on which to base their decisions. Corporate deregulation does not lead to better products or lower prices; it leads rather to greater inequality and increased suffering (Piketty 2014). In recent years, for example, a period of financial deregulation and underenforcement of existing regulatory rules against Wall Street led to a painful recession that resulted in 8 million people losing their jobs. The anti-regulatory drive, ironically, is now rationalized with the assertion that regulation on corporations that protect the public's health and well-being are "job-killers" (Weissman 2011).

The ever-stronger corporate turn in healthcare in the US, and its causes, were not unanticipated. When Paul Starr (1982) wrote his widely read examination of the medical profession in the 1980s, *The Social Transformation of American Medicine*, he titled his final chapter "The Coming of the Corporation." There he described the movement within the healthcare industry toward "higher levels of integrated control" within an increasingly privatized set of institutions (Starr 1982: 429). The key features of corporatization Starr indicated were: (1) the movement, already described, toward for-profit hospitals; (2) a shift from locally controlled hospitals with community connections toward complex companies with multiple individual hospitals distributed across diverse locations, often at great distance, geographically and socially, from the company headquarters; (3) vertical integration of functions like financing and purchasing, and policies, across institutions, and (4) ongoing growth that produces ever larger multi-unit conglomerates with ever-steeper top-down management systems.

When the U.S. healthcare system is compared with the systems of other wealthy nations, one item that stands out is how much more the U.S. system costs than countries like Australia, Canada, Denmark, France, Germany, Japan, the Netherlands, New Zealand, Norway, Sweden, Switzerland, and the United Kingdom, without producing any superior results in terms of overall population health (Squires 2012). A number of factors have been identified to help explain excess spending in the U.S. healthcare system: (1) more use of high-tech interventions, which, as shown in Chapter 2, is driven by the intense lobbying and influence-buying efforts of the high-tech medical industry; (2) greater emphasis on specialty care over primary care, despite the fact that primary care helps prevent illness and death and contributes to a more equitable distribution of health in populations (Starfield, Shi, and Macinko 2005); (3) higher drug prices produced by the effective efforts of the pharmaceutical industry to block pricing regulations, as detailed in Chapter 2; and (4) notably higher physician fees compared to other wealthy nations. Importantly, these differences are not explained by the tuition costs of medical education or higher practice costs in U.S. medicine (Laugesen and Glied 2011). One additional force driving up the cost of healthcare in the US is hospital administration costs. This was first documented in the early 1990s by Woolhandler and Himmelstein (1991) who found that that healthcare administration consumes 19–24 percent of the total healthcare spending in the US and that this administrative burden helps explain why U.S. healthcare costs are so much higher than in Canada or the United Kingdom. In a follow-up to this study, Himmelstein and colleagues (2014) report that administrative costs now consume 30 percent of healthcare expenditures, while the share of the healthcare labor force employed in administrative (as opposed to care delivery to patients) has grown by 50 percent and now comprises more than one of every four workers in the health sector. Within hospitals, the proportion of costs devoted to administration is highest in the US, at a rate that is more than twice the percentage in Canada and Scotland. In the US, for-profit hospitals have higher administration costs than non-profit or government-owned hospitals. High administration costs, moreover, were not found to be associated with better care. The role of insurance companies in the U.S. healthcare system, however, does appear to be a critical factor driving up administrative costs, because of the amount of time and effort hospitals, or even office-based healthcare providers, must spend on reimbursement requirements, as well as the time they spend trying to get the greatest reimbursements possible in light of insurance company pay-for-performance policies. Himmelstein and co-workers (2014) consequently recommended reforming the U.S. healthcare system "so that it operated on a single-payer basis [which would] result in large savings on administration."

One of the ways the heavy weight of administration and corporatization have drilled down into clinical examining rooms is through the implementation of electronic medical records (EMR) systems. Today it is standard for doctor–patient interactions to be mediated by a third party, the ubiquitous computer screen, on to which the doctor and other care providers type in patient history and examination information at every encounter. Observes Bruce, "the data should be amazing [from the standpoint of patient care], but EMRs were not designed for [improving] the clinical encounter, they were designed to capture billable events and compliance." In a study of 57 U.S. physicians in four specialty areas—family medicine, internal medicine, cardiology, and orthopedics—who were observed for 430 hours, and in which 21 of them also completed after-hours diaries, Sinsky and colleagues (2016) found that within the clinic day, for every hour physicians provided direct clinical face time to patients, nearly two additional hours of their time was spent on EMR tasks and desk work. Outside office hours, physicians spent another one to two additional hours of personal time each night doing computer and other clerical work related to their jobs. As this suggests, increasingly doctors' direct interaction time with patients is minimized as doctors are transformed into expensive data entry clerks, and patients are turned into itemized lists of coded services for scrutiny and payment by insurance companies. Rather than patient care per se, doctor–patient interactions are directed at the completion of a billable document, which may account for why there is no demonstrated link between EMR records and patient outcomes. Doctors complain that EMRs are annoying and have made the patient encounter far more complex. Additionally, they are faulted for constraining the independent decisions of highly trained practitioners, and for erecting barriers between doctors and their patients (Chesanow 2014). As Rajeev Alexander, an Oregon physician, has noted, "Real life is all about the narrative . . . It's sitting down and talking about bowel movements with a 79-year-old woman for 45 minutes. It's not that interesting, but that's where it happens" (quoted in Scheiber 2016). With growing pressure to see more billable patients, and the insertion of EMRs between doctors and patients, the ability to collect a detailed patient narrative disappears. A physician satisfaction study sponsored by the RAND Corporation and the American Medical Association (Friedberg et al. 2013) found that while physicians like being able to remotely access patient information through EMRs, the majority of doctors who participated in the study found EMRs to be cumbersome and time-consuming, difficult to manage because of non-intuitive data entry screens, interference with face-to-face patient care, frustrating because information does not flow freely between systems, the cause of an information overload triggered by automatic email alerts sent to physicians from the system, out of synch with important aspects of patient care, and degrading of what should be useful clinical documentation. EMRs contribute to why many physicians feel marginalized and on uneven ground with insurance companies, with the latter having the upper hand when it comes to how they treat their patients. In the words of one physician who participated in a survey conducted by Medical Economics: "Insurance companies have planted themselves between the patient and doctors and on top of the money pile" (Bendix et al. 2014). In short, EMRs meet the needs of medical institutions to get as much billable reimbursement as they can, and those of insurance companies to increase profits by controlling expenses, but they do little for improving patient health, nor do they contribute to patient or physician satisfaction. Then again, that is not what they were designed to do—they are about making money, not improving patients' health. Hence there was little physician input in their development

In an effort to respond to the pressure of the increasing demand for electronic documentation and patient health screening—demands that narrow doctors' ability to thoroughly examine their patients and focus on their narratives—Bruce and colleagues developed and tested a patient self-screening tool:

> The amount of required screening a patient is supposed to have yearly is mind boggling! It's no longer possible to accomplish the number of things you are supposed to cram into a 15-minute visit. But now, a lot of the screening which used to be obtained orally on history, like smoking, drinking, depression, risk of STDs, risk of heart attack—are on validated survey instruments with scoring algorithms where you get so many points for this, and so many points for that. The number of variables makes you crazy, and often makes it difficult to determine what to do next. The scoring systems that calculate a patient's risk, are based on sensitivity specificity, positive and negative predictive value, etc.—which I have taught in the past—but are not commonly well understood among clinicians. We took a lot of those screenings recommended by the U.S. Preventative Services Task Force [2016]—and we reduced it to 17 questions. We put it on a touch screen tablet in the waiting room, and rather than have the doctor trying to do it in the 15-minute visit, the patients do it themselves. The tablet zaps the information to a server behind the front desk, which then analyzed it and printed out a risk report card on that patient—that not only said that they were at risk for STDs, PTSD, pre-homelessness, and depression, but told the team the recommended action. If a patient was at risk of domestic violence, it suggested a referral to our social worker—it would actually tell the doctor and unless they knew better—this is what they should do . . . The ultimate goal was to take a lot of the screening out of the doctor's hands—to free them up to do the other things that only they can do. We tested it at both Burgdorf and one of the community health centers, and we proved the concept. I didn't believe that an 85-year-old, inner-city patient who'd only made it through eighth grade would be able to do a touch screen survey accurately. And I was wrong. They can. We also had earphones, so that if the patient was illiterate, the computer would read them the survey in English or Spanish. Our ultimate plan was to have the patient do the survey from a smartphone, or telephone, from a home or library computer, or from the EMR portal. You could even do it twice a year or yearly, and use it as an indicator of quality improvement. If we look at a cohort of individuals that have taken it for three years, one can argue that if we are doing our job as providers, then the rate of depression should go down, barring a societal disaster, something like a 9/11 event where everyone is depressed. We were also looking at it from the public health standpoint; that if all the clinic waiting rooms in Hartford are doing this survey, then the Department of Public

> Health can utilize the data as indicative of the ambient rates of depression, post-traumatic stress disorder, or other risks untreated in the community and use that as a way to direct public health efforts, or improve access to certain resources. We proved that our patients could do the screening using touch tablets, and generate the patient-specific risk report, but integrating the screening into the clinical process was tougher because we ran up against IT issues. Solving those issues just wasn't a priority for the institution. We did a chart audit comparing the rates of diagnoses we got on screening to what those patients had already been diagnosed with in the clinic over many years. We found that roughly 5 percent of people have post traumatic stress disorder, but zero percent had it diagnosed in the chart. Thirty plus percent were depressed, but only 10 percent had it in their chart, or had been treated for it. A significant opportunity for improvement!

Corporate Practice of Medicine Laws and the Health Insurance Industry

The question has been raised in public discourse about the propriety of corporate entanglement in the practice of medicine and whether, because the health insurance industry is now in a position to both control physicians' compensation and negatively influence patient care, it is in some sense involved in the practice of medicine. This is of importance because of the existence of corporate practice of medicine laws (CPM) at the state level that specifically prohibit corporations from practicing medicine or employing physicians to perform professional services. As Silverman (2015: 2) explains, while state laws vary, and are variously enforced, the doctrine of corporate practice prohibition "is rooted in the perceived evils that corporations and laypeople motivated by profit will exert control over physicians, tainting the fiduciary role of physicians . . . and compromising the medical judgements of physicians." This doctrine dates to an effort during the 1930s by the American Medical Association to establish ethical principles for the practice of medicine.

In the view of some physicians:

> The corporate practice of medicine is overwhelming American health care . . . This is why doctors are marginalized in decision-making, yet the public has not grasped this reality. On the horizon, medical care will only deteriorate as these health care corporations further erode protective CPM laws. (Dorio 2015)

As Bruce comments: "In the past, as a physician, you were less of an employee; you had much more control; you had some choices in your professional life. I'm not sure that's true anymore." Common is the experience of a Texas physician who told a reporter about his social interactions with other physicians (Swartz 1995):

> At hospitals, over coffee, at cocktail parties, the docs gathered in groups and whispered among themselves. They couldn't treat people the way they needed to anymore because of the insurance companies. They were on the phone all the time, haggling with insurance company clerks instead of practicing medicine. They were referring patients to doctors they didn't know or didn't trust because of insurance company rules.

In an op-ed published in the largest newspaper in the city where Bruce practices, a physician described how he and 2,000 other physicians were summarily dismissed as approved medical providers by a major insurance company:

> This was done presumably to protect its profits by eliminating those doctors who did not follow their rules, which are supposed to protect their profits . . . This is only one example of what can happen when insurance companies amass too much power and dominate the health system, controlling physicians and patients. (Volpentesta 2015)

There are various ways the power of doctors to treat their patients has been eroded by the power of insurance companies over what practices, tests, and treatments are permissible. As Kathleen Sebelius stated during her confirmation hearing as Secretary of Health and Human Services:

> as an insurance commissioner [in Kansas], where I served for eight years, [I] saw [rationing] on a regular basis by private insurers, who often made decisions overruling suggestions that doctors would make for their patients that they weren't going to be covered. (Quoted by Armbruster 2009)

Adds family physician and author, Linda Giris (2015), insurance companies now

> hold free rein in what they approve and disallow. They ignore the medical advice doctors give their own patients and override their decisions. Yet, they are protected from liability. As more and more care gets denied, the quality of our entire health care system is degraded . . . When the insurance company overrides my clinical acumen based on their predetermined guidelines, medicine and science is tossed out the window to contain costs.

Not that overall medical costs ultimately are contained, those keep rising; the issue for insurance companies is not cost containment for the patient, but profit enhancement for the companies. Corporatization of this sort, in both dealings with insurance companies and in the practice of medicine within hospitals and hospital conglomerates, and even in private offices, has become the norm, a norm that is exacting a great toll (O'Rourke 2014).

Battling to Serve the Poor

Over the years, and increasingly over time, Bruce has tried to challenge corporatization on behalf of patients and co-workers. After he became the Medical Director at Burgdorf Clinic, he reported

> the [new] CEO of St. Frances came to meet me at the Burgdorf. He said he needed a chairman of ambulatory services at St. Frances Hospital, told me he viewed me as young and ambitious and so I also became Chief of Ambulatory Services at St. Frances and ran their outpatient service [the Gengras Clinic], which was twice as big as the Burgdorf, and ran the Burgdorf at the same time.

As a result, to a degree, Bruce felt pulled in two directions:

> At that time, half my salary came from UConn [University of Connecticut], because historically the Burgdorf was UConn's outpatient service, and this position of Director of the Burgdorf was funded half by Sinai [before it was taken over by St Francis], half by UConn; the two institutions were afraid [that if one of them] paid more, I would be more loyal to them. At that point in time, it seemed I was doing more work for St. Francis [Hospital]. I was concerned whether that was fair to UConn but no one at UConn seemed to care. Clearly what I was doing at the Burgdorf was more than they expected. And to be honest being able to coordinate the two outpatient services with overlapping catchments made sense . . . and both sites were UConn medical student teaching facilities.

Before long, however, in dealing with St. Francis Hospital, Bruce began to encounter problems:

> I'm a quality improvement guy [focused on trying to improve outcomes of health care services]. I ran both facilities, Burgdorf and Gengras, till '94 or so . . . that was for four plus years. It feels like a lot longer. That's when things started to go crazy at St. Francis. The atmosphere became overbearing, and a pretty hostile place to work, in my view, if you're caring for the poor. They began cutting, always cutting, always cutting. I understand "no money, no mission," but I could never depend on [whether] the budget number that they gave [me] at the beginning of the year was going to be the number I'd have to work with. Quality care requires quality staff and staffing is dependent on the budget. You make plans to improve how you do things, workflow, team care and then all of a sudden employees were gone and the changes don't happen. I complained: our volumes were up and was told [by St. Francis], "you can't make it up on volume, if you sell below cost," and my patients [at Burgdorf] just didn't bring in money.

As this comment indicates, exemplary of the problems that haunted Bruce's efforts to sustain and even expand healthcare for the poor, St. Francis Hospital "downsized" its staff at Burgdorf Clinic, as well as at another of its North End sites (on the original Mt. Sinai hospital campus), upon its absorption in 2015 by a larger medical conglomerate, as discussed in the next chapter. The result was a significant drop in patient visits. Notes Kovner (2015), "As the hospital has reduced clinical staff in north Hartford, it has expanded its services in the suburbs by opening several walk-in clinics in the stores of a major supermarket chain." In 2014, St. Francis stopped providing obstetric and gynecological services at Burgdorf, but these were restored in response to intense community complaint. Dental services also were closed at the Burgdorf, and moved to the main hospital two miles away. As Frolich (2015) points out, "Partly as a result of the residents' poor financial situation, more than two in five Hartford residents did not own a vehicle in 2013." Without a car, two miles can be significant, given the facts that lack of car ownership and reliance on a hampered public transportation system are common problems faced by the poor in Hartford.

Another example of the effect of hospital corporatization noted by Bruce was a dramatic change in the way his patients were admitted and cared for. In his early years at Burgdorf, he and his colleagues had their own service at Mt. Sinai. He, the other physicians at Burgdorf, as well as the doctors at a nearby federally qualified community health center (FQHC) would take night and weekend calls, admit patients to the hospital and then follow them until they were discharged. During the week and when he was on call on weekends, he would go "make rounds" of his patients in the morning before clinic hours at Burgdorf and again in the evening after clinic. Moreover, he noted, "whenever something went wrong, I would get a call from the nursing staff." By contrast, today, in an effort to improve efficiency and outcomes, in most hospitals, patients are no longer cared for by their primary care doctor that cared for them before being admitted. They are treated by "hospitalists," doctors that specialize in inpatient medicine who pick up their patient as they enter the hospital, care for them while they are in the hospital, and end their involvement in the patient's care when they leave the hospital. Bruce notes:

> Hospitalists and the hospital are under such enormous pressure to crank patients through, to get them in and out in as short a time as possible that often there is no communication with the primary care physician or team. So a patient that I've been caring for twenty years gets admitted to the hospital, no one gives me a call and says, "Bruce, Mrs. Jones came in. What's going on [with her case]?" When they did call, I could say, "Well, yeah, I've been caring for Mrs. Jones for a long time, these are her health problems, and these are the mitigating circumstances that should influence her care in the hospital. I could ask that 'before you send her home, if you don't want her to bounce back, be aware that XYZ' . . . and fill them in on pertinent history . . . important history." But few ever call because they're busy and it's much quicker and easier to take care of somebody if you don't know all

> those details [about their past history]. It's not better [medicine], but you can get 'em in and get 'em out more quickly! And so, I do still try to go over to the hospital, if my patient is in the hospital just to show my face. It's better care for them. It's therapeutic for my patients to know I'm watching. It gives them a sense of security. When you care for someone over years and decades you're more than their doctor. You become an honorary trusted family member. It seems that for those caring for my patients in the hospital, it may just be a distraction, more noise. And there are times when I will step in because they are getting ready to discharge the patient, and I will tell them, "You know the patient came in with X, Y, and Z. The clinical questions on admission were such and such. That's why they were admitted to the hospital and you're going to send them out and we still don't have the answer? So they're in the hospital, figure it out." Or they came in with heart failure with 60 pounds of fluid, and they still have 60 pounds of fluid on board. I can do it with oral agents [diurese them with medication that make them urinate] as an outpatient but often it is much more difficult and may not be successful once they're at home. And especially with poor patients, we're not yet willing to pay for the systems to effectively monitor patients as they pee their brains out at home, to make sure they don't lose dangerous amounts of potassium or magnesium, that you don't overdo it and cause their blood pressure to drop. Whereas, in the hospital, every day you are monitoring blood pressure, heart status, and labs, at least then, you know what you are doing and then, can judge when it's safe to release the patient. And yet, patients often get sent home without answering the primary questions sufficiently related the admitting issues. And that is bad medicine.

In another case, involving an 88-year-old man who was still working as a bricklayer, Bruce recommended a colonoscopy which led to a diagnosis of colon cancer, surgery, and a colostomy. A year later, the patient developed anemia, and Bruce had him have another scoping that found polyps, which were removed. The patient went home afterward, but a few days later Bruce found him and his daughter waiting for him in the parking lot of the Burgdorf. The man was complaining of abdominal pain. Bruce examined him in the parking lot and suspected a bowel perforation. He sent the man to the emergency room. When Bruce called the hospital later, he learned that his patient was being sent for a computerized tomography (CT) scan. Bruce felt the patient was in good hands but decided to drop into the hospital that evening to see how he was doing. He was startled to find his patient sitting in the corner of the emergency room receiving saline through an intravenous drip. Said Bruce, "They forgot about him. He kept getting bumped for the CT scan. The shifts had changed. And I had a tantrum. I don't usually have tantrums, but I was really upset" (quoted in Meldrum 2010: 95). As a result, within the hour his patient was operated on for the perforation, an operation that was a success. But the man was never able to go back to work and wound up in a nursing home. Bruce subsequently wondered: "Should I have been more suspicious?

I thought I had handed off [the patient to the hospital]. In fact I had. But someone needed to turn the light on. And it didn't happen. He died a year later" (quoted in Meldrum 2010: 96). This experience affirmed Bruce's belief that every patient needs an advocate if they are to successfully navigate our broken healthcare system. This perspective was further highlighted in his own life as he believes both his mother and Lisa's mother would have died earlier than they did if he had not been their advocate, as they struggled with receiving good healthcare.

Bruce's continued advocacy for resources at the Burgdorf in the face of ongoing cuts did not endear him to hospital administration. Relations with his superiors became increasingly contentious and unproductive. His ineffectiveness led him to consider leaving the institution. He sought counsel from Eugene Sigman, emeritus Dean of the Medical School who had hired him five years before. Dean Sigman was surprised that no one had called Bruce to tell him he had been appointed as the first Associate Dean for Primary Care at the University of Connecticut School of Medicine, a position created to address a predicted shortage of primary care practitioners in the state. Bruce would remain as Director of the Burgdorf Health Center half time, but would assume the associate deanship with the other half of his time. Although his salary would remain a 50:50 split between UConn and St. Francis, his check would come from UConn rather than St. Francis. He was now a state employee. Following his transition, the President and CEO of St. Francis called him into his office for a meeting. He told Bruce that he was

> decommissioning the Department of Ambulatory Services. You will no longer be chairman of the department at St. Francis, since there will be no department! "Why should I trust you with one of my departments, if I don't control your salary?" He was no longer my paymaster, and to a degree he was right. From a business standpoint, unless an institution is controlling your remuneration it has a lot less control over you. So that's how I ended up moving back to the Burgdorf. By 1995, I was no longer the Chair at St. Francis. They went back to having their own leadership there. I went back to the Burgdorf and now was also the Associate Dean for Primary Care [at UConn] and then Director of AHEC.

The University of Connecticut: The Struggle Continues

The nature of the fight Bruce was engaged in for years to expand or at least maintain health services for low-income individuals and families in Hartford also was described by fellow Burgdorf physician Patricia Joyce:

> I think for a lot of the time that we were there [the Burgdorf], we felt like we were fighting adversity because primary care is—especially [in a] Medicaid and uninsured patient clinic—a money loser, a leading money loser for a hospital, and so we were always fighting the good fight to make our case with the institutions [St Francis and UConn] . . . The most recent effort that

> the university and St. Francis made to further the demise of the clinic was to try to concoct a plan to give us to CHS [Community Health Services, a non-profit federally qualified health center servicing low-income patients that is located about two miles from the Burgdorf]. There was a slow pulling away of service after service after service and sort of a dying by neglect, really. I dug out close to thirty years of records of clinic visits and [patient] volume, and Bruce was able to match that on a graph to demonstrate that first the staffing would get cut, then the volumes would fall, then the staffing would be cut again, then the volumes would fall. The hospital and the other institution [UConn] would try to say, "Well, your volumes are down; you don't need as much staff." Bruce did this big spreadsheet that he presented at the university so that he could back up our claim that, no, we actually do need these services and if they had not made these cuts then our volumes would actually be still preserved and it would be very clear that we need the services. Not that it worked, but that was what we tried.

Adds Bruce:

> In 2007, the contract that governed the resources that each institution was required to provide at Burgdorf was allowed to lapse and cuts were accelerated. In about 2011, St. Francis, UConn, and CHS met, and the decision was made to close the Burgdorf and to sell the UConn physicians at the Burgdorf to CHS as contract physicians. No one talked to me about it because they knew I wouldn't have been happy. To be fair, from a strategic business standpoint, it was the right thing to do. "We'll keep Bruce out of this until the end, because he may try to screw it up." They were right. The problem was that the loans taken to build the [new Burgdorf] building were HUD loans, Housing and Urban Development, federal loans, and the city was involved. I heard there were promises made in writing by St. Francis that there would be health care delivery to the North End of Hartford from that building for the duration of the loan, and beyond, which was at least twenty years. We were on year 15 or 16. So they had to go to the Mayor's office to ask permission so they would support a change in the status of the building . . . they were planning to knock the building down. The federal government had given them money to build the building and St. Francis' premise was that they had only built the building for twenty years and it had reached the end of its life cycle. Not to say that the building was in great shape . . . it wasn't . . . the roof leaked, the carpets were worn, the wall paper falling off, due to deferred maintenance. They suggested it was somehow a disposable building. So, they went to the Chief of Staff of the city, Juan Figueroa, but they hadn't done their homework. Juan was the Founding Director of the Universal Health Care Foundation, a health care advocate and a civil rights lawyer, [and, over time, both Assistant Attorney General and a member of the Connecticut General Assembly from Hartford's Third District].

After the meeting ended, Bruce explained

> Juan calls me and says, "there were fifteen people from St. Francis, CHS and UConn in here today talking about closing the Burgdorf to improve access to care. I asked them two questions and the first one was 'How does that work?' They didn't have a clue. They had not thought that far ahead. They assumed that the city would just say 'sure.' And the second question I asked was 'Does Dr. Gould know about this, he's the Medical Director for the Department of Health and Human Services?' He said, 'I thought they were going to lose [it]. Their jaws just hung open, and it was the end of the meeting. They had not done their homework and I told them that they could do whatever they want–with their building, their faculty–but that the city would not give them cover." They left and he thought that might be the end of it, but he asked me, "Bruce, should we let them close the Burgdorf?" And my gut reaction was to say, "Hey, that's where I've lived," and "that's my baby." But I thought about it and decided, "It's not right for me to make that decision based on my own my staff's needs and emotions."

As a result of this realization, Bruce initiated an assessment at the city health department to determine if the Burgdorf was an irreplaceable part of the health safety net in the city. A geo-mapping of healthcare providers showed that the Burgdorf was the only provider north of Albany Avenue, a main thoroughfare on the North End in Hartford in a highly residential neighborhood. Notably, the North End of Hartford is one of the poorest neighborhoods in the entire state of Connecticut:

> Does it make public health sense to tell people that they should just walk a couple miles, knowing that a couple of miles crosses neighborhoods and people don't cross neighborhoods on foot. Without the Burgdorf, many people, including people who were acutely ill or with debilitating health problems, would have to ride a bus for an hour to access health care. If a mother without a car wanted to take her child to a clinic, she would have to take all of her kids on the bus if she could not afford childcare . . . and buses cost money.

Based on the data that he and co-workers compiled, Bruce felt confident that he could say, "this is not a good idea," the safety net would be in shreds "lying on the pavement."

One product of this effort to save the Burgdorf was an initiative Bruce started to strengthen the city's safety net by improving communication and data sharing among healthcare providers, including data on hours of operation, cross-credentialing of safety net providers between sites to allow access to patient records across providers, and an info-line to help people find the health and social services addressing wellness, social determinants of health, and self-management of chronic disease, and connect them to these services. This response to adversity is typical of how Bruce has continually sought new and innovative ways to improve services for the poor in an unsupportive, increasingly corporate environment.

Bruce admitted that because of his battles to retain healthcare at the Burgdorf:

> I'm sure that there are lots of folks out there that started to look at me as a barrier to "change," and clearly St. Francis thinks of me that way cause they wanted to close the Burgdorf and it didn't happen due to community support though I think they give me much of the credit. If they closed the Burgdorf, its patients would be cast to the wind. Some would find another doctor. Would it be as effective? Who knows? What the Burgdorf has is a reputation for not just caring for its patients, but caring about its patients. We've taken care of generations. I have grandmothers who had their babies with our Ob-Gyn doctors. Forty-five years—that's incredible. And, you know, I've been there 27 years, others have been there 25 years, but lately it has been trimmed and trimmed and trimmed. A lot of the nursing staff have been there forever because they are dedicated to the mission. The problem is that it's becoming harder and harder to do what we do. And more and more frustrating. At some point people get tired. I'm getting tired. But I stuck it out and I was going over to St. Francis and I was trying to play the game and fight the fight, but it became more and more difficult. And again, my makeup is such that lying is not my thing. You know, if you tell me to do "X" and I don't think it's right on a very visceral level, I'm not going to do it. So, it's been a tough 27 years, because I have often disagreed with corporate decisions and when you're in an organization, you are expected to accept decisions from those above you. You may have the freedom to argue, and if it's a good organization they encourage both line staff and middle managers and upper management to express their views honestly without repercussions so that they can get all sides. At the Burgdorf and the system that it's part of, most individuals did not feel that they could honestly say "I'm not sure that this is the right thing to do," because they'd get their heads handed to them.

Subsequently, Bruce had another opportunity to work with Juan Figueroa on health issues. This time the effort involved developing a single-payer universal healthcare system for Connecticut. While Juan was at the Universal Health Care Foundation of Connecticut, he directed an initiative to implement a coverage system that would provide healthcare and financial protection to all Connecticut residents. The state legislature passed the bill but it was vetoed by then Governor Jodi Rell. Figueroa then organized a coalition that successfully lobbied the legislature to override Rell's veto. A nine-member board was established and charged with coming up with a specific plan for a statewide public health insurance plan that would be called SustiNet. Before this was finalized, however, Figueroa took a leave of absence to launch a campaign to be governor of Connecticut (Keating 2010). The rationale for the SustiNet program was recognition that medical costs were rising to unsustainable levels, many people in Connecticut could not afford health insurance, including, especially the poor and ethnic minorities, and even people who did have health insurance often were unhappy with the quality of the healthcare coverage they received for their premium. When Figueroa lost his bid for the governorship, the single-payer plan was not implemented in Connecticut, due to opposition from the newly elected Governor Dan Malloy. The state then passed a watered-down version of SustiNet that eliminated the single-payer approach but, like the federal Affordable Care Act, ensured that low-income residents would receive financial help in getting healthcare coverage, ended discrimination in access to health insurance for people with preexisting health conditions, and sought to implement a slowdown on increases in healthcare costs in the state. Noted Bruce:

> I was on the Sustinet committee but it failed. I spent two years helping design a health system and then when Governor Malloy took over—I voted for him, but when he took over he nuked it. Because we were taking all the power of the dollars—a lot of money—for all this employee insurance—and putting it under a quasi-governmental board that would make the decisions for this quasi-single payer system, rather than have the insurance companies have control of health coverage. It's unfortunate because we would have been the first state with a public option for health care and that would be very cool. But it didn't happen and some of it was overreach and I found myself in the surprising position of working closely with the representative of CBIA—which is the Connecticut Business and Industry Association. He was very conservative. He really did not support a public option for health insurance. But we found ourselves teaming to assure that the plan would be comprehensive but not overreach and have a chance of implementation.

Medical Director for the Hartford Department of Health

In addition to his other responsibilities, Bruce agreed to become the Medical Director for the Hartford Department of Health:

> I'm at the Burgdorf. The first floor of the Burgdorf is the Hartford Department of Health and Human Services. I've always been involved with them. I served on the Task Force for the Uninsured, etc., etc. I have to walk through the department to get to my car. They had a medical director but he could no longer do it. The medical director signs for vaccines, whatever—it's never been a robust position. And so they called me and just said, "Bruce, will you be the Medical Director for the Health Department?" "What does it entail?" "Oh, signing for vaccines and whatever else you want to make of it." So "sure, OK!" It started off with Ramon Rojano, who was the Director of Health, and then the games began—because my predecessor had been a St. Francis doc—St. Francis didn't want a UConn doc to be the Medical Director of the

> Health Department. So there was an enormous amount of political jockeying. And it wasn't until Carlos Rivera took over, a year or two later, as the Director of Health that things moved forward. He had been the Administrator of my clinic for years. So, we knew each other. He had worked with me and he made it happen [for me to be appointed]. A pro bono position—I don't get paid—the health department medical director establishes protocols for vaccines, and signs for vaccines, sits on the advisory board for the Department of Health and Human Services for the city [of Hartford], all very routine, but as medical director for the health department, I could venture beyond the Burgdorf, see how the health system functions within the city and how to better coordinate it. I initiated the Safety Net Without Walls effort.

Safety Net Without Walls is a project designed to identify creative solutions and resources to improve healthcare delivery to underserved communities in the greater Hartford area. In 2015, the group working on developing the project with Bruce received a $25,000 grant from the Connecticut Health Foundation to begin bringing together key individuals with experience in improving healthcare delivery to begin mapping out the service components of the planned safety net.

Confronting Challenges: AHEC and the Farm Worker Clinics

As he began his new position as Associate Dean for Primary Care, Bruce encountered tensions with other doctors:

> I got a lot of push back from my primary care colleagues at the University that probably came from me becoming Associate Dean for Primary Care. I was an outsider from the Burgdorf, not from the Farmington campus. They didn't want to work with me, even though they had been my friends for five years. It was a little [sad]. I took a step back, realized that the primary care landscape at medical school was evolving, and I didn't need to control it or to control my colleagues. One door closes, another opens. That's when I was approached about AHEC [Area Health Education Center]. And later, after a request for a summer project from two students, I became aware of the migrant farmer worker population in Connecticut. My career has been this pattern of following need and following serendipitous opportunity and not turning down challenges.

Connecticut has had a long history with the AHEC program, as Bruce explained:

> Back in the '70s, the first urban AHEC in the country was in Hartford. It was funded for 6-plus years. Out of that came the Med School primary care rotation and some of the community health centers. It did a lot of good, but at the end of that time it folded because it had never gone beyond Hartford. It had never [been] extended to a state-wide program.

Nationally, the AHEC program is credited with increasing the supply and geographic distribution of healthcare providers, as well as enhancing the quality of care provided (The AHEC Bulletin 1983). And then, in 1995, Connecticut Governor Lowell Weicker charged Steve Bongard, PhD, with starting another AHEC in the state. Bongard had been Weiker's former healthcare legislative advisor when he was U.S. Senator, and returned to Connecticut when Weicker became governor, to be chair of the state Commission on Hospitals and Health Care. But, he had had a heart attack and so was transitioned to the medical school, away from the stress and politics of state government. Adds Bruce:

> The legislature had appropriated about a quarter million dollars, a chunk of change especially in 1995 dollars. So I arrived in Farmington, and I'm a little forlorn . . . my feelings were hurt and was trying to plot a course for primary care at UConn. Steve Bongard comes up to me and says, "I'm not a clinician, you are. I'm trying to start this AHEC thing." I really didn't know what AHEC was at that point. He said, "I need a clinician to do road trips with me." My father had died, a few years before and I was still licking my wounds, and here's this older guy who was a tough cookie but a sweetheart underneath. He was a warrior and became a mentor. And he would say, "Bruce, you've got to get up in the morning, you've got to gird your loins and ask 'who am I going to battle today?'" And to Steve, it was war and he loved the fight. That's not the way I wanted to live, but it was helpful for me to learn at the feet of a master, because I had fought many battles and would fight so many more and Steve prepared me well. Steve cut to the chase: "Our charge is to rebuild this AHEC system." I didn't realize that AHEC would be the focus of the next 20-plus years of my life!

The national AHEC program was developed by Congress in 1971 and charged with recruiting, training, and retaining a healthcare workforce committed to the well-being of underserved populations. The AHEC program was designed to help bring the resources of academic medicine to meet local community health needs. Today, there are 54 AHEC programs with one in almost every state and the District of Columbia. Approximately 120 medical schools and 600 nursing and allied health schools work collaboratively with local AHEC initiatives. After folding during the 1970s, the Connecticut Area Health Education Center was re-established in 1995 with funding from the Connecticut General Assembly. Today, there are four AHEC centers in Connecticut affiliated with the CT AHEC Program Office at the University of Connecticut School of Medicine. Each center is an independent non-profit organization. The mission of the Connecticut AHECs is to improve access to basic healthcare by linking local community groups with the resources of the UConn Health Center and other health professions training programs across the state. For example, when two rising second-year medical students approached Bruce to "do something for the summer," he used the CT AHEC program as a vehicle to bring UConn medical students and faculty together with the Community Health Center Association and several other community-based organizations to establish the migrant farm worker healthcare program in Connecticut. The Connecticut AHECs also try to improve access to healthcare by recruiting minority students into the health professions, teaming up with community organizations to address locally identified healthcare issues, provide continuing education designed to improve the care received by vulnerable populations, and develop and support community training opportunities for students in the health professions.

Through the farm-worker initiative at AHEC, Bruce was able to launch the Migrant Farm Worker Clinics and remains the faculty advisor to the program. Although Connecticut is not usually thought of as an agricultural state, the Connecticut River, the longest river in New England, produced a fertile river valley of sandy loam soil that is well suited to agricultural production. The state's largest crop is tobacco, especially shade-grown tobacco, a high-quality but labor-intensive commercial crop. The harvested leaves of this plant are used for two outside aromatic layers of cigars, the binder and the wrapper, into which is poured filler tobacco that is grown primarily in Latin American countries. Shade tobacco fields are distinctive because they are covered with white gauze or cheesecloth hung on wires to mimic a tropical environment and protect the plants from humidity and exposure to direct sunlight. This growing strategy was adopted in the early twentieth century to compete with a fine-grained leaf that was being imported from Sumatra. At the height of the industry, 20,000 acres of land in Connecticut were planted in shade tobacco, although today the area covered by the white tents and red drying sheds of the industry is about 2,000 acres. In 2010, Connecticut produced about 4 million pounds of tobacco (Gammell 2014), largely for export to the Dominican Republic. Connecticut ranks first in New England for tobacco acreage and production, and tobacco has had a significant economic and cultural impact on the state.

Because the leaves of shade tobacco are delicate, and must remain undamaged to be of value in the cigar industry, Connecticut's tobacco fields are largely unmechanized and farmers depend on a large influx of seasonal farm workers to plant, tie wires and string to the ceilings of the tents, tend and trim plants, harvest the crop, cure the final product by hanging it in the sheds to dry, and packing the cured leaves in crates for shipment. This kind of work requires that farm laborers must crawl on their hands and knees through row after row of closely grown tobacco stalks that can grow to a height of 10 feet. This labor is performed at the height of the Connecticut summer under hot, breezeless conditions for long hours. The fast-growing plant can be harvested as early as six weeks after planting (Boynton 2007). In addition to tobacco, Connecticut farms produce various other crops, including grains and beans, potatoes, vegetables, berries, orchard fruits, and ornamental plants, many of which also pull migrant laborers to the state. Connecticut's agricultural labor force constitutes a multi-ethnic blend of approximately 7,000–20,000 Mexicans, Puerto Ricans, Jamaicans, as well as a smaller number of Central Americans (UConn Migrant Farm Worker Clinics

2016). Most are recruited to the state through the efforts of the farms' owners. As discussed further in Chapter 5, farm workers in Connecticut, like those living elsewhere in the country, endure significant hardships rooted in discriminatory policies and practices. Farm workers are explicitly exempted from national labor laws designed to protect workers' health and safety and despite the vital work that they do, are among the lowest-paid group of workers in the country.

The clinics initiated by Bruce provide medical services to about 300–600 patients each summer season. The program provides free medical and dental screenings, medications for mild and self-limiting health problems, and treatment for both acute and chronic conditions on farm sites to migrant farm workers who otherwise might not have access to care. Preventive education is also provided. Services are provided by medical students and physicians three nights per week from June to October each year. According to Bruce, the clinics are not only good for the patients but for the providers as well:

> We've got 30–40 community and university physicians with us and a lot of them have regained their souls. Some of them are specialists, nephrologists, and they have forgotten why they went to med school, they bemoan the fact that the health care system has devolved to its present state, and they come out one night to the fields, and they remember why they went to med school. (Quoted in Meldrum 2010: 98)

The most common health problems seen at the clinics are musculoskeletal disorders, pesticide-related problems, traumatic injuries, respiratory conditions, skin problems, infectious diseases, and eye problems. The clinics work closely with the Connecticut Migrant Health Network and their outreach workers. Other partner outreach workers are provided by the state Department of Labor and the federally qualified community health centers. These outreach workers provide transportation to farm workers who need follow-up health services at participating community health centers. Explains Bruce, "it's a way to provide health care to underserved populations. It also provides our students lessons in social consciousness and advocacy" (quoted in Migrant Farm Worker Clinics Video 2016). The program exemplifies the way Bruce seeks to bring the considerable resources of the university to meet the needs of underserved low-income populations.

Quality Improvement Initiatives

As noted, Bruce has long considered himself to be "a quality improvement guy." His enduring commitment to QI is reflected in his participation, through his role as the Associate Dean for Primary Care, in the implementation of a comprehensive multi-component quality improvement curriculum for medical students at the UConn School of Medicine. Successfully launching and improving this training program has proven to be a serious challenge, as students have not always been enamored with aspects of the program, Bruce has stuck with it however, doggedly trying to improve the program and prepare students for a medical world in which outcome assessment and cost-cutting initiatives are the norm.

Building on earlier efforts to teach QI in medical schools (e.g., Barbaccia 1976, Weeks et al. 2000), the UConn QI curriculum, which was added to the medical school's Human Development and Health course, included a specially designed training module for continuous quality improvement and patient chart abstraction (Gould et al. 2002, Gould et al. 2004, Shea et al. 2004). The latter component of the training involved familiarizing students with the process of collecting important information by reviewing patient medical records and entering it into discrete fields on a computer spreadsheet. Formal training in chart abstraction was followed during the second year of medical school by hands-on practice with a sample of patient charts (that had patient identifying information removed), including the use of an answer key that provided students with immediate feedback. This component was part of Student Continuity Clinic (SCP), an established UConn Medical School training, during which students see patients at a community-based primary care physician's office one-half day per week for the first three years of medical school.

As part of the QI initiative, a random sample of patients with Type 2 diabetes at 24 participating clinical sites around Connecticut was developed using billing data. Students abstracted 20–30 patient charts from each site and turned in their completed abstractions to the Area Health Education Center Program, coordinated by Bruce, for data entry by his staff. A feedback report was subsequently returned to students and their clinical site preceptors identifying how each provider site fared on each quality indicator relative to the aggregate performance of all the clinical sites. Each site used this information to identify opportunities for improvement and developed local interventions to enhance outcomes of care. Alternately, sites could choose appropriate interventions from a toolkit that was provided, which included items like diabetes guideline-based care tracking forms, patient reminders for foot care, and patient home glucose-monitoring materials. Students and their site preceptors implemented the selected interventions at the end of the students' second year of medical school. To assess improvements six months after implementing the interventions, students abstracted another random sample of patients from the same clinical practices. Following analysis of their findings, students and their preceptors received a report containing pre- and post-intervention data with aggregate data for comparison. During the second year of medical school, students also received lectures and participated in seminar sessions on clinical outcomes and quality measurement, clinical protocol development, additional information on chart abstraction, and the enactment of clinical-process change using continuous QI interventions. All students also participated in a 2½-hour seminar that reviewed the history and theory underlying continuous QI methods and compared the similarities and differences between continuous QI and clinical outcomes research.

To evaluate the effectiveness of the training program, participating students completed both a pre- and a post-training questionnaire comprised of forty questions organized into six continuous QI domains: the nature of this approach, its specific focus, its underlying principles, its key concepts, its use of a team approach, and the student's perceived personal confidence in performing continuous QI activities. Each item was rated on a five-point Likert scale. The nonparametric paired Wilcoxon signed-rank test was used to compare the pre- and post-test knowledge, attitudes, and beliefs scores for all students. Attitudinal assessment with formative feedback was obtained after the abstraction experience. The effects of the project on both process and outcome indicators at the practice level were assessed using baseline and remeasurement performance data. Students selected their responses from a Likert scale (e.g., strongly agree to strongly disagree) and also answered some open-ended questions. Pre-/post- test comparison showed that student knowledge of the nature, concepts, and principles of continuous QI improved significantly. In two areas, however, analyzing data and using data to identify the root causes of problems and develop solutions did not improve. Disappointing to Bruce, students were either neutral regarding the overall value of the chart audit learning experience (43.4 percent) or did not find it to be a valuable learning experience (41.6 percent). About half of the students (45.3 percent) either agreed or strongly agreed that the chart audit was of benefit to the clinical practice they worked in during the project. About a third of the students (34.6 percent) felt that the experience was beneficial to patients, while almost as many (30.8 percent) reported they saw no benefit to patients. It was evident as well that students were frustrated with the tedium of the chart abstraction process and they provided useful feedback for improving the project (e.g., schedule the chart audit during less intense portions of the medical school curriculum, make chart-audit less time-consuming and onerous). Pre-/post-intervention comparisons at participating sites found that the rate of documentation of performances of foot and eye exams increased significantly from baseline to remeasurement. Moreover, the mean value for patient blood sugar levels dropped significantly at remeasurement. Based on the findings, the project evaluation team concluded that medical students can successfully initiate continuous QI activities

> at practices in which they participate with positive effects on the quality of care delivered. The use of medical students to initiate these efforts may represent an underutilized resource in efforts to improve the quality of care afforded the public . . . Getting learners to embrace the process of quality measurement and improvement, however, will be challenging as long as data collection remains tedious. Creative approaches to data collection and measurement (use of available managed care organization claims data) and active involvement of students in the planning process will be necessary to improve student experiences. (Gould et al. 2002: 1017)

In subsequent years, medical students were given a choice of studying diabetes, hypertension, or pediatric asthma (Gould 2004). Despite this change, the UConn Medical School classes of 2002 and 2003 were even less enthusiastic about the project than the initial cohort. Based on this feedback, and in an attempt to decrease the workload associated with the initiative, in the classes of 2004 and 2005, students and their clinical preceptors were given insurance company health plan employer data on their practice sites, that included quality indicators for diabetes care, well child care, mammography and pap smear rates, early periodic screening, diagnosis, and treatment compliance, and use of inhaled steroids in asthma. Despite these adjustments, the new configuration of the program also ran into problems and student evaluations again were not favorable. Many complained that by using health plan data, the project put them in the adversarial position of attempting to be a "change agent" in clinical practices that were not necessarily ready for change. These experiences led to the decision to move the continuous QI experience to the third year of medical school and to integrate it into the six-week internal medicine ambulatory care medical student rotation. Additionally, the clinical practice sites now are limited to facilities that generally embrace and have implemented a continuous QI program and can integrate and mentor students in program activities onsite.

Bruce also has participated in other research over the years designed to improve physician performance. In one study, designed to upgrade residents' readiness to engage their patients in smoking cessation activities, residents were provided with a three-hour training on a patient-centered counseling approach. The program emphasized questioning and exploring feelings, rather than providing information. Pre-/post-test questionnaires and videotaping of changes in resident knowledge about smoking, attitudes concerning smoking intervention, and intervention skills found a significant increase in knowledge and perceived ability to positively influence their patients who smoke (Ockene et al. 1988). In a subsequent study at the University of Connecticut, Bruce worked with colleagues to evaluate a training package for alcohol screening and brief intervention (SBI) in primary care settings. In the study, three groups of medical personnel—44 physicians, 88 medical students, and 41 other medical staff—were compared before and after SBI training. The researchers found that physicians and medical students acquired increased confidence in performing screening procedures, and increased self-confidence in conducting brief interventions. Non-physicians perceived fewer obstacles to screening patients after training. Individuals who participated in the program reported conducting significantly more SBIs than providers who were not involved in the program. Both of these studies reflect Bruce's long-term involvement in improving the quality and impact of clinical encounters.

Sustaining Commitment

Bruce sees his approach as one of encountering community need and trying to address it:

> That's how a lot of these programs got started over the years. People, groups, came to me with unmet [human] needs. I don't know if it's a passion for change, or I just can't help myself. I think it's that I can't say no . . . when

> people make me aware of an issue, an unmet need, it becomes a puzzle [to be solved]. You start to problem solve, to see the issues as part of a larger system . . . and then think "oh wow, if we just pulled it together and wrapped it up in a different way" [we can address that problem]. It is being able to see how disparate resources and efforts and groups can come together to solve things together.

Sometimes the commitment can start to feel overwhelming. On occasion, Bruce gets concerned that he takes on too much

> and assumes it will happen [i.e., his efforts will succeed], and most of the time it does. I'm very, very busy right now and I'm starting to worry . . . get a bit anxious about getting things done. Despite the humor and being able to rise above it, to take a deep breath, I am also very responsible . . . which I guess isn't really a negative, but the combination of being sensitive to unmet need, not wanting to miss the opportunity to do good, and an innate sense of responsibility to fulfill promises made, creates the perfect storm to generate anxiety.

The significant work level that he has taken on challenges Bruce's longing to stay orderly. He notes:

> I'm not as organized as I'd like to be. I'd love to be perfectly organized with everything filed and prioritized, but I just don't have time. It's one of the things that I decided early on that I would not have time for. If I spent more time organizing and maintaining that clear desk that some of my colleagues have . . . it would mean that I'd have to say "no" to other projects, issues, things that need to get done. And so, I'm a little less organized than I should be but somehow things do get done. I have a system, part of it's a Moleskine notebook in my pocket where I jot things down. Then I look at it every week or two, check things off, cross off some that just are never going to happen and then focus on the ones I forgot. But most of it has gotten done just by Brownian motion. I do wish I had more help. They laid off my secretary 10–15 years ago and they gave me a half-time person back six years ago, then laid her off four years ago, and so I don't have dedicated help. I have to ask people for assistance and make administration feel guilty that they balanced the budget on my back, which in essence they did. A bit of hyperbole . . . a secretary doesn't get paid that much. But I'm probably the only associate dean not to have at least a half-time secretary. Luckily, my ego's not that big, so I laugh it off. But sometimes in the wee hours of the morning, I get a bit paranoid and wonder, "Is this a message?" And certainly, at academic institutions, taking your help away, your office, closing your clinic, things like that send a message that they'd just as soon have you move on. But thankfully, one of my better attributes is that I'm hard of hearing when it comes to those messages.

> And I absorb abuse well and let it roll off my back . . . but it takes its toll. The hospital wants full productivity . . . 15 minute visits, despite the complexity of our patients and the enormous educational responsibilities that we have for residency training and medical student training and they will squeeze every drop of juice out of you, if they can. On the other hand, if I were given free rein, the Burgdorf would become an interprofessional education center within an FQHC (Federally Qualified Health Center) environment. That would be incredible but the system would need to want to see that happen and be willing to support it, instead of trying to balance their budgets by cutting services where they're most needed.

Federally qualified health centers, as Burgdorf will become, are outpatient clinics that receive federal grants through Section 330 of the Public Health Service Act. These provider organizations, which are found coast to coast, qualify for enhanced reimbursement from Medicare and Medicaid, as well as other benefits. They must provide healthcare to an underserved area or population, offer services to all persons regardless of the person's ability to pay, offer their patients a sliding fee scale, provide a comprehensive array of services, maintain a quality assurance program, and have a governing board of directors at least 51 percent of whom must be patients.

Given Bruce's history of challenging and confronting some of the major local healthcare institutions over their desire to retreat from providing care to the underserved, he wonders if all of the battles he has fought have taken a toll on his health:

> From a personal health standpoint, the stress, the environment, the adversity, can't be good for me. I should have left a long time ago but it's my nature to see things through. The trend in health care is toward corporatization, whether for profit, or not for profit, and that transition is not driven by community needs or educational needs but by competition and bottom line . . . I get it! My job is making sure that those needs are identified and presented, and that institutions lose their "plausible deniability," as they make their economic decisions. At times the interactions with the institutions get so nasty, so ugly, so contentious, that I get angry . . . and can't believe that we're all on the same team. But I take a deep breath, reconnoiter, dig my heels in, and remind them that our decisions affect our patients, their neighborhoods, our students . . . shame on them. But in the corporate model, there is no shame, only bottom line and corporate survival. For that, as forgiving as I am . . . I can't forgive them. They should know better. I often have to say "no" to the things they want me to do, which doesn't make the job easy, but it's important that they hear it.

In recent years, St Francis has worked consistently towards separating itself from the Burgdorf Clinic, and hence from much of the non-emergency healthcare services it provides to the low-income community of the North End of Hartford.

The process has been both protracted and secretive, and has involved a steady, often painful, reduction in the clinic's budget. Explains Bruce:

> Cut, cut, cut, cut, cut. The hospital is making decisions, not talking to any of the staff that are actually delivering the care. Not sharing those plans with their own employees at the facility resulted in increasing anxiety. In the three years they were negotiating to close and, when that failed, to give away the Burgdorf, they never had an administrator come over and speak with the staff. It would have been both human kindness and respect. It also would have been good human resource management. So I was put in the position of being told not to say anything, but the staff had heard rumors and staff would come up to me and ask "what's going on Bruce," and, I don't lie. I would tell them, within reasonable parameters, what was going on . . . without giving away any company secrets. Often I would just tell them that final decisions had not yet been made . . . as simple as that. And knowing what was going on, what was real and what was rumor . . . actually calmed everyone down. I was honest. You need to be very careful going through life to maintain your own self-respect and moral compass.

Facing these wearing conditions, Bruce has waged a long strategic struggle to hold on to healthcare services for the low-income patients of Burgdorf Clinic. He notes:

> I realize that my judgment, in fact, may not be correct. Or I may not agree with cultural or business norms; I have to do what I think is right. But once I feel that something needs to get done, I am strategic in figuring out how to get there and sometimes that means working with people and sometimes that means working around certain people. And sometimes that means, yes, asking someone and getting "no," but then knowing how to influence that individual and convince them to say "yes," or to back up, change the plan and go around them, or how to wait them out, knowing that they won't be in that position forever. I have never . . . destroyed anyone. I've had colleagues try to do that to me. I've seen colleagues do it to other people. I like people, I respect people but there are times when I've raised my voice, I'm only human . . . but I can count those times on one hand and, frankly, I know it doesn't work. I've found staff and colleagues respond to leadership by example and kindness rather than fear. Unfortunately, not everyone agrees with me.

The challenges Bruce has had to confront in recent years also have, at times, been confounded by the university:

> For the first 20 plus years at Burgdorf, the University always had my back, was always supportive of what we did at Burgdorf. But deans and leadership change, state budgets get cut, and the University was not immune to the

> push toward the corporatization of health care. I get it . . . no money, no mission. I have no delusions about absolute loyalty or absolute commitment to service [to the North End]. It's a balance between mission and bottom line. It's not just here in Connecticut, it's not just the university, it's not just St. Francis, it's the corporate mentality, which is part of the reason why Americans are the most productive work force in the world . . . less vacation, more work hours at home, working on the weekends, always being at the end of a phone. Even when we are on vacation, we're still available. The last two weeks I was away, I kept up with my email because I really can't afford not to. I'd never catch up. So, I'm a good employee. They get far more hours out of me, certainly, more than a 35- or 40-hour work week. But I also have no illusions that the moment that I ask for anything they may well say "no." I'm really an optimist by nature, but as one ages, as one gets a little older, you can call it pessimism or realism but you don't get a sense of being valued. You realize that the day you die, they put your stuff in a box and put it out on the curb, and the hole you left behind, quickly closes up behind you, and life moves on. If you're lucky, you become a vague memory. So the payoff has to be the work itself, the people you help and not the legacy you leave behind.

While those in the local healthcare hierarchy may not always appreciate Bruce or his strong-willed commitment to the underserved, he is well respected in the community, by patients, and by those who work closely with him. Noted one medical colleague:

> His cause is serving the underserved . . . with the most excellent care in the most respectful manner, preserving dignity, and then trying to really engage everyone else to do the same. He wants to build a system that does that, and I agree with him on that, as opposed to just depending everything on charity care. You want to actually build a system that takes care of the least . . . A couple of different times now he has given a gift to the staff at the Burgdorf. He gives a Christmas present to everybody every year—a Jewish doctor—and the most recent one it's a mug says "Burgdorf" on it and Martin Luther King's quote that says, "Of all the forms of injustice, inequality in health care is the most shocking of them all." Because he's done it twice, I think that's his philosophy.

5

STRUGGLING FOR HEALTH EQUITY FROM THE INNER CITY TO RURAL FARMS

> Medicine is a social science and politics is nothing else but medicine on a large scale. Medicine as a social science, as the science of human beings, has the obligation to point out problems and to attempt their theoretical solution; the politician, the practical anthropologist, must find the means for their actual solution.
>
> *Rudolf Virchow*

Poverty and Health: Place Matters

In 2016, the U.S. Census Bureau's annual report (Proctor, Semenga, and Kollar 2016) revealed that the percentage of people living below the federal poverty line fell to its lowest level in seven years. The median income of U.S. households jumped by 5.2 percent from $53,718 in 2014 to $56,516 in 2015. Additionally, the poverty rate for children dropped slightly to 19.7 percent from 21.1 percent the previous year. This news was greeted with great excitement by the Obama administration, as it suggested the success of its efforts to recover from the punishing recession of 2007–09. While the change was certainly important for those households that were able to raise their socioeconomic standing, the poverty rate in 2015 was still higher than before the recession. Despite the improvement, 43.1 million people, including 14.5 million children, were still impoverished in the US. A much more significant drop in poverty occurred in 1974 when the rate fell to 11.2 percent from 19 percent ten years earlier. What fuelled this dramatic decline in poverty? Studies indicate that it was the federal War on Poverty that was responsible, including the creation of Medicare and Medicaid, the availability of food stamps and housing subsidies, and the strengthening of Social Security (Wimer et al. 2013). By contrast, contemporary efforts to address poverty stress getting people into jobs, which would be an excellent solution if most of the jobs currently available to less-skilled workers actually paid enough to lift a household out of poverty. This is not the case, however. As Hoynes, Page, and Stevens (2006: 48) pointed out, "Increasing income inequality—in particular stemming from declining wages for less-skilled workers—may have limited the poverty-fighting effects of economic growth." In short, the strategies for significantly reducing poverty—jobs that pay adequate wages and provide sufficient health and other benefits, on the one hand, and social welfare programs including healthcare coverage, for those who cannot work, on the other, are well known. Lacking has been the political commitment to actually end poverty in a country that produces more than enough wealth to achieve this goal.

Importantly, in the US, poverty finds differential expression in rural and urban areas. Many of the features of inner-city urban poverty have been described in previous chapters. Notably, in the social construction of the contemporary inner city in many parts of the US there have been impactful changes that began to have a noticeable effect in the 1980s and 1990s. During this era, many inner-city areas, already struggling economically, experienced a dramatic intensification of concentrated poverty due to globalization, the flight of capital and production, and the loss of jobs in urban centers (Singer 2009). As Bourgois (2003: 319) notes:

> The economic base of the traditional working class has eroded throughout the country. Greater proportions of the population are being socially marginalized. The restructuring of the world economy by multinational corporations, finance capital, and digital electronic technology, as well as the exhaustion of social demographic models for public sector intervention on behalf of the poor [e.g., the welfare state] have escalated inequalities around class ethnicity and gender.

Increasingly, as a result of these changes, poor individuals and families are isolated in neighborhoods populated by other poor people. This pattern of concentrated poverty has come to typify the core areas of many urban areas across the country. These inner-city zones often are disconnected from the job market, as larger companies avoid locating in these areas. Moreover, educational systems have deteriorated as lack of government support led to high student-to-teacher ratios, decline in the quality of school buildings, poor educational preparation, plummeting test scores, and elevated dropout rates. As stressed by Kati Haycock, as director of the Education Trust, "we teach different kids different things. Poor, minority kids are often separated early on from other kids, either in separate schools or on separate tacks and are systematically taught less. They get less rigorous curricula from elementary through high school" (quoted in Freel 1998: 18). Research, for example, shows that mathematics classes in high schools in severely distressed areas are twice as likely to be taught by a teacher with a credential in a topic other than mathematics as are classes taught at high schools in non-distressed areas. Similarly, the teachers in high school science classes in inner-city areas are three times as likely to be credentialed in a field other than science compared to those who teach science in wealthier areas (Wirt et al. 2004). Moreover, teachers in schools in impoverished areas are more likely to report having to use outdated textbooks, outmoded computers, obsolete educational tools and technologies, and inadequate or non-existent science equipment and laboratory spaces. College-preparatory or advanced placement classes in inner-city schools are significantly weaker than in schools serving more advantaged students (Freel 1998).

Economic pressures, school failure, and lack of employment, in turn, have contributed to high rates of males in inner-city areas who are unattached to the job market as well as high frequencies of one-parent families that are often headed by females. Between 1990 and 2000, the number of people who lived in severely distressed neighborhoods increased by 19 percent (Jargowsky 2003). The concentration of poverty in these neighborhoods, moreover, is highly racialized, with African American and Latino children being much more likely to live in distressed neighborhoods. By 2000, 55 percent of children living in distressed neighborhoods were African American, 29 percent were Latino, and only 1.4 percent were White (O'Hare and Mather 2003).

Consequently, the U.S. inner city, a sociocultural and experiential space that Wacquant (2002) has termed the "hyperghetto," today has come to function as a kind of ethno-class prison "in that it encloses a stigmatized population with its own distinctive organizations and culture." This development reflects a broader societal pattern involving the devaluation of physical labor, continuing shrinkage of working-class salaries, and a dramatic loss of working-class jobs. This pattern is revealed by the fact that in the years between 1973 and 2003 the productivity of U.S. labor increased by 72 percent while the average worker's income grew by only 35 percent. Workers simply were not able to maintain their share of income in the country as wealth flowed upwards to the richest sectors of society (Mishel, Bernstein, and Allegretto 2005). The end result was a slide of middle-class, often unionized workers, into less secure, non-unionized, and lesser-paying jobs, the transformation of a strata of the working class into the working poor, and, especially for ethnic minority workers, a fall into the status of the nonworking very poor. While in 1979, the average poverty rate in the U.S. inner city was 16 percent, by 2007 it had risen to 17.5 percent (Currie 2007). During the 1980s, author Gore Vidal (cited in Adams 2008) observed of Ronald Reagan's economic policies that "The U.S. government prefers that public money go not to the people but to big business. The result is a unique society in which we have free enterprise for the poor and socialism for the rich." This pattern continued in ebbs and flows until the present and is now on the ascendency again in the Trump administration. While economic gains are privatized in the hands of the wealthy, and the wealth gap between the rich and everyone else widens, the social costs of wealth generation (e.g., air pollution, release of greenhouse gases) are socialized (and to the degree they are addressed at all, it is with public tax dollars).

Two processes have contributed to the dramatic loss of working-class jobs in the US. The first is the movement of manufacturing jobs to other countries, enabling corporations to reap higher profits from the use of cheaper labor, as well as the economic benefits of weaker job safety and environmental protection laws and enforcement. Data from the U.S. Department of Commerce show that

"U.S. multinational corporations, the big brand-name companies that employ a fifth of all American workers . . . cut their work forces in the US by 2.9 million during the 2000s while increasing employment overseas by 2.4 million" (Wessel 2012). Because of overseas outsourcing by U.S. corporations:

> Manufacturing employment collapsed from a high of 19.5 million workers in June 1979 to 11.5 workers in December 2009, a drop of 8 million workers over 30 years. Between August 2000 and February 2004, manufacturing jobs were lost for a stunning 43 consecutive months—the longest such stretch since the Great Depression. (Working America 2010: 13)

The government has not attempted to stem the agonizing flow of jobs overseas nor the hollowing-out of American manufacturing industries because of the powerful lobbying voice of industries that benefit from the global hunt for profits.

The second process that is eliminating jobs in the US is mechanization. The replacement of workers by machines, which already has jettisoned millions of jobs, is likely to eliminate an ever-growing number of blue-collar and even white-collar jobs in coming years. The beginnings of this trend were well described in 1982 in a set of eight articles published in a focused issue of *Scientific American.* In one of the articles, "The Distribution of Work and Income," which was republished in the volume *Input-Output Economics*, Nobel Prize-winning economist, Wassily Leontief (1986), argued that a growing number of jobs are being lost to the growing mechanization of work. At the time, the jobs that were being taken over by machines, again as a strategy by corporations to increase their profits, were dispersed across an array of industries, including manufacturing, coordination of manufacturing, agriculture, mining, and information-based office work. Stressed Leontief (1986: 364):

> With the advent of solid-state electronics, machines that have been displacing human muscle from the production of goods are being succeeded by machines that take over the functions of the human nervous system not only in production but in the service industries as well.

While mechanization has reaped billions for some, it has destabilized the lives and futures of millions of people. Thus, those in a position to push for increased automation of jobs, the companies that grow their profits by decreasing their labor forces, are highly motivated to continue to expand the technological process. But those whose jobs are now being done by machines are paying for mechanization with their livelihoods. As Frase (2017), an editor at *Jacobin* magazine, stresses, the key issue: "Who benefits from automation, and who loses, is ultimately a consequence not of the robots themselves, but of who owns them." In addition to jobs that already have been lost, it is estimated that 45 percent of work activities, across various industries that traditionally have provided salaries to millions of workers, can be automated with existing technologies. In the US, these job-producing tasks represent about $2 trillion in at-risk annual wages (Chui et al. 2015). Political solutions to the dilemma, such as direct government subsidies to lower-income workers to augment their wages and increased public spending on schools and other social and recreational facilities, public transportation and other basic infrastructure, and the reversal of environmental degradation, are opposed by the rich because it is their sizeable incomes that would have to be taxed to pay for these job-creating initiatives.

Wacquant asserts that, as a consequence of these kinds of sweeping structural changes and damaging loss of jobs, including employment not directly in manufacturing but dependent on it, the contemporary inner city lost many of its earlier communal features and acquired a social structure and cultural climate that parallels those of a prison. Unlike the more communal ghetto of the mid-twentieth century, a place where the church, cultural and social organizations, and kin-based social networks provided a degree of stability and an interconnected sense of community involvement even in the midst of poverty, the population of the contemporary hyperghetto is dominated by the most precarious social sectors including the unemployed, drug use and street violence have escalated, and people's feelings of security have diminished. Economically, while in the past the ghetto provided a reservoir of cheap labor that could be mobilized as needed by the wider society, including to bring down wages of other workers and to break strikes, the hyperghetto, like the prison, warehouses a surplus population with limited market value in most sectors of the changing economy. Further, as described in Chapter 2, there has been a loss of public institutions and services involving a process of urban social desertification combined with intensification of policing and other social control measures. Research affirms that the social conditions in neighborhoods, including

> the quality of public schools; the age, density, and size of housing; availability of medical care and healthy food; availability of good jobs; levels of exposure to environmental degradation and violence; and availability of exercise options . . . powerfully predict who is healthy, who is sick, and who lives longer. (Joint Center for Political and Economic Studies 2012: 1)

Being overweight or obese, for example, is known to be linked to perceived neighborhood safety (Lumeng et al. 2006). Without question, the hyperghetto is an unhealthy place with multiple expressions of health disparity. In short,

> it is reasonable . . . to describe the U.S. as constituting . . . two separate if intertwined societies: people of the inner city and everyone else. While poverty is by no means confined to the inner city, and neither are all oppressed ethnic minorities or people of color, the intersection of urban poverty and socially devalued ethnicity . . . have proven to be a particularly unhealthy combination (Singer 1994: 931)

While rural poverty has many of the same negative health outcomes as urban poverty, it also has some unique features. The rural poor tend to have even less access to healthcare than people living in impoverished urban areas, even in those areas where major hospitals have closed. Public transportation often is lacking in rural settings, making it difficult for the poor to reach the widely dispersed healthcare facilities that do exist. Traditionally, rural areas have been tied to agricultural production and in the US there is a large population, totaling about 3 million, of both settled and migrating farm workers that toil for the multi-billion dollar food industry, harvesting the food everyone eats, but for miserable wages and often under risky conditions. Farm workers have limited protection under U.S. labor laws and face health threats from exposure to pesticides, heat-related diseases, and living in substandard housing. A study of demographic, socioeconomic, and health variables for almost 800,000 patients of 164 Migrant Health Centers carried out in 2012 found that 80 percent of migratory and seasonal agricultural workers had family incomes below 100 percent of the federal poverty level line. The most common diagnoses for patients at these clinics designed to serve the healthcare needs of farm workers were hypertension, Type 2 diabetes, and mental health problems. Seventy-one percent of these workers were found to be uninsured (Boggess and Bogue 2016).

The health toll from pesticide exposure alone is significant for agricultural laborers. The U.S. Environmental Protection Agency estimates that between 10,000 and 20,000 physician-diagnosed pesticide poisonings occur every year among U.S. farm workers, with acute effects ranging from rashes and nausea to serious respiratory conditions and death. Cumulative long-term exposure to pesticides increases the risks of cancer, birth defects, and neurological impairment (Greene 2012). Working outdoors in direct sunlight and humidity, farm workers also are at higher risk for heat-related illnesses than workers in most other occupations. Illnesses that arise because of high core body temperature, including heat edema, heat cramps, heat syncope, heat exhaustion, and heatstroke, occur when the body is exposed to and/or produces more heat than it can dissipate into the air. Moreover, exposure to certain pesticides, especially organophosphate insecticides, can produce sweating which contributes to the onset of overheating (Rao 2007).

Anthropologist Sara Horton (2016), who has studied farm worker health in California, argues that heat stress, intensive physical exertion, dehydration, and kidney disease (which, based on a series of health studies among farm workers in Central America, are linked to pesticide exposure and recurrent heat stress and dehydration) constitute a syndemic of adversely interacting and progressively debilitating diseases. In syndemics, co-occurring diseases or other health conditions in interaction facilitate the development and promote the advancement of health deterioration, resulting in an increase in the overall health burden of a population. Syndemics, she stresses, do not occur in a social vacuum, but are directly conditioned by structural factors that put people at risk for disease clustering and make people vulnerable to disease onset and progression (Singer 2009).

The structural factors of concern with regard to farm workers are multiple. In addition to occupational pesticide exposure, studies have shown that while housing among farm workers is somewhat variable, overall it is of poor quality. Living in poor-quality housing is known to have a negative impact on health (Jacobs et al.

2009). Adverse physical characteristics of subpar housing, including mold, insect or rodent infestation, structural damage, and unsanitary facilities, have been found to be associated with respiratory disease, skin disease, infectious diseases, and injuries (Krieger and Higgins 2002). A survey of farm worker housing sites conducted by the Housing Assistance Council (2001) found that over half of farm worker housing was crowded; 22 percent of housing units had a broken toilet, bathtub, stove, or refrigerator; 22 percent suffered from serious structural damage; 36 percent had broken windows or torn screens; 29 percent had evidence of water leakage, and 19 percent showed signs of rodent or insect infestation. Similarly, a survey of 43 randomly selected farm worker camps (Vallejos et al. 2011) found that all of the dwellings in camps had at least one exterior housing problem and 93 percent had at least one interior problem, and, further, that housing conditions tend to grow worse across the agricultural season.

While the national statistics for farm workers indicate this population suffers from many health risks and comparatively poorer health than the country as a whole, there are important regional differences among farm workers in the US as reported in the Regional Migrant Health Profile (National Center for Farmworker Health 2014). Those living in the western parts of the country were found to be somewhat older and less migratory than those employed in the eastern US. Unlike those in the West, farm workers in the East were much more likely to travel without their families. Moreover, eastern farm workers had a higher proportion of individuals with incomes below 100 percent of the federal poverty line. Significant health problems among eastern farm workers were hypertension, diabetes, and tuberculosis.

The National Agricultural Workers Survey (Carroll, Georges, and Saltz 2011), based on a nationally representative random sample of farm workers sponsored by the U.S. Department of Labor, found that 78 percent of farm workers in the US were foreign-born, had an average level of completed education of the eighth grade, and often (30 percent) had a total family income that was below the official national poverty line. The average individual income of farm workers in 2005 was between $10,000 and $12,499, with total family income averaging between $15,000 and $17,499. By comparison, the median household income overall in the US at the time was $46,343 (Webster and Bishaw 2006).

Additionally, farm workers rarely have access to worker's compensation, occupational rehabilitation, or disability compensation benefits, as they are often specifically excluded from occupational protection laws, a legal exception successfully lobbied for by big agricultural companies. Similarly, while many farm workers qualify for federal Medicaid and the Food Stamp Program, very few are able to actually receive these benefits because of various state-level eligibility requirements. Also, Social Security has proven difficult for farm workers to access (U.S. Department of Labor 2005).

While farm workers and their allies have fought valiant battles for improved wages, working conditions, and union representation, they remain a super-exploited sector of the working poor. Their urgent health needs drew Bruce into

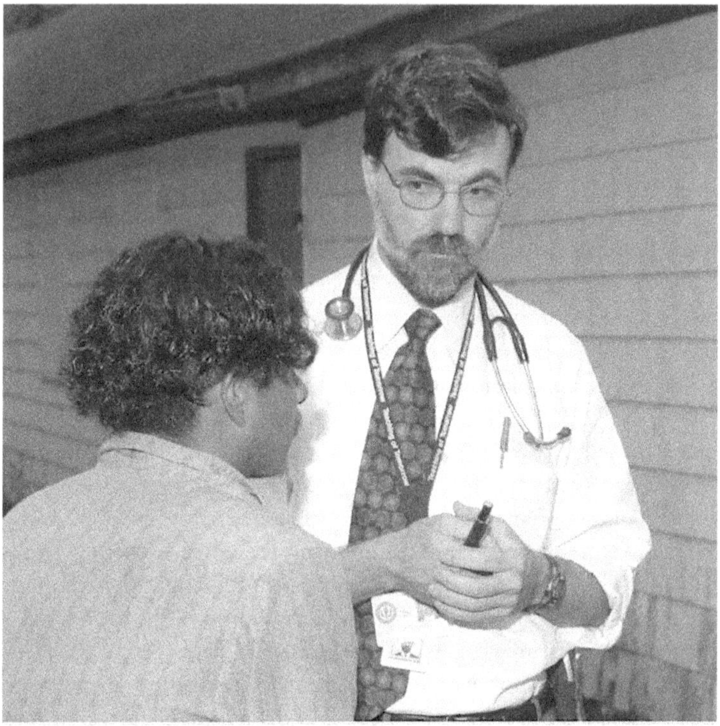

FIGURE 5.1 Bruce with farm worker patient

the effort to bring healthcare directly to rural areas of Connecticut and to the places farm workers in the state live and work, just as his efforts in an inner-city clinic address the barriers to addressing the pressing health needs of the urban poor.

These efforts are needed because there is a yawning gap between often-repeated celebratory statements about the nature of our society and the actual lived experience of many people at the lower rungs of the socioeconomic ladder in the US today. While people may no longer read his books, the official view of American society, repeated often by politicians but reiterated and reinforced by primary social institutions including schools and churches, is the story told by nineteenth-century novelist Horatio Alger. The creator of fiction for young adult readers, Alger wrote at least a hundred books, like the widely sold *Ragged Dick*, about young impoverished boys who rise up from very humble backgrounds to middle-class success through their own hard work, angelic honesty, and unwavering determination. His theme came to be labeled "the Horatio Alger myth." Notes Weiss (1988: 3):

> Tradition has it that every American child receives, as part of his birthright, the freedom to mold his own life . . . this idea that ours is an open society, where birth, family, and class do not significantly circumscribe individual possibilities, has a strong hold on the popular imagination.

The Culture of Wealth and the Poverty Trap

The Horatio Alger myth is a core element in what might be called the "culture of wealth" in the US. It is predicated on the notion that if we support the healthcare and social needs of the most vulnerable people in society, we weaken the economy, and economy is king. Stemming from this is the idea with regard to anything that can be made into a commodity and sold for a profit—which is almost everything—private is good and public is bad. Moreover, in the culture of wealth, anything that enhances and concentrates wealth is good, anything that equitably distributes wealth or promises to do so is labeled as a threat to society, as ungodly socialism, or demonized under some other accusation. Also privatized is failure, at least for those at the bottom of society. The poor are responsible for their own poverty because of an endless stream of defects of character, morals, family structure, values, and sometimes genetics. Indeed, societal problems are not caused by social inequalities and structural violence, but by those who want to live off of but not contribute to society.

Further, as macroeconomist and co-director of the Center for Economic and Policy Research, Dean Baker (2017) observes:

> There is a widespread belief that spans the political spectrum, that rich people are somehow especially insightful. The idea is that the process of accumulating money is some sort of vetting process. The more money you make, the more you have established yourself as an intelligent person whose insights should be sought on important matters of public policy.

Baker points out a glaring example of this attitude in the frequent interviews with Bill Gates seeking his views on multiple public and social issues having nothing to do with his business experience. The underlying assumption seems to be that being one of the richest men in the world makes Gates one of the most knowledgeable. Similar patterns are found with other wealthy businessmen like Jeff Bezos, Warren Buffett, and Mark Zuckerman. When the wealthy fail, however, their knowledge or individual characters is rarely impugned. Case in point, despite a long list of "[l]ost contracts, bankruptcies, defaults, deceptions and indifference to investors," failures documented by "regulatory, corporate and court records, as well as sworn testimony and government investigative reports" (Eichenwald 2016), Donald Trump remained sufficiently unmarred to be elected the 45th president of the United States. Trump is very much an advocate of the culture of wealth, touting his claimed success as a product of his own skills, acumen, and work effort, while downplaying the considerable financial support (amounting to millions of dollars to bail Trump out of various business setbacks) provided by his father. Trump has long styled himself as an authority on many issues, a claim brought to unimaginable heights during many of his campaign speeches, and a factor in people's decision to vote for him because his wealth proves he can solve the challenges faced by the country.

In his book *Corporation Nation: How Corporations are Taking Over Our Lives and What We Can Do About It*, Charles Derber (1998: 28) likens the current era—and it can be argued especially the period unfolding during the Trump administration—to the time of the robber barons of the Gilded Age of the early nineteenth century. During both eras, wealth came to be equated with virtue, while greed was disguised as evidence of responsibility. He observes:

> Today, as in the Gilded Age, we live in a world where morality of personal responsibility rubs shoulders with a culture of greed and a flagrant social irresponsibility. Now as then, business has shed its collective responsibility for employees—just as government has for citizens. Yet, this threat to the common good is organized in the name of nurturing responsibility itself. The politics of personal responsibility offers a public moralism that does not disturb the culture of greed or existing relations of power. Making money is again a sign of personal responsibility while failure to do so suggests a moral lapse.

From the perspective of the culture of wealth, programs to assist the poor in the US have become a poverty trap that makes people dependent and blocks them from upward social mobility. In the words of Congressman Paul Ryan of Wisconsin: "we don't want to turn the safety net into a hammock that lulls able-bodied people to lives of dependency and complacency, that drains them of their will and their incentive to make the most of their lives" (quoted in Delaney 2012). This assumed group of permanently dependent people were the ones Republican presidential candidate Mitt Romney had in mind in his infamous (but secretly videotaped) speech to wealthy contributors at a private fundraiser in Boca Raton, Florida in 2012. Romney, who was running against the eventual winner of the election, Barack Obama, stated:

> There are 47 percent of the people who will vote for the president [Obama] no matter what. All right, there are 47 percent who are with him, who are dependent upon government, who believe that they are victims, who believe the government has a responsibility to care for them, who believe that they are entitled to health care, to food, to housing, to you-name-it. That that's an entitlement. And the government should give it to them. And they will vote for this president no matter what . . . These are people who pay no income tax. (Quoted in Corn 2012)

Of course, as U.S. tax laws are now written—under the political influence of very wealthy people—among those who do not pay taxes, or pay at a strikingly low rate, including Romney (14.1 percent on an income of $12.7 million in 2011), and Trump (zero income taxes for many years), are the super-rich (Sahadi 2012). These individuals instead pay top-drawer tax accountants to make use of every available loophole Congress has written into the law to benefit this well-heeled social stratum. As reported by the IRS in 2015, as one goes from being quite wealthy (the top 1 percent in the country) to extremely wealthy (the very top 0.001 percent), a person's average federal income tax rate declines (Ingraham 2015). Of note, the adjusted gross income of the richest 0.001 percent is $62,000,000 annually, and they pay taxes at the same rate of people earning $85,000 a year. As widely read author and journalist, Malcolm Gladwell (208:33) comments, "We cling to the idea that success is a simple function of individual merit and that the world in which we all grow up and the rules we choose to write as a society don't matter at all."

The Welfare Fraud Hoax

A significant subtheme in the poverty-trap narrative is the issue of welfare fraud. This idea was given voice by Ronald Reagan while running for and serving as the 40th U.S. president. Reagan sought to undercut support for the existence of a financial safety net for the poor by creating the stereotype of the welfare queen, often portrayed as an African American women who duped the government by receiving multiple welfare checks while driving around town in an expensive Cadillac. Reagan built up in the popular imagination a picture of poor people who feel entitled to the benefit of other people's hard work. This image of the lazy welfare cheater was actively mobilized as a trope for undeserving people of color in efforts to gut welfare programs. Exemplary of his demonizing comments about the poor, on the campaign trail Reagan talked about an alleged welfare queen in Chicago:

> She has eighty names, thirty addresses, twelve Social Security cards and is collecting veteran's benefits on four non-existing deceased husbands. And she is collecting Social Security on her cards. She's got Medicaid, getting food stamps, and she is collecting welfare under each of her names. Her tax-free cash income is over $150,000. (Quoted in Loder 2013)

This grand tale was concocted from a relatively minor case of welfare fraud involving about $8,000. In their book, *The Mommy Myth*, Susan Douglas and Meredith Michaels (2005: 185) pointed out the nature of Reagan's verbal strategy:

> He specialized in the exaggerated, outrageous tale that was almost always unsubstantiated, usually false, yet so sensational that it merited repeated recounting . . . And because his "examples" of welfare queens drew on existing stereotypes of welfare cheats and resonated with news stories about welfare fraud, they did indeed gain real traction.

In fact, very few individuals engaged in significant welfare fraud have been accused, arrested, or tried, as Douglas and Michaels report, yet polls from the period show that many people in the US, influenced by the sensationalized language and frequent stories about welfare scams reported in the media, vastly overestimated the actual incidence of welfare fraud, which actually pales in comparison with the size and regularity of white-collar fraud committed by wealthy individuals. Some polls at the time found that respondents believed that 40 percent of those on welfare were cheaters, although the Department of Health and Human Services estimated less than 4 percent of individuals receiving welfare lied about their financial situation on their applications.

None the less, support programs for the poor, including food stamps which have been demonstrated to make a significant contribution to the nutritional health status of children living in poverty, remain under constant attack. Donald Trump, for example, a few years before running for the presidency asserted:

> The really infuriating thing is that the Obama administration doesn't seem to care about how taxpayers are being shaken down by this outrageously mismanaged government program. The blatant waste of taxpayers' dollars doesn't bother Obama because it's all part of his broader nanny-state agenda. (Trump 2011: 113–114)

Downsizing the Safety Net

As a result of the success of the wealth culture in redefining assistance for the poor as, in effect, the cause of continued poverty, and the poor as an unworthy and undeserving group, the government has enacted "reforms" that have severely restricted the availability of aid for the poor and turned the social safety net into a punitive gauntlet. Under President Bill Clinton, Aid to Families with Dependent Children (AFDC), which was enacted during the Franklin D. Roosevelt administration, primarily to assist poor White women (and only later opened to ethnic minorities), was replaced by the far more restrictive Temporary Assistance for Needy Families (TANF) program. TANF policies include time limits on assistance, linking benefits to work effort, and a block grant structure that gives states greater leeway in how to distribute resources (including to programs that do not help the poor). As a result, welfare caseloads have contracted and the program no longer provides assistance to a majority of the country's poor population. While in 1996, 68 percent of poor households received TANF, this had dropped 23 percent by 2014. The actual size of welfare rolls has dropped dramatically, falling from 4.4 million families in 1996 to 1.6 million in 2014. Moreover, those admitted to the program received significantly fewer benefits over time. The overall appropriation of federal funds for TANF, set at $16.5 billion a year, has remained stagnant for twenty years, which means that because of inflation the actual level of benefits fell by one-third (Cramer 2016). Despite these patterns, the number of families living in poverty has not dropped and the number of especially poor families, those described as being in deep poverty, has increased. Today, most poor families (about 75 percent) do not receive welfare.

Moreover, under TANF, states have considerable discretion in how they spend federal welfare allotments, and some have figured out ways to spend it on those who are not poor, or on budgetary items that do not involve helping the poor (Esch 2016). In 1997, after the introduction of TANF, approximately 80 percent of welfare funding went to providing basic assistance, promoting work, and supporting child care. By 2014, only about 51 percent of TANF dollars went to these core-related activities for relief from poverty. State expenditure for TANF dollars vary but in some states this money is used to counsel women who are desirous of an abortion (to convince them not to have one), to financially support middle-class college students at private colleges, as well as to open the public marriage and family counseling programs (Clark and Esch 2016). TANF, in short, is less and less a program to help the poor and more of a program to allow states to spend federal dollars any way they please. This is the great danger of turning funding to address specific social needs, like fighting poverty or helping people pay for health insurance, into block grants to states. This is why block grants are frequently supported by politicians who embrace the culture of wealth.

Research and analyses have accumulated information suggesting that, in the words of Nobel Prize-winning economist Paul Krugman (2014), "the whole poverty trap line is a falsehood wrapped in a fallacy" (e.g., Ben-Shalom, Moffitt, and Scholz 2011, Parrott 2014, Smedley 2006); the culture of wealth is so embedded in the U.S. social system and so often repeated that it has the feel of naturalness about it, rather than looking like something conveniently invented by (some) people to serve their (narrow) personal interests. Deconstructed as a culture that reflects and serves the interests of the wealthiest and most privileged members of society, the cracks in this ideology become evident. For example, the notion that the economy is king and growth in the economy is good for everyone is undercut by data showing that half or more in the rise in income between 1992 and 2012 went to the wealthiest 400 people in the country, and 93 percent went to the wealthiest 5 percent of the population. The other 95 percent of the population received only 7 percent of the total and even this tiny amount was not equitably distributed (Freeman 2012).

The gap between the rich and the poor has been growing and this is one of the most important economic developments of modern times. The wealthiest 1 percent of people in the country are now worth more than the entire bottom 90 percent of the U.S. population, with upper-income families having a median net worth that is almost 70 times greater than that of the country's lower-income families. Only the richest 10 percent of Americans are now seeing their wealth grow, while the bottom 90 get a smaller piece of the pie each year (Fry and Kochhar 2014). This development was one of the most important forces that rallied voters around Donald Trump's campaign for the presidency in 2016, ironically given that he claims to be a multibillionaire, has been rich his whole life, and has no direct experience of the lives of poor and working people in the country. Still, despite announcing he would implement tax cuts that strongly favor the wealthy and cut back restrictions placed on Wall Street that were implemented to block another punishing recession that cost many working people their jobs, Trump, using bluster, showmanship, and the claim to being an outsider to the Washington establishment, convinced working people that he is on their side, including many people who had voted previously for Barack Obama. Once elected, however, Trump nominated a cabinet composed of many billionaires and comprised the richest group ever nominated to these positions in U.S. history—not a group likely to challenge the increasing growing unequal distribution of wealth in the country.

The Color of Income Inequality

Entwined with but somewhat distinct from the class wealth divide that separates the social strata of the U.S. society is the ethnic wealth divide that separates Whites from people of color. The intensity of the ethnic wealth divide is affirmed by a recent study entitled "The ever-growing gap: Without change, African-American and Latino families won't match White wealth for centuries" (Asante-Muhammed et al. 2016). The study found that over the last thirty years, the average wealth of White families (which, of course, was not actually equally distributed among White families) grew by 84 percent, which was 1.2 times greater than Latino families and three times greater than African American families. A glimpse at the wealth of the richest people in the US further illuminates the extent of the ethnic wealth divide. The Forbes 400 is a list of the richest people in the US. Getting on the list is so difficult that in 2015 145 billionaires did not have a net worth that was big enough to gain entry. Some well-known, massively wealthy people, like Bill Gates (net worth $76 billion), Warren Buffet (net worth $62 billion), and Larry Ellison (net worth $47.5 billion), were worth enough to top the list (Doland and Kroll 2015). During the last 30-year period, the wealth of individuals included on the Forbes 400 grew by an average of 736 percent, or about ten times the rate of growth of wealth among Latinos and 27 times the rate for African Americans. Currently, the top hundred people included on the Forbes list own approximately as much wealth as the entire African American population. If African American family wealth continues to grow at the same pace it has over the last thirty years, it will take African American families another 228 years to accumulate the amount of wealth that White families have today, a time span almost as long (240 years) as the history of the US as a nation thus far.

Wealth Management

Connecticut, where Bruce lives and practices medicine, has the largest income gap in the nation between the top 1 percent of taxpayers and the bottom 99 percent. While the wealthiest 1 percent earn an average of $2.4 million, the other 99 percent receive a mean income of $56,000, a startling ratio of about 43 to 1 (Sommeiller, Price, and Wazeter 2016). Since the recovery from the recession began in 2009, the income of the top 1 percent in Connecticut grew by 35 percent (through 2012), while the bottom 99 percent of state taxpayers saw an average real income decline of 5.4 percent. Among the richest of the richest in Connecticut, the top 0.01 percent, the average income is $83,891,599. While the half century after the Great Depression was a period of slow decline in income inequality, during the twenty-first century there has been a sharp reversal of this pattern. In short, the world is not the same place as in the past when it comes to wealth inequality, and in the immediate future, at least, the gap between the rich and everyone else, and especially the very rich and the very poor, threatens to reach massive, unprecedented proportions.

Furthermore, the total income and wealth of the elite rich is not clearly evident in reported taxable income, the source used in the discussion above. This is because many wealthy people spend some of their money to hire attorneys and financial advisors to dodge income taxes, including using offshore tax havens (registering a company's headquarters in a place with low tax rates), building shell companies (firms that only exist electronically that are used to funnel money away from tax collection), shell trust funds (disguising income as loans), and incorporation (in which a person registers as a company, retains his/her wealth, and receives a salary at a far lower rate than their actual income). It is estimated that $60 billion a year in taxes is lost through these schemes on individual income and another $90 billion on corporate income (Baxandall and Smith 2013).

Peter Lindert and Jeffrey Williams, economics professors respectively at University of California, Davis and Harvard (emeritus), have carefully traced the patterns of income inequality throughout the history of the US. In their provocative book, *Unequal Gains: American Growth and Inequality since 1700* (2016), they report that income inequality may be higher at the present moment than at any time in the history of the country. There has occurred, in the words of noted broadcast journalist Bill Moyers (2016), a "heist of the economy" by the corporations and super-wealthy of the country at the expense of everyone else, from the shrinking middle class to the expanding community of the impoverished. How did this all occur? It is a product of an economic system that promoted the growth of ever-larger, ever-wealthier, ever-more powerful corporations, which, acting in general concert, flexed their bulging muscles and grabbed control for themselves. As Moyers (2016) expressed it:

> Capitalism produces winners and losers big time. The winners use their wealth to gain political power, often through campaign contributions and lobbying. In this way, they increase their influence over the choices made by the politicians indebted to them. While there are certainly differences between Democrats and Republicans on economic and social issues, both parties cater to wealthy individuals and interests seeking to enrich their bottom lines with the help of the policies of the state (e.g., loopholes, subsidies, tax breaks, deregulation). No matter which party is in power, the interests of big business are largely heeded.

The price of gross economic and social inequality, as identified in epidemiological research, is the rising rates of mental health problems, a significant level of infant mortality, high rates of teenage births, mass incarceration, loss of social mobility, and daily uncertainty about an imperiling future (Wilkenson and Pickett 2011).

Despite the significant gains already achieved by the economic elite in shifting wealth to themselves and away from the poor and working classes, the campaign to further cut benefits for the poor continues every day. As Speaker of the House, in 2016 Paul Ryan, for example, proposed further welfare reforms. In the assessment of Massachusetts Senator Elizabeth Warren (quoted in Caldwell 2016), Ryan's proposal

> looks more like an agenda for creating poverty than reducing it . . . In fact, if you look closely, Paul Ryan's new plan is just a shiny repackaging of Paul Ryan's old plan: Keep huge tax breaks and special loopholes open for billionaires and giant corporations, gut the [controls] on Wall Street, then say there's no money for Social Security, for Medicare, for education, or anything else that will help struggling working families.

Slate senior business and economics correspondent, Jordan Weissman (2016), particularly critiqued one aspect of Ryan's plan, repeal of the Obama administration's fiduciary rules (which require financial advisors to provide retirement advice that is in the best interest of their clients), but his comments, in fact, apply well to the entire proposal, namely that "Trying to cloak it in the language of an anti-poverty effort is as sad as it is hilarious."

Social Immobility

These economic factors underlie the low level of upward social mobility now occurring among the poor in the country. Analysis of the economic data by the Hamilton Project of the Brookings Institute (Greenstone et al. 2013) concludes that children born into wealthy families are disproportionately likely to remain wealthy during their lives, while the children of poor families are very likely to remain poor. For example, a child born to parents who have an income in the lowest 20 percent of the population is more than ten times more likely to wind up being poor as an adult than those born into the richest one-fifth of the population (43 percent versus 4 percent). A child born to parents in the richest 20 percent of the population is five times more likely to be rich as an adult than a child born into a family in the lowest sector of the population (40 percent versus 8 percent). These results contradict the ethos of equal opportunity that is a key pillar in the US's dominant ideology.

Working for many years with people who live in the kinds of conditions that spawned Alger's mythic heroes, Bruce recognizes the glaring hole in the prevailing ideology: "the problem is, if you're here [now], and you're poor, and maybe of color I'm not sure you can really make it. Or if you make it, it's only because somebody helped you a little bit along the way." Exemplary of the social challenges faced by his patients; Bruce brought up the case of a young woman:

> She's a nurse aid now, in a care facility; she was in college but she ran out of money. So here you have a reasonably bright kid who has gotten through the gauntlet of inner-city life, and was on her way towards getting the credentials she would need to be successful And she's a nurse aid. There's nothing wrong with that, but the point being that you want people to fulfill their potential, her potential was a lot higher.

Moreover, Bruce finds that getting people to get involved in making a difference in really addressing the social burdens of the poor or marginalized minorities is becoming harder. Part of the problem, as Bruce sees it, is a shrinkage in the number of people taking social responsibility and feeling a sense of social solidarity. Instead, they are taught to have a narrow focus on their own needs with limited understanding of the life experience of others:

> In some ways, it's a lot tougher to get [young doctors] to volunteer for [work in] the homeless shelter clinics. I find that some of my younger colleagues are much [more] protective of their time and I understand that, they have families.

He understands because Bruce has worked hard to stay very active in teaching, clinical practice, community activism, and family life, although finding a balance has been a daily challenge.

Through the Prism of the Diabetes Epidemic

Health disparity in the US finds expression across multiple health problems. The rate of HIV infection among African Americans is eight time that of White Americans. African Americans, Latinos, and Native Americans are two or three times more likely to develop lupus than Whites. People of color also are two to four times more likely than Whites to reach end-stage kidney disease. Non-Latino African American children suffer the greatest burden of asthma (16 percent versus 8 percent among non-Latino White children (Kelly Report 2015). Diabetes, one of the most devastating chronic diseases in the US, however, both as a result of its growing prevalence and its cacophony of serious bodily harms, stands out as a threat to the health of the poor and ethnic minorities.

Diabetes, a chronic disease that combines the presence of a high level of glucose in the blood with a breakdown in the body's ability to produce or properly make use of insulin, has become a significant epidemic among the poor. Insulin—a hormone that evolved to help convert sugars in the diet into useable energy—is produced by specialized cells located on areas of the pancreas known as the islets of Langerhans. When bodily cells do not recognize the presence of insulin in the blood system, it is not absorbed by fat, liver, and skeletal muscle cells, resulting in a rise in blood glucose levels. This, in turn, triggers a reduction in insulin production, contributing further to mounting blood glucose levels. At the same time, cells that need energy to function do not receive adequate supplies (Alonso-Magdalena, Quesda, and Nadal 2011). The progressive development of these interrelated dysfunctions constitutes diabetes, a serious threat to well-being. By 2012, almost 30 million people in the US had developed Type 2, or adult-onset, diabetes. This comprises just under 10 percent of the U.S. population, although it is far from equally distributed across all sectors of the population. The incidence and prevalence of diabetes are two to four times greater among individuals with lower incomes and less education than among more economically and socially advantaged individuals (Saydah and Lochner 2010).

Symptoms of diabetes include damage to the retina of the eye; tingling, pain, and numbness in the hands or feet; fatigue; reduced ability to fight infection; increased healing time for bodily injuries; gastrointestinal problems; and increased urination (American Diabetes Association 2016). Diabetes exacts a significant toll on sufferers. It has become one of the primary causes of blindness, kidney failure, stroke, and gangrene and limb amputations among U.S. adults (Mayo Clinic 2016). For example, the largest study to date of emergency department admissions for diabetic foot-related problems found that the disease takes a substantial clinical and economic toll, especially among the rural and working poor. The study also found that rural patients do much worse than their urban counterparts, with a 40 percent increase in the risk of major amputation (Skrepnek, Mills, and Armstrong 2015). Moreover, it is the seventh leading cause of death in the country (CDC 2014). Diabetes causes more deaths per year than breast cancer and AIDS combined. Also, diabetes commonly interacts with and promotes depression, stroke, several types of cancers (pancreatic, liver, breast, bladder, and colon and rectal), high blood pressure, and heart problems (Giovannucci et al. 2010). Death rates from heart disease are two to four times greater among adults with diabetes than those without it. The risk of stroke is similarly high. (Minkel 2007). In short, as a disease of poverty, diabetes is a loathsome threat.

With many poor diabetic patients, Bruce confronts the downward spiral that diabetes can become:

> for clinicians, diabetes represents a variety of vicious cycles that if unaddressed, leads to catastrophe. Peripheral vascular disease is one example. An uncontrolled diabetic develops poor circulation in their toe, gets gangrene, and the toe dies. If we're not aggressive in addressing their diabetes, hypertension, and assuring proper fitting shoes, they can lose the forefoot. Eventually, they can lose the whole leg and become unable to ambulate. I have a number of patients that are in wheelchairs, on walkers. The key is to control their diabetes and hypertension to prevent the arterial disease from developing in the first place.

In the past, Bruce would have sent patients at risk for the development of diabetic foot problems to the podiatry clinic within the Burgdorf Primary Care Center, but the hospital that partially funds the Burgdorf—St. Francis Hospital and Medical

Center, which since 2015 has been part of Trinity Health, one of the largest multi-institutional Catholic healthcare delivery systems in the nation—closed down its podiatry program. This is not a uniquely Hartford issue. Bonnie Tesch, a physician in Milwaukee, notes her own experience in this regard

> I've worked at six different Milwaukee clinics that closed, including a clinic for the homeless and several low-income neighborhood facilities . . . Usually, it was because of political things, funding . . . The last one, honestly, no one told me it was closed. I arrived one day and there was a sign on the door, and that's how I found out, like the patients. (Quoted in Thomas 2014)

As a result of defunding and underfunding, Bruce explained

> Now we have to send people out, and you're less able to find spots [to refer them to], and you can't get them in, and then they don't want to go because it's not at the Burgdorf. They're used to coming to our building, and they feel safe in our building, they trust us. And so when you send them over to the hospital or another clinic, there's a parking fee, or an extra bus, or there's all sorts of little challenges and barriers that make someone less likely to keep their appointment. I have patients that are religious in keeping their appointments with me, but somehow they won't keep their [referred] appointment with the podiatrist, the endocrinologist, etc. Which is a little upsetting.

Another slippery slope involves eye care:

> I have patients with retinopathy. Diabetics [can] get vascular growth in the back of their eyes, and then it bleeds, and then they can go blind. That's treatable now with laser surgery. But again, if someone's not showing up, they're not getting care, they don't have a dilated eye exam, you can miss it and people can lose their sight.

Another involves heart problems:

> I have a lady who has been in and out of Hartford Hospital probably five times in the last six months with heart attacks. She's a non-adherent diabetic. She doesn't keep appointments. But she's poor, she's got other fish to fry. Her husband died a year ago, she's still in the grieving process. She's raising her grandkids and brings them to the visits . . . and her 9-year-old granddaughter, tells me she doesn't take her insulin. The pharmacist tells me she's not filling her prescriptions on time, which means she's not taking her medications. You can work through that with someone, and you can assess them for depression, and treat their depression, and everything else. You can counsel your patients, troubleshoot their barriers, get them their meds but, in the end, you can't necessarily make them take their meds.

For the most part, standard diabetes treatment focuses on trying to get patients to lose weight, adopt healthier diets, reduce sugars and foods like carbohydrates that are converted into sugar in the body, increase regular exercise, practice blood glucose monitoring, and provide medication. Physicians, however, often find diabetes patients, especially lower-income patients, hard to treat, noncompliant, and extremely frustrating. As a result, in treating this patient population, physicians report feeling inadequate and overwhelmed (Beverly et al. 2011). As one physician expressed this frustration on a website for medical students:

> Is it just me or is diabetes the most frustrating condition to treat? At least 25% of my [patient] population is totally unmotivated to make real changes to potentially cure themselves of this ailment, and at each visit when they're 3–5 lbs heavier, it always nothing but salad and water that they've had . . . no idea how I gained that weight doc. (Student Doctor Network 2004)

Diabetes is a frequent issue in the patients treated by Bruce and his colleagues at Burgdorf Clinic. He stated:

> most of the patients I see have diabetes or pre-diabetes and it's actually relatively rare for me to see a patient without diabetes, amongst my long term patients . . . My sense is that in our dedicated patient population . . . the prevalence of diabetes is very, very high. In part, [this is] because our patients are inner-city poor, are overweight, have poor diets high in carbs and fast food because it stretches your budget. I have some patients that aren't that obese and aren't yet diabetic, but still their A1C [average level of blood glucose over a three-month period] is elevated, meaning they're pre-diabetic, and if we don't aggressively address their lifestyle, diet, exercise and weight, they will be.

Bruce's comments about the relationship between poverty and obesity, a condition defined by nutrition scientists as having a Body Mass Index (BMI) > 30, is well documented (U.S. Department of Health and Human Services 2000). BMI is a measure of body fat based on a patient's height and weight; specifically, it is a person's weight in kilograms divided by the square of their height in meters. The highest rates of obesity—a condition that in its most severe forms is linked to an estimated 5–20-year reduction in life expectancy—are found among sectors of the population with the greatest poverty and the lowest levels of education (Kumanyika 2005, Olshansky et al. 2005, Wardle 2002). Stemming from this, rates of obesity and diabetes in the US adhere to a socioeconomic gradient in which the greatest burden of this disease falls disproportionately on the poor and people of color (Mokdad et al. 2003).

One aspect of physician frustration with diabetes involves cultural factors. Explains Bruce:

> So . . . I have very heavy . . . morbidly obese, women [patients]. When I suggest they take a few pounds off . . . they say "well no, I'm just curvy." In their culture, women are desirable with full figures. I've had, not one, but a number of patients when I've talked to them about dieting and decreasing their BMI they say that their significant other wouldn't be happy if they lost weight. From a white middle-class cultural perspective, we somehow imagine these thin, emaciated models that we see on the covers of fashion magazines as the ideal. Each population, each cultural group, has their own norm, as well as health beliefs, around what a good size, a healthy size, an attractive size should be. What we, the doctor, would consider a healthy weight for a child, in some cultures they would consider that kid to look sick because they don't have rolls [of fat].

One aspect of the cultural element at play is reflected in a study of about 390 women by Marian Fitzgibbon and colleagues (2000) which found that White women began expressing discontent with their bodies at a BMI score of just under 25, which, according to the international definition is defined as the starting point for being in the 'overweight' category. According to this system, someone who is 5 feet 4 inches tall and weighs 150 pounds has a BMI score of 25.7. By comparison, African American and Latino women did not express concern until they were close to a BMI score of 30 (29.2 and 28.5, respectively), which is the beginning point of the heavier 'obese' category. Notably, neither level of income or education was significant in the findings. While culture is a factor in obesity, Bruce recognizes as well the critical role of structural factors in body weight.

The Political Economy of Diabetes, Obesity, and Related Ill Health

Key structural factors in obesity, Bruce noted, are poverty, racism, and structural violence in myriad forms, as well as failures of the healthcare system:

> The system may not want to equip itself to most effectively teach and teach back, you know, make sure the patient has heard what you think you told them. [This is] because of cuts in funding, and just lack of interest on the part of institutions, or lack of know-how. Patients with diabetes are time-consuming and the sicker, the less well-controlled their diabetes is, and the less educated an individual is, the more time consuming they are. And in an understaffed environment, it becomes more and more of a challenge serving the poorer and more needy patient . . . There's a million details and you can't necessarily treat one little piece of it and expect to be successful . . . It's not just their diabetes, it's not just their [blood] sugar, it's not just the food, it's the complexity of having other diseases, and the long-term organ damage they may have from having diabetes, which then increases the complexity of managing their diabetes. You really have to have an integrated program

> that's going to address both the multiple needs of a diabetic patient, the education, making sure they can easily get their medications, that they know how to use them, and that they can both understand what diet is preferred or recommended, as well as get their hands on the right foods. If they can get their hands on the right food, can they cook it in a healthy way? It's a million details, foot exams, and self-exams, and if they go on insulin, can they effectively check their blood sugar and regulate their insulin? To be a well-controlled diabetic is not that simple. It takes a motivated, individual willing to learn and to own their disease . . . and it takes a team of dedicated caregivers, to teach and support that patient!

Diabetes control, in short, is not easy for anyone, but it is much harder for people struggling with poverty, discrimination, dangerous neighborhoods, lack of access to healthy diets, and the multiple stressors of living in the hyperghetto, or as farm workers who must migrate to make a living: "We have to address poverty, and living conditions, and we have to address institutional racism, and health disparities and access to care."

How is racism a factor in diabetes? The relationship of bigotry to a chronic condition like diabetes reveals the important pathways that link lived experience to disease. As psychology researcher Monica Williams, who studies African American mental health and discrimination, points out:

> Correlations between perceived discrimination and symptoms of PTSD have been documented across a number of studies, and minorities have higher rates of PTSD. Negative physical health outcomes include obesity, hypertension, and heart disease, such as one sees from chronic stress. Negative mental health outcomes include depression, anxiety, traumatization, substance abuse, binge eating, and even psychosis . . . there is evidence to suggest that even watching news accounts of violence on television can contribute to traumatization, which is particularly relevant to the current African American experience (e.g., media coverage of unarmed Black people being killed by police). (Sawyer et al. 2016)

It is possible to treat PTSD as an individual mental health problem, but to only handle it in this way ensures the social production of more PTSD sufferers, as well as the range of health conditions that follow from exposure to trauma and chronic stress, including diabetes.

Further, Bruce asserted

> we also have to look at healthy living environments in cities, and access to walking groups, and bike trails, and access to food, and food security, and education, and all of those other resources. Someone living in a very rural area or in an urban area that is in a lower socioeconomic group finds it very difficult to impossible to adhere to what we consider a healthy

> lifestyle. And then you add advertising on cigarettes and alcohol and fast food, all stacked against someone trying to live in a manner that would keep them healthy, with a reasonable weight and being reasonably active throughout the day.

In short, Bruce maintains, the cards are stacked against the poor both when it comes to developing diseases like diabetes and in terms of maintaining the careful regime of home care needed to effectively manage a complex chronic disease. Under such conditions, the choice seems clear to Bruce: as part of the medical response, doctors must address the social production and progression of disease.

An important part of the disease social production process has been the restructuring of labor that has occurred in the US over the last five years. As the Pew Research Center reports: "Since it was last raised in 2009, to the current $7.25 per hour, the federal minimum has lost about 8.1% of its purchasing power to inflation" (Desilver 2015). In terms of actual spending power, Pew analyses found that U.S. workers were making more in 1968 than they do today. Over 20 million people (or 30 percent of all hourly, non-self-employed workers who are 18 years of age and older) have salaries that fall near to minimum wage. Of these, 18 percent are working in the restaurant and food service industry. Because of falling purchasing power, many individuals working in low-wage jobs receive an inadequate income. To assess the actual minimum wage needed to live in communities across the US, Amy Glasmeier (2016), professor of Economic Geography and Regional Planning at the Massachusetts Institute of Technology, developed the Living Wage Calculator. For Hartford County, where Bruce works, the calculator indicates that a living wage needed to support a single individual is $11.40 an hour (compared to the existing minimum wage of $9.15); for a family of four with one wage earner (and one stay-at-home parent), the needed living wage is $25.03 an hour; and for a family of four with two wage earners, the needed living wage is $19.27 an hour.

Despite the fact that many workers do not earn a living wage, there has been strong opposition to increasing the minimum wage by conservative forces in and beyond Congress. The Cato Institute (2013), an ultraconservative policy think tank, argues there are four reasons not to increase the minimum wage of U.S. workers: it would cause a loss of jobs as employers cannot afford to pay their workers more than the existing minimum wage; it would especially hurt low-skilled, less educated workers; it would have little effect on reducing poverty, and it could result in high prices that consumers pay for the things they buy. All of these arguments are brought up whenever the issue of the need to increase the minimum wage has been laid on the Congressional policy table. Speaker of the House, Paul Ryan, for example, opposes increasing the minimum wage because "it will do more harm than good" by causing job loss (quoted in Fitzgerald 2016). When he became Speaker of the House, Ryan's personal salary, however, went up from $174,000 to $223,500 a year, over ten times per hour more than the rise in the minimum wage he opposes for U.S. workers (Wattles 2015). The standard of living and access to health and other resources experienced by Paul Ryan's three children is dramatically superior to the life experience of the children of families struggling to make ends meet on the existing minimum wage or even less, as is their probable longevity and lifetime standard of living. Currently, 16 million children in the United States—22 percent of all children in the country—live in families with incomes below the federal poverty level (National Center for Children in Poverty 2016). Additionally, very informed voices question the Cato Institute's arguments. In a letter sent to President Obama and Congressional leaders in support of a minimum wage increase in 2016, over six hundred economists, including seven Nobel Prize winners wrote:

> In recent years there have been important developments in the academic literature on the effect of increases in the minimum wage on employment, with the weight of evidence now showing that increases in the minimum wage have had little or no negative effect on the employment of minimum-wage workers, even during times of weakness in the labor market. Research suggests that a minimum-wage increase could have a small stimulative effect on the economy as low-wage workers spend their additional earnings, raising demand and job growth, and providing some help on the jobs front. (Quoted in U.S. Department of Labor 2016)

Notably, the Department of Labor reports that since 1938, the federal minimum wage has been increased 22 times. For more than 75 years, real GDP per capita has steadily increased, even when the minimum wage has been raised (U.S. Department of Labor 2016).

Improving the minimum is not just an economic issue, it is a public health issue as there are important health effects of both underpaying workers and working in an environment with little job security. As Bruce emphasized:

> The productivity that's expected out of American workers is very high, and because their union system has been undermined in the last several years, there are relatively fewer protections against layoffs. With layoffs, additional work is transferred to the remaining workers, so that they're working longer days and longer hours. More and more jobs are becoming increasingly sedentary, and workers are being paid relatively less so you have very little free time to do the cooking that allows you to eat healthier foods and the exercise that leads to better outcomes. Whether it's the food industry or agribusiness or fast food or city government, there has to be a basic floor below which we won't allow people to fall and we're just not there. We need a living wage law in this country, I don't mean a minimum wage law, but a living wage law.

Bruce's assertion that the decline in unions has negatively impacted both blue-collar income and health is supported by several studies. While much public and media attention has focused on the decline in jobs in manufacturing in the US and their partial replacement by low-wage jobs in the fast food industry, in big-box retail chain stores, and elsewhere in the service industry, less attention has been directed at changes in wages in the remaining manufacturing sectors of the economy. In "Producing poverty: The public cost of low-wage production jobs in manufacturing," a report by the Labor Center at the University of California, Berkeley, Jacobs and colleagues (2016), for example, found that a third of non-management production workers toiling on factory floors and in related occupations are so underpaid that they now are forced to apply for some form of public assistance, such as food stamps or the Earned Income Tax Credit. Many manufacturing workers are temporary hires recruited by staffing agencies, and this labor category now accounts for an ever-larger share of factory employment. The Labor Center study found that between 2009 and 2013, the federal and the state governments spent $10.2 billion a year on public safety net programs for employed workers in manufacturing jobs and their families. This includes both workers directly hired by manufacturing companies and those employed through staffing agencies. The high utilization of public safety net programs by manufacturing workers is primarily a consequence of low wages, rather than less than full-time work schedules.

In the past, workers employed in the manufacturing sector earned wages that were significantly higher than the U.S. average, but this has changed dramatically in recent years. By 2013, the average manufacturing production worker was earning 7.7 percent below the median wage for all occupations. The average hourly income for production workers in the manufacturing industry in 2013 was $15.66, but 25 percent of these workers earned $11.91 or less. During this same time period, productivity in the U.S. manufacturing sector increased at a rate one-third higher than in the private, non-farm economy overall. For people without a college education, jobs in manufacturing still pay better salaries than most jobs available to this sector of the population, but this is not true for many such workers. Hidden by the averaging of salaries across labor categories is the fact that long-term workers make significantly more than those entering newly created jobs in manufacturing, which tend to pay less than the current average. Additionally, there are important regional variations. In Michigan, manufacturing workers earn about $2 more per hour than those in South Carolina (Casselman 2016). Why? The answer is unions. In southern "right-to-work" states, unions were never strong compared to the Midwest and other areas of the country. In Michigan, for example, 23 percent of manufacturing production workers were still union members in 2015; by contrast, in South Carolina, less than 2 percent belonged to a union.

Unions, moreover, also help account for why the middle class is comparatively healthier in the Midwest than in the Southeast, an area where non-unionized, lower-paying manufacturing jobs have been steadily increasing in recent decades. Analysis by the Pew Research Center (2016) shows that the middle class is shrinking in urban areas across the country. This decrease is substantial, measuring six percentage points or more in the 53 metropolitan areas included in the study. In many midwestern cities, 60 percent or more of households are considered middle-income by the Pew definition (i.e., households making between two-thirds and double the national median income, after controlling for the local cost of living); by contrast, in some southern cities, even those that now have large manufacturing bases, middle-income families constitute a minority of households. Lower income translates directly into lowered ability to purchase quality healthcare, or even any healthcare coverage at all; it also may mean having to work a second job for many workers, and, with a loss of union protection, more stressful and less safe working conditions. As Ben Casselman (2016), a senior editor and the chief economics writer for *FiveThirtyEight*, comments:

> When politicians pledge to protect manufacturing jobs, they really mean a certain kind of job: well-paid, long-lasting, with opportunities for advancement. Those aren't qualities associated with working on a factory floor; they're qualities associated with being a member of a union.

Thus, he concludes, what workers in the US who previously had dependable middle-class incomes miss is not manufacturing (which is still going on but pays less than in the past), but unions. Ironically, it appears to be the case that workers who have been most adversely affected by the corporate and state effort to weaken unions were an important voting bloc for Donald Trump in the 2016 presidential race, despite Trump's expressed preference for non-union workers in his businesses (Gabriel 2016). The term "false consciousness" has been used to label situations like this, when members of a subordinated social class, like current and former manufacturing employees relative to their employers, perceive the world through dominant frameworks that systematically obscure the existence and nature of their subordination. False consciousness entails more than a lack of specific information, such as details about the enormous income gap between Trump and many of his supporters, as well as the cause of this gap—it constitutes a fundamental misunderstanding of the nature of the structure social relationships in society. Ratner (2013), director of the Institute for Cultural Research and Education, cites an example involving employer-based health insurance:

> American corporations are transforming health coverage for their employees. They are refusing to pay into health insurance plans for employees, and they are instead giving employees a fixed stipend with which they are to shop for their own health coverage . . . However, employees have no input into the amount of the stipend that companies give them. Nor do employees have any control over the premiums that insurance companies charge. The stipends will be lower than the premiums which the companies formerly paid into employees' health plans, which leaves employees paying more than before. Corporations are freed from the vagaries of rising insurance rates while employees are subjected to them. Consequently, the vaunted control, empowerment, and responsibility of employees over their [new] health plans is specious . . . and serve the economic interests

of employers (cutting costs), not the healthcare needs of employees who assume that the stipend system increases their freedom of choice. While the utility of false consciousness as a diagnostic concept has been debated in recent years, the 2016 presidential race is likely to strengthen arguments in support of its soundness as an analytic tool.

Ignorance is Bliss

Another factor in diabetes and related conditions is people's perceptions of their neighborhood, which, as noted in Chapter 4, involves the impacts of emotional reactions people have to the immediate world around them. Thus, one of the ways structural violence impacts diabetes is through institutional withdrawal and hospital closings, loss of services, landlord neglect of housing quality and building abandonment, built environment structural decay, hazardous dumping in poor neighborhoods, lack of employment, and related onerous features of the hyperghetto as a place of residence. Research by Moreno and colleagues (2014), for example, used medical record reviews of a random sample of 250 adult Latinos with Type 2 diabetes and a survey involving patient ratings of neighborhood problems (e.g., crime, trash and litter, lighting at night, and access to exercise facilities, transportation, and supermarkets) to assess the relationship between neighborhood perceptions and the control of cholesterol levels, A1C blood glucose levels, blood pressure and BMI. Perception of neighborhood problems was found to be independently associated with higher BMI and BP levels.

By ignoring these structural issues—a dynamic that has been called the "ignorance is bliss" attitude of social elites—the health of poor and working people is allowed to progressively decline (Polk 2008). In the case of diabetes, from Bruce's viewpoint:

> [It is] putting Band-Aids on by treating their diabetes once they have it [and thinking] that somehow the incidence is going to go down. [We need] to develop an intersectoral plan identifying and prioritizing the issues in Hartford, education, poverty, living conditions, housing. [We need to] develop a plan with people living in Hartford's neighborhoods, that identifies evidence-based actions that we could implement with the population of Hartford, in their neighborhoods, to impact the conditions at the street level and actually create a healthier city . . . We need more integrated approaches that go beyond the doors of the clinic [and address] social determinants. I think the health care system has sufficient dollars to do the job. The problem is they're very much mal-distributed . . . There is a lot of waste in the system, fraud, all of those things. The pharmaceutical companies take a disproportionate percentage of the health care dollar and too much of that dollar goes to Wall Street in the form of dividends.

Also of concern are

> the way we live, and where we live, and the way our cities are designed, or not designed, how our food supply is processed and distributed, and the marketing of that processed food to children and other vulnerable populations, and the educational system's relative lack of content on health and nutrition. The food industry is to a large degree unregulated as far as salt content, sugar content, chemicals and other additive in our food supply.

Beyond the Clinic: Where Life Is Lived

From a clinical standpoint, to deal with complex issues that are intimately tied to the social and experiential lives of patients and the broader social structure that shapes their lives, Bruce emphasized the need to find ways for the healthcare system to reach beyond the walls of the clinic and into struggling communities:

> Community health workers certainly are one method of going beyond [the clinic], creating a health system without walls to improve effectiveness . . . We are still treating our patients in a monolithic way and not necessarily targeting approaches to what's going on in the neighborhoods and in the homes in which they live, that might be a factor in their diabetes, in their asthma. If someone has asthma, you may never get to their home, and never know that there's mold, and leaks, and dirty rugs, and bedbugs, and cockroaches. Maybe that's what's exacerbating their asthma, and that's why you never quite get on top of it. We hand patients written instructions, but there's no community health worker to actually go over it with them and drop in and say "how are you using that inhaler? Why don't you do it for me, let me check." Or looking at their food cupboards, nutrition, and what is in their refrigerator at home? And if it's all the wrong foods, then why is this the case?

The ultimate goal, said Bruce, is this:

> I want to fix Hartford. But people get upset when I say it . . . they tell me that people don't think it's broken. I believe if you think it's not broken then you're living under a rock. We need to rebuild the health care system and have adequate resources in places that serve underserved populations so you can assure that people have access, access to housing, to quality food, to medications, to care, that you're addressing social determinants, that you're looking at where they live, and that you can assure that people have the tools that they need educationally, as well as resources to actually self-manage their chronic diseases.

For example, in pointing to the challenges presented by corporations seeking to make a profit from vital resources, Bruce commented:

> We're getting fatter as a nation. And the food industry has gotten more adept at influencing us to eat more carbohydrates, more processed food, The lower-middle class and working class have, compared to 1980, fewer disposable dollars for buying things like food.

He cites the case of high-sugar fruit drinks that are marketed especially to lower-income populations, beverages that parents think of as real fruit juice. While the sugary soft drinks consumed by children is an issue, in fact, fewer than half of sweetened drinks consumed by toddlers in the US are carbonated; much of the rest is fruit drinks, although they may not contain much if any actual fruit juice (Wang, Bleich, and Gortmaker 2008). A study in Los Angeles Country found that overall 28.6 percent of children age 5 years and under consumed one or more sweetened drinks or sodas every day, with the percentage climbing to about 50 percent for African Americans and Latino youth of this age (Los Angeles County Department of Public Health 2007). Han and Powell (2012) studied the changing prevalence of heavily sugar-sweetened beverage consumption (≥500 kcal/day) by examining data from the National Health and Nutrition Examination Survey for the years 1999–2000, 2001–02, 2003–04, 2005–06, and 2007–08. Consumption increased more among African American children and adolescents, especially of fruit drinks, than Whites. Low-income children had a higher odds of heavily sugar-sweetened beverage consumption and a higher caloric intake from such drinks than did high-income children. Lower socioeconomic status also was associated with a higher likelihood of heavily sugary-sweetened drink consumption among adults.

How did this dietary pattern and the alleged cultural factors driving it develop? According to a policy brief developed for the California Center for Public Health Advocacy:

> Children are especially targeted in the [soft and sugar drink] industry's drive to gain new sugary drink customers. Soda companies spend $500 million dollars a year, including fees to highly trained psychologists and marketing experts, to promote their products to children . . . Marketers exploit . . . human vulnerabilities by tapping into what research has shown about hard-wired automatic decision-making processes that cause our instinctive attraction to foods high in calories . . . Marketers also delude consumers with images of colorful fruit or attractive athletes on labels leading them to believe the product is healthful and rich in nutrients the body needs when in reality the opposite is true. (Giancoli and Soto 2011: 4–5)

In other words, there is nothing traditional or inherently cultural—in the sense of a social group's unique and historically developed set of life-organizing values, norms, beliefs, and behaviors—in the consumption of sugar-laden beverages. Rather, there has been an active, well-funded, and skillfully developed marketing crusade designed to deceive in the interest of profit. And it has worked. While sweetened drinks date to the eighteenth century, it was only during the second half of the twentieth century that sugar-sweetened beverages became a prominent U.S. dietary component (Morrison, Busby, and Wells 2010). After World War II, the soft-drink industry jumped on the increasing availability of televisions to become a prominent advertiser of their products to the general public. The presentation of these sugar-sweetened beverages emphasized celebrity endorsements, the use of catchy slogans and jingles, tie-ins with Hollywood movies, and other forms of mass marketing that were particularly focused on young consumers. Examination of TV watching times shows that viewing for four or more hours per day is highest among African American boys and girls and lowest among Whites of both genders (Eisenmann, Bartree, and Wang 2002). Related to this finding, White boys and girls reported the highest rates of both moderate and vigorous physical activity each week and African American and Latino girls reported the lowest rates of both levels of activity.

Introduction to high sugar content can precede ingestion of fruit drinks and sodas and begin with marketed baby foods. A study by the Rudd Center for Food Policy and Obesity at the University of Connecticut (Harris et al. 2016) found that advertisements for baby food and drinks often promote the idea that these commercial products are healthier for infants than either breast milk or homemade food. The study pointed out that the period from birth to age 2 is a critical period for establishing lifelong dietary preferences, including eating habits that influence teen and adult bodyweight and related health status. There is widespread agreement, including in both the World Health Organization (2001) and the American Academy of Pediatrics (2012), that breast milk is the healthiest diet for children under six months of age but continuing for at least to the age of 1 year or more. Further infant health experts stress that children under age 2 should not be exposed to added sugar in the foods they consume (American Academy of Pediatrics 2012). Research reviewed by the Rudd Center shows the use of marketing strategies by commercial baby-food producers, primarily involving television, magazine, and Internet advertisements, that could mislead parents to believe that infant formulas have superior dietary benefits not present in breast milk, while, in fact, there actually are high levels of added sugar, as well as glucose syrup and honey (and salt) in some well-known toddler formula products such as Similac "Go and Grow," Nestlé's "Nido 1," and Pediasure "Grow and Gain" (Cogswell et al. 2015, Elliot and Conlon 2014). Notably, the study also found increasing advertisement by baby and toddler food manufacturers targeted to Hispanic populations.

In a public health policy response to the health risks of sugary drinks, some local governments have implemented a tax on sugar-sweetened beverages. The first jurisdiction to do so was Berkeley, California, which implemented a $0.01/ oz excise tax in March 2015. To assess the effectiveness of this approach from a public health perspective, Falbe and colleagues (2016) conducted a cross-sectional comparison study in low-income neighborhoods of Berkeley, and also Oakland and San Francisco, using an interviewer-administered beverage frequency questionnaire. The questionnaire was administered to 990 participants before the excise tax went into effect and to 1,689 participants four months after implementation.

These researchers found that the consumption of sugar-sweetened beverages decreased by 21 percent in Berkeley but increased by 4 percent in the nearby comparison cities. Additionally, they found that water consumption increased in Berkeley more than in comparison cities. What has been the industry's response to government efforts to promote public health like the excise tax in Berkeley? According to an industry spokesperson: this kind of policy

> won't make any measurable difference when it comes to combating obesity . . . At the end of the day, such regulation will limit choice, and add an extra burden, and will fail to deliver on the promise to help health. In other words, it's a misguided policy. (Quoted in Sustain 2014)

As the Berkeley study shows, and as other research affirms (Malik, Schulze, and Hu 2006), from a public health perspective, such policy is supported by research. By contrast, the consistent actions of the sugar and related industries is motivated by profit, even if its fiscal gains come at the expense of the health of the public, including those least able to access healthcare.

In recent years the public health struggle has gained global momentum. On October 11, 2016, which has been dubbed World Obesity Day, the World Health Organization (WHO) elevated its campaign against high sugar consumption. It issued a call to member national governments to introduce subsidies so that people could afford and would be encouraged to buy fruits and vegetables, and it proposed the taxation of unhealthy foods, with a particular emphasis on sugary drinks. Previously, the WHO had issued a health guideline entitled "Sugar Intake for Adults and Children," which noted that the growing consumption of sugar-sweetened beverages "may reduce the intake of foods containing more nutritionally adequate calories, leading to an unhealthy diet, weight gain and increased risk of NCDs [noncommunicable diseases]" (World Health Organization 2015). The new WHO recommendations were based on global expert opinion on health and diet, as well as on a set of systematic reviews of the literature on the effectiveness of fiscal interventions in improving diet and preventing NCDs like those associated with high sugar consumption. To underline its message, the WHO ended the provision of sugary drinks at organization functions held at its headquarters in Geneva (*Lancet* Editorial 2016).

Sugary drinks, in fact, are only the beginning of the sugar problem in the general population and specifically in low-income household diets. As the Union of Concerned Scientists (Bailin, Goldman, and Phartiyal 2014: 2) points out: "Many unlikely products contain surprising amounts of added sugar. These foods include crackers, pasta, sauces, salad dressings, yogurts, and a wide variety of other processed foods." While the health risks of excessive sugar consumption are well known, and despite repeated research-based recommendations to curb sugar consumption, "deceptive and exploitive marketing strategies of sugar interests" and the food industry (Bailin, Goldman, and Phartiyal 2014: 2), including aggressive advertising, continue to influence consumer behavior. Blatant use of false information—such as touting products as being far healthier than they are—is common in well-funded industry advertising campaigns. Accompanying these are public relations efforts by industry trade groups designed to obscure the link between added sugar consumption and health consequences. The packaging of high sugar products often is designed to obscure their sugar content. Industry code words, such as "naturally sweetened," "healthy," and "lightly sweetened" are used to hide sugar content in products that exceed recommended daily sugar intake by public health institutions (World Health Organization 2015).

Additionally, the sugar industry has attempted, with considerable success, in manipulating nutrition science by funding researchers to produce results that diminish the adverse health effects of high sugar consumption, shape scientific evidence to blame fat and exonerate sugar as the dominant dietary cause of heart disease, and aggressively criticize the integrity of scientists whose findings are deemed undesirable by the sugar industry. This effort began in the 1950s, when evidence began to emerge suggesting a relationship between sugar consumption and coronary heart disease (CHD), the leading cause of death globally. By the 1960s, two alternative views emerged of the dietary agent most implicated in heart problems: added sugar and total fat, especially saturated fat and dietary cholesterol. Over the next twenty years, however, sugar came to no longer be seen as playing a significant role in the development of heart-related disease, as dietary research and education focused primarily on fat consumption. An examination of internal sugar industry documents by researchers affiliated with the Philip R. Lee Institute for Health Policy Studies in San Francisco found that the sugar industry sought to "downplay early warning signals that sucrose consumption was a risk factor in CHD" (Kearns et al. 2016: 1683). Central to the industry's strategy was an attempt to increase sugar sales by getting people in the US to eat a low-fat diet that relied on sugar as a source of calories. Included in industry tactics was an effort to discredit the findings of British physiologist John Yudkin on the role of sugar in CHD. To promote its work, in 1965, the industry's Sugar Research Foundation invited Fredrick Stare, chair of the Harvard University School of Public Health Nutrition Department and an expert in dietary causes of CHD, to join its scientific advisory board. The connection between Stare's industry-favorable positions and his financial ties to the industry only came to light in the 1970s, when it was revealed that over thirty scientific papers authored by members of his department were funded by the Sugar Research Foundation in the years between 1952 and 1956. Similarly, the industry paid almost $50,000 (in 2015 dollars) to Mark Hegsted and Robert McGandy, two members of Stare's department whose prior work had suggested that blood glucose levels were a better predictor of atherosclerosis than blood cholesterol or hypertension, to write a review of the scientific literature that downplayed the role of sugar in heart disease. The industry was pleased with the two-part review, which was published in 1967 in the *New England Journal of Medicine*, because it concluded that the only dietary change needed to prevent CHD was to reduce dietary cholesterol and substitute polyunsaturated fat for saturated fat in the diet (McGandy et al. 1967a, McGandy et al. 1967b). The influential review exonerated sugar as an important factor in heart disease. As the Union of Concerned Scientists (2016) asserts, "Stare's department at Harvard is a key example of how industry funding can influence academic science, with dangerous consequences for public discourse and public policy."

Targeting Children

Omnipresent advertising of high-sugar processed foods targets specific population segments, including children, women, minorities, and low-income populations. Advertising for sugary cereals, for example, is targeted specifically at children who are not experienced in discerning the sophisticated persuasive intent of advertisers (Ferguson, Munoz, and Medrano 2012). Research on the use of fantasy characters in the promotion of sugary foods to children (e.g., Tony the Tiger, the Lucky Charms leprechaun, the Keebler elves) has shown that it produces positive associations and low perceptions of manipulation among 8–10-year-old children (Rose, Merchant, and Bakir 2012).

Sports figures also are used to market unhealthy consumables to children. In 2012, for example, the McDonalds corporation spent a reported $98 million to extend its Olympic sponsorship, which began in 1976, until 2020. Coca-Cola's contract as a sponsor of the Olympics, which runs until 2020, is thought to be worth $43 million for each four-year Olympic cycle (Tylee 2016). In a report published by the Rudd Center for Food Policy and Obesity in the journal *Pediatrics*, researchers studied a hundred professional athletes and their product endorsement contracts. The researchers used the Bloomberg Businessweek's 2010 Power 100 report, a ranking of athletes based on their endorsement value and prominence within their given sport and found that among the 512 commercial brands associated with the athletes, the most common were sporting goods, followed closely by food and beverage brands (Bragg et al. 2013). Sports drinks, which commonly are high in sugar and calories, comprised the majority of the consumables advertised by the athletes, with soft drinks and fast foods making up most of the rest of their endorsements. The study noted that of the 46 beverages that were endorsed by athletes, 93 percent relied exclusively on sugar for their calories. The researchers also reported that children between the ages 12 and 17 saw more athlete-endorsed food and beverage brand commercials than adults.

Music celebrities also are sought as advertisement symbols to youth markets because endorsements are known to enhance brand desirability among consumers (Kamins 1989). A study of music celebrities using the performers with songs on the 2013/2014 Billboard Hot 100 Chart list identified 590 product endorsements made by 163 musical celebrities. While consumer goods (e.g., fragrances, makeup) were the largest endorsement category (26 percent), the second largest were food and beverage products (18 percent). Analysis of these items concluded that "music celebrities who are popular among adolescents endorse energy-dense, nutrient-poor products" (Bragg et al. 2016). As these examples reveal, common-sense contradiction (e.g., using athletes to sell unhealthy consumables to children) has not been a barrier in efforts to use all means possible in averting people's eyes from the chemistry of the products they regularly see advertised as desirable goods to ingest. The consequences are seen in the obesity crisis and the high rates of potentially lethal chronic diseases.

Blocking the Right to Know

The commitment of the food industry to keeping sugar content in their products hidden has been revealed by the intense battle it has waged to block Food and Drug Administration efforts to add a new line to food labels on packaged products that would indicate the number of teaspoons of sugar that have been added. Major food trade associations, including the American Bakers Association, American Beverage Association, American Frozen Foods Institute, Corn Refiners Association, International Dairy Foods Association, and National Confectioners Association, launched a vehement publicity and lobbying effort to preserve the existing, limited, food label (Ferdman 2016).

The consumer's right to know what is in the products they eat is a contentious issue for the food industry. In November 2012, for example, giant chemical companies (Monsanto and Dupont) and a number of large food producers (including PepsiCo, Kraft, Coca-Cola, Nestlé, General Mills, Kellogg's) teamed up to successfully wage an expensive effort to oppose Proposition 37, a California ballot initiative that would have required the package labeling of genetically modified foods (GMO) and blocked manufacturers from advertising foods made from GMO plants or animals as "natural." Many processed foods contain genetically modified soybean oil, corn syrup, refined sugar, and cottonseed oil, and hence anything that might threaten profits is fought forcefully by the industry. In 2013, an array of companies raised millions of dollars to try to defeat a similar initiative in Washington state, and were successful in 2014 in both Oregon and Colorado blocking consumer legislation (Center for Food Safety 2016). When Vermont, Connecticut, and Maine successfully implemented GMO labeling laws, President Obama signed into law a bill passed by Congress overriding these state initiatives and denying consumers the right to know what they are eating. The bill would allow digital access (e.g., through a smartphone) to information on food content for any products that met a set of very difficult requirements to mandate GMO labeling. This is an example of structural violence, in that the new federal law overlooks the fact that over

> 50 percent of America's low-income and rural populations—a disproportionate number of which are minority communities—and more than 65 percent of the elderly don't even own smartphones—and for those that do, many cannot afford monthly payments, or live in areas lacking internet access. (Kimbrell 2016)

Food Insecurity

A key element in the appeal of sugary drinks and foods, and calorie-heavy diets generally, among the poor is food insecurity, a concept developed from work by the Food and Agriculture Organization of the United Nations. In 1995, the U.S. Department of Agriculture incorporated food insecurity into its Current Population Survey. Food insecurity was defined as "limited or uncertain availability of nutritionally acceptable or safe foods" (Carlson, Andrews, and Bickel 1999). The survey found that 11.9 percent of U.S. households were food insecure. Not all food-insecure households showed evidence of hunger, and the relation between poverty, food insecurity, and hunger is complex, as programs like food stamps impact levels of actual hunger. The third National Health and Nutrition Examination Survey, which covered the years 1988–94, defined food insufficiency as "sometimes" or "often" not having enough to eat (Alaimo et al. 1998). The survey found that 14 percent of low-income respondents met this definition. Additionally, women, but not men, living in food-insufficient households were more likely to be overweight than were women living in food-sufficient households (58 percent compared with 47 percent), a paradox that stimulated research on food selection among the poor. This point aside for the moment, over 10 million people in the US were experiencing some level of food insecurity by the end of the twentieth century. Households with children were twice as likely to report food insecurity as those without children. In addition to poverty, food insufficiency was found to be associated with single-parent families, lacking health insurance, and having a family head with less than twelve years of education (Andrews et al. 1999).

But what of the paradox of obesity among the food insecure? Do the poor make poor food choices from a health standpoint? Is it a question of lack of education, unhealthy cultural patterns, or a poverty-driven search for comfort foods? Or, in fact, is the selection of energy-dense foods a rational response to having limited resources in an environment of focused advertisement and ready availability?

Research shows that the diets consumed by the poor in the US provide cheap, concentrated energy from sugar and fat. As Drewnowski and Spector (2004: 10) indicate, "energy density (MJ/kg) and energy costs ($/MJ) are inversely linked, such that the selection of energy-dense foods by food-insecure or low-income consumers may represent a deliberate strategy to save money." In other words, people with limited resources to devote to food purchases tend to select calorie-dense but palatable foods, like sugary beverages, to ensure dietary energy at the least cost. Seemingly recalcitrant people with diabetes from low-income families, while making food choices that in the long run have significant health costs, must handle the immediate and pressing social and economic issues they face each day to even have a chance to address longer-term issues like diabetes and its progressive symptomatology. Healthier eating, in fact, is more expensive than simply meeting energy needs (Aggarwal, Monsivais, and Drewnowski 2012). Confronted daily with multiple challenges, the poor behave in a way that suggests recognition of a simple truth: if you do not survive in the short run, the long run is irrelevant.

This leads to a pattern of actions that is confusing to and even contemptible from the perspective of the non-poor, who do not face similar challenges and often have little understanding of the realities of being poor. In a powerful essay entitled "This is why poor people's bad decisions make perfect sense," Linda Tirado (2013), until recently a night cook in an inexpensive restaurant, writes about the myth of longer-term planning based on her own experience of poverty during a period of her life:

> It does not matter what will happen in a month. Whatever happens in a month is probably going to be just about as indifferent as whatever happened today or last week. None of it matters. We don't plan long-term because if we do we'll just get our hearts broken. It's best not to hope. You just take what you can get as you spot it.

Examination of the social determinants of diabetes, suggest that:

> For disadvantaged individuals, the constant scramble to make ends meet results in high levels of chronic stress, spurring both psychological and biologic responses . . . Chronic stress can lead to increased depression and anxiety, reduced self-esteem, and decreased energy and motivation, which amplify the likelihood of self-destructive behaviors and choices (e.g., tobacco use, excessive alcohol intake, and consumption of unhealthy foods). (Hill 2013: 68)

Thus while Tirado is well aware of the health risks and expense of smoking, she admits to being a smoker. Her reason is that like many poor people she is often exhausted:

> When I am enraged and beaten down and incapable of accomplishing one more thing, I can smoke and I feel a little better, just for a minute. It is the only relaxation I am allowed. It is not a good decision, but it is the only one that I have access to.

And so, for her, it makes perfect sense. So too, all of the patterns of behavior among the poor—the issue simply is fully understanding the day-to-day if not hour-to-hour contours of life on the hard-to-climb-above lower rungs of the socioeconomic ladder. Unfortunately, politicians who make social policy usually have never known poverty and their understandings of it are skewed by their own more privileged life experience and by social ideologies rooted in the culture of wealth. Of note, the median net worth of a member of Congress in 2013 was $1,029,505, while the net worth of the average American household was $56,355. The majority of members of Congress, in fact, are millionaires (Rappeport 2015). Stresses Rappeport, "while lawmakers like to talk about . . . poor and middle-class Americans, few of them can relate financially."

Marketing and Disease Promotion

As noted, corporate advertising targeted to the low-income shopper, an aspect of industry market segmentation, is another influential factor in the construction of poor people's eating habits. Studies on this issue that were summarized in a report from the Institute of Medicine (2005) entitled *Food Marketing to Children and Youth: Threat or Opportunity?* which documents a pervasive pattern in how food is marketed differently to rich and poor neighborhoods in the US. One expression of this marketing strategy is the distribution of advertising circulars with discount coupons. Harkinson (2013) notes the case of Walmart pledging to offer healthier grocery options and then sending out a circular

> aimed at low-income customers [which] included discount coupons for a two-liter bottle of Coca-Cola, a 10-pack of Kool-Aid Jammers drinks, and a 9.5-ounce bag of Cheetos. Only three of the 36 discounted items in the ad were labeled "Great for You [Walmart's official healthy food label]" while ten of them touted high-sugar, high-sodium, or high-fat junk foods. The ad did not include any coupons for fresh fruits or vegetables.

The coupons sent to non-poor homes, by contrast, included discounts for yellow onions, whole carrots, and Bartlett pears. This is a typical pattern in the food industry.

Another expression of marketing to the poor and ethnic minorities involves advertisement placement. An analysis of 2004 Nielsen Monitor-Plus data on food and beverage advertising found that advertisements placed in African American media showed significant spending by food and beverage companies to promote high-calorie and low-nutrient foods and beverages. The three most frequently advertised categories of food and beverage products that appeared in magazines targeted to African Americans (e.g., *Jet*, *Ebony*, *Black Enterprise*, *Essence*, *Vibe*, and *Savoy*), were for carbonated soft drinks, cookies and crackers, and fruit juices and fruit-flavored drinks. Similarly, advertisement spending for the top three food and beverage categories on Black Entertainment Television were regular carbonated soft drinks, candy and gum, and fruit juices and fruit-flavored drinks (Williams 2005). Moreover, several content analyses of the types of food and beverage advertisements seen by children and youth of different ethnic backgrounds found that food advertisements aired on prime-time television programs directed to African American households more often were for high-calorie and low-nutrient food and beverage products than prime-time programs directed at White audiences (Henderson and Kelly 2005, Tirodkar and Jain 2003). While the food and beverage industries assert that their advertisement merely reflects differences in preferences across subgroups, a systematic and carefully structured review of 123 published empirical studies, mostly of television advertising, found that there is strong evidence that television advertising influences the food and beverage preferences and purchases of children age 2–11. Thus researchers conclude "television advertising influences children to prefer and request high-calorie and low-nutrient foods and beverages" (Institute of Medicine 2005: 307).

This outside-of-the-clinic reality is the dilemma of the physician, even the social medicine physician: when there is so much working against the health of poorer patients, where do you focus your energies? When it comes to children and sugary foods, there are some short-term issues at hand that have both short- and long-term consequences. Bruce notes one of these:

> we try to teach parents that it's important early on in life to feed children when they're hungry, but that snacks and things like that don't have to be high sugar. Then there is "bottle mouth" . . . Kids won't go to sleep so you stick [a bottle with] apple juice in their mouth, so they can suck on it and it puts them to sleep. They are falling asleep with their mouth filled with sugar around their teeth. It's a fact that within in seconds of a sugary meal, the bacteria start eating away your teeth.

Poor teeth are a stigmatizing mark of poverty, a badge of shame in a society that privileges beauty and equates bad teeth with bad people; it is also a significant health issue (Horton and Barker 2010). The National Hospital Ambulatory Medical Care Survey (Wall and Nasseh 2013) found that the number of emergency room visits for dental problems increased from 1.1 million in 2000 to 2.1 million in 2010. Also, there was a statistically significant increase in the proportion of dental emergency room visits of the total number of emergency visits during this period. Many poor patients with serious dental problems go to the emergency room rather than to a dentist because they either have no dental insurance or they have insurance coverage that is restricted to emergency care, and they cannot pay for dental treatment out of pocket (Carrion et al. 2011, Castaneda et al. 2010). Obamacare does not address this issue because it excludes dental care from coverage, one of many concessions that were made to industry lobbyists to get the bill passed.

Journalist Sarah Smarsh knows well the health and social problems of having poor teeth. She was born to a working-class family in Wichita, Kansas, a family without dental coverage that suffered with decayed, infected, and pulled teeth. Her father almost died of heart failure at age 50 from an infection that began in an abscessed tooth. She writes (2014) about the "psychological hell of having poor teeth in a rich, capitalist country: the underprivileged are priced out of the dental-treatment system yet perversely held responsible for their dental condition." Additionally, she notes, "Poor teeth, I knew, beget not just shame but more poorness: people with bad teeth have a harder time getting jobs and other opportunities. People without jobs are poor. Poor people can't access dentistry—and so goes the cycle" (Smarsh 2014). Indeed, the dental crisis of the poor is emblematic of the larger built-in structural causes of poverty that are hidden by the individual and group-blaming accounts of poverty that circulate within the culture of wealth and are embraced by many of the non-poor (Kluegel and Bobo 1993).

Diabetes and the Wider Community Environment

Also contributing to the increase in diabetes among the poor is a lack of access to healthy food. A study in New Haven, CT that compared food availability across stores and neighborhood, for example, found that "stores in lower-income neighborhoods (compared to those in higher-income neighborhoods) stock fewer healthier varieties of foods and have fresh produce of much lower quality" (Andreyeva et al. 2008). On this issue, Bruce stressed, that

> working against prevention is the fact that many of my patients lived in what might be called "food deserts," that lead to lack of access to healthy food, including economic access to fruits, vegetables, and other things [that] people can't afford [because] they run out of money and food stamps and just about everything else by the end of the month. We make recommendations to our patients that often they cannot fulfill. And it's not that easy to "follow the doctor's instructions" because it can all be quite confusing, even for me as someone who teaches nutrition. When I was shopping for my mother with diabetes, and hypertension, and heart failure, I really needed a PhD in nutrition. I would literally spend hours in the soup aisle just trying to figure out what she could eat that would be both palatable and not kill her.

While culturally and interpersonally sensitive care is vital, as is having a community-based setting like the Burgdorf Clinic in which to provide such care, there is a critical need, Bruce stressed, to go beyond the individual patient to the wider community:

> There are certainly community interventions that we might implement that would make our patients healthier, but no one wants to pay for them. I thought about it and we clearly didn't have the money for an educational counter-marketing campaign to influence folks to buy healthier food, so that's when we decided to plant a garden [on the grounds of the Burgdorf]. There is a Chinese proverb: if you're planting for a season, plant rice; if you planting for a decade, plant fruit trees; if you're planting for a century, educate your children. A garden is a commitment, certainly for at least a season. But then we also planted fruit trees with the hope that we would use it to educate our patients and their children. Planting a garden, with all the work that that entails, is an act of nurturing for the community, and that, hopefully, it's a commitment to the community, beyond what the politics of health care and medicine might be telling them.

The garden, billed as a joint initiative of the Hartford Department of Health and Human Services, St. Francis Hospital, the UConn School of Medicine, Hartford Food System and Knox Parks Foundation, opened in June 2011. Symbolically, the garden—planted with tomatoes, bok choy, collard greens, broccoli, green peppers, green beans, callaloo, jalapenos, eggplants, and cabbage—embodied

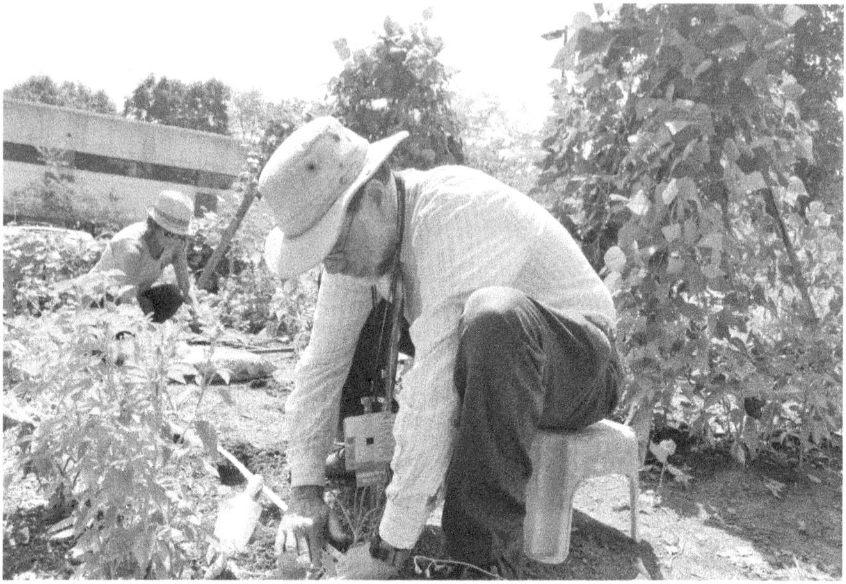

FIGURE 5.2 Bruce working in the Burgdorf Clinic garden

Bruce's social approach to medicine involving breaching the clinical/community divide to serve patients as people with full lives, experiences, and diverse needs. Produce grown in the garden is distributed to patients and North End residents through the Women, Infants, and Children program (WIC) office at the Hartford Department of Health and Human Services, the medicine and pediatric clinics at the Burgdorf, and the emergency food bank also located at the Burgdorf. For Bruce the garden is also a metaphor:

> We've put roots down in the community, and we've been nurturing and strengthening those roots . . . What we have here is an opportunity to produce food for our patients and to teach them about healthy eating. It's all part of primary care and community health. (Quoted in DeFrancesco 2014)

6

PUTTING PEOPLE FIRST: ENVISIONING A HEALTHY SOCIETY

Qui bono – who benefits?

> We can change the world and make it a better place. It is in your hands to make a difference.
>
> *Nelson Mandela*

People of a Struggling City

Working at the local level, it is Bruce's dream to build a healthier society, beginning with the city in which he practices medicine, Hartford, Connecticut. Founded in the early 1600s on the banks of the Connecticut River by a small band of restless Puritans, Hartford, named after Hertford, England, developed to become a center of abolitionist organizing in the mid-1800s. Harriet Beecher Stowe, author of the famous anti-slavery novel *Uncle Tom's Cabin*, and her sister, Isabella Beecher Hooker, a woman's rights activist in the suffragist moment, called Hartford home (Frank 2015). The Stowe sisters, as well as Mark Twain, lived in Nook Farm, a vibrant neighborhood of the city and a hub of New England literary life. Other well-known residents included abolitionist Francis Gillette, and Joseph Hawley, governor of Connecticut and U.S. Senator, and Susan Lee, who helped to establish the Hartford Philharmonic Orchestra. Expressive of the nature of Hartford in the mid-1800s, it became home to the Wadsworth Athenaeum, the first public museum in the U.S. Bushnell Park, the oldest publically funded park in the country, is located nearby. The park was conceived of by Reverend Horace Bushnell as a pastoral escape from the grimy downsides of the fast-moving Industrial Revolution, including increasingly polluted water and air, the emergence of local poverty among those who could not find jobs, and inadequate sanitation. Nowhere in the city were these problems more evident than in the space that Bushnell proposed for the park. The area was home to two leather tanneries, a soapworks factory, numerous pigsties and other livestock corrals, crowded tenements, and a garbage dump. Bushnell himself described it as "hell without the fire" (Bushnell Park Foundation 2016). Local businessmen opposed the park, arguing that it would remove taxable property from the tax rolls. Nonetheless, the city council approved the Bushnell proposal and the park was built, an achievement that inspires Bruce's vision of making Hartford a livable and equitable place for its residents.

Despite emergent problems, Hartford grew rapidly and became a prosperous and vibrant municipality, with one of the strongest economies in the country. The city developed into a center of banking and manufacturing, as well as publishing and shipping along the Connecticut River, and eventually acquired the nickname of "Insurance City" because of the many insurance companies first founded there. It also became home to the booming Colt Manufacturing Company, which produced, among other guns, the Colt Single Action Army Revolver (also known as the Colt 45), the weapon that claims the title as "the gun that won the West" (Spencer 2015). Unmentioned in this motto is who the West was won from, namely indigenous Indian people and the sovereign nation of Mexico of which the West was a part.

From early in its history, Hartford was not a monocultural city. African Americans have lived in Hartford since the seventeenth century, and sites of early African American presence have been identified in an area that was once called Hog River (which is today a stream that flows underground but surfaces to feed the pond in Bushnell Park). James Mars, a former slave who moved to Hartford in 1815, was active in pressing for African Americans to gain voting rights and helped to influence the Connecticut State Legislature to ban slavery in 1848. In the post-Civil War period, many freed slaves migrated to Connecticut and made their homes in a section of the city called the Bottoms, a place where some of the early dwellings that housed this community still stand. After World War II, African Americans from the South and people from the Caribbean began moving to Hartford in large numbers in search of factory jobs and farm employment nearby. As a result, the city's Black population grew to about 55,000 by 1990. In more recent years, beginning during the mid-1990s, middle-class African Americans, like middle-class Italians, Jews, French Canadians, and others before them, initiated a movement out of Hartford into neighboring suburbs that are part of other towns (Swift 2001). Puerto Ricans began to be attracted to Hartford in the period after World War II.

The percentage of the population of Hartford with a Latino identity has grown steadily since then, especially during the latter decades of the twentieth century. While in 1980, Latinos represented 20.3 percent of the city's population, by the year 2000, Latinos comprised 40.6 percent of city residents. Today, Hartford has one of the highest percentage of Latinos in the US (after Miami) (Trinity College 2014). US. After World War II, many Puerto Ricans moved to the Hartford area in search of employment, which, as U.S. citizens, they could freely do without visas. By 1959, the Puerto Rican population of the city reached 6,000 and continued to grow. Other Latino subgroups, including Cubans, Peruvians, and Mexicans, have also contributed to the size of the city's Latino population (Vasquez 2003).

The population of Hartford reached a height of more than 177,000 in 1950 but has declined since then, dropping in size by over 50,000 people (Sterner 2012). Today it is an impoverished and struggling city in fiscal crisis, a city that Bruce both loves and endures. The city, comprised of just 18 square miles, now has a population of about 124,000 people living in approximately 43,500 households (U.S. Census Bureau 2015). Among non-residents living far from its boundaries, Hartford often conjures an image of a white-washed Yankee hub set among deep-hued New England foliage. But of far greater import for its residents, Hartford ranks 33rd in terms of income inequality in U.S. metro areas with at least 100,000 population. Thirty-eight percent of the city's residents live at or below the federal poverty line (Connecticut by the Numbers 2014). While the state of Connecticut is populated by residents who have higher incomes (the fourth highest in the nation), lower unemployment rates, and more years of education than the nation as a whole, the same is not true of its capital city, Hartford. Among the poorest cities in the US, Hartford was one of only a small number that saw an increase in the rate of poverty between 1990 and 2000 (Connecticut Department of Public Health 2002). The average per capita income in Hartford is $16,619, the lowest of any city in the state (Connecticut Department of Community Development 2013). As Hartford's mayor announced in 2016, "the structure is broken" (Haar 2016), with a deficit of over $30 million. What is the reason for this crisis? Some would blame the people of Hartford, as the poor often are blamed when things go wrong. But, as long-time commentator on the city, journalist Tom Condon (2016) asserts:

> Hartford cannot be blamed for decades of [federal and state] government-aided suburbanization that took tens of thousands of middle-class residents out of the city . . . The real problem, as has been obvious for years, is the almost exclusive use of property taxes to fund local governments . . . Hartford is forced to play a game it cannot win. It is small to begin with . . . and more than half of its property—schools, churches, government buildings, [hospitals,] arts institutions [many of which serve the whole region or the whole state]—is tax exempt, a hole only partly filled by state . . . reimbursement.

In short, Hartford is an impoverished island in an otherwise largely wealthy sea. And the wealthy residents of the state, and their representatives in state government, have not been inclined to implement statewide solutions to this disparity. Rather, the trend has been to allow the state to remain divided into wealthy suburbs and poor cities, with little regard for the damage this approach inflicts on the poor, including poor children who will likely never know or even see the lavish wealth found elsewhere in the state.

As this discussion indicates, "Wealth and poverty are highly concentrated in Connecticut—more so than in many other large metropolitan areas [in the US]. And often, those neighborhoods are racially and economically segregated from each other" (Buchanan and Abraham 2015). Findings of a DataHaven study of rising neighborhood inequality in Connecticut by Buchanan and Abraham reveal that 10 percent of all Connecticut residents live in racially concentrated, affluent areas, three times the average found in a national study by University of Minnesota researchers. The study also showed that in Connecticut a substantial portion of the population is exposed to very high rates of neighborhood poverty. These researchers found that "Statewide, 15 percent of Connecticut's poor population lives in a racially concentrated, poor neighborhood. Poor residents . . . face among the highest levels of segregation in the nation, similar to the experiences of those living in Greater Detroit and Philadelphia." Buchanan and Abraham (2015) emphasize that an important indicator of concentrated poverty in a region is the percentage of poor residents who live in a neighborhood of concentrated poverty. This condition, which well describes the challenges of people living in Hartford, has been called "double jeopardy," because of considerable research evidence suggesting that exposure to multiple layers of disadvantage is significantly more risky to health, child achievement, and overall well-being than enduring any single indicator of poverty. Moreover, neighborhood segregation of this sort promotes the perpetuation of poverty as it tends to inhibit the development of regional solutions to inequality. The geographic concentration of wealth and poverty diminishes shared regional identity and lessens understanding by the wealthy and most influential segments of the population of the lives and needs of poorer residents. According to Douglas Massey (1996: 409) "The social worlds of the rich and poor . . . diverge . . . [divorcing] the interests of the rich from the welfare of the poor."

With such a high concentration of poverty, social conditions in Hartford overall are tenuous: 58 percent of families with children are headed by a single female; 39 percent of adults lack a high school degree, and unemployment is three times that for the state (Trinity College 2001). Teen birth is notably high, a statistic that is understood (by some) to be a marker of social disadvantage; the issue is not which teens (from which social strata) have sex but which teens have babies. In some of Connecticut's poorest cities, the number of children born to teenage mothers is more than twice the state average. In Hartford, however, the teen birth rate approaches three times the state average (Charles 2014). Moreover, findings of a DataHaven study (2016) of 16,000 people in Connecticut found that living in a highly distressed, impoverished neighborhood often means that you are quite unhappy. The study revealed that approximately 40 percent of African American and Hispanic participants and 33 percent of White participants living in distressed neighborhoods were either not happy at all, only a little bit happy, or somewhat happy. Similar percentages of people (42 percent of African Americans and 33 percent of Whites) living in distressed neighborhoods reported feeling down, depressed, or hopeless very often, fairly often, or sometimes. All of these factors put Hartford at high risk for poor health indicators. Sexually transmitted diseases are higher in Hartford than in any other city in the state. The city's preterm birthrate and infant mortality rate are both above the state average. The asthma-related emergency room visit rate among children is high and 11.5 percent of public school students in the city report having asthma. Diabetes also is more frequent in Hartford than in Connecticut as a whole (Hartford Department of Health and Human Services 2010). In short, compared to the wealthy areas of Connecticut, Hartford is not a healthy place to live, an issue that has been of highest concern to Bruce since he arrived in the city.

Reaching Toward Change

These multiple undesirable indicators in Hartford clarify Bruce's motivation for wanting change. In his view, in working for change:

> Your motivation has to be that you want to help people, or addressing an injustice, or because there is an unmet need. Not because you want to be famous or make your Mom proud. Because the fame infrequently happens and when it does, it tends to be evanescent, very brief.

His approach to bringing change involves finding a way to place the health and well-being of his patients above the constraints imposed by the medical-industrial complex, even though this often leads to conflict with the local powers that be. Noted Raul Pino, the Connecticut Commissioner for Public Health, during an interview about Bruce:

> I think [his] belief [is] that the collective good can enrich the individual good, that the health of your neighbor is as critical to you as the value of [your] property, that we should all have access to a minimum standard of care. [He asks] why this country being the richest in the world cannot offer what others a lot less rich than we are can offer to their citizens, a quality of care for all, and [there is] his passion for the individual—not just for health care but the individual as a whole. [He had] the ability to comprehend this very early that all these factors are critical to individual health: the stress, the housing, the employment, the ability to provide . . . He believes in continuum of care. I think he believes that care doesn't end when you get discharged. Care doesn't end when you were seen by your provider last time, after you get diagnosed, treated, and cured. I think that he understands that care is a continuum, that . . . involves the community.

Bruce's orientation is badly needed in the neighborhood where he works. Community Solutions (2016), a community organization that focuses on the issue of homelessness, describes the area around the Burgdorf clinic in these words:

> A place of contradictions, seemingly equal parts opportunities and obstacles. Walking through the neighborhood, one stumbles along crumbling sidewalks under broken streetlights, then finds groups of engaging young people gathered at street corners, energetic but bored. A large historic park provides hundreds of acres of green space, but it is seldom used, as fear of crime keeps residents traveling their own well-worn routes. Two and three-family homes line the streets, many long in need of repair. Six out of seven houses are occupied by tenants, who wield little power to fix their homes. Rates of foreclosure and eviction are among the highest in the City, and the instability that is a fact of life for so many families contributes to pervasive health issues. Though the neighborhood is vibrant with many cultures, it is also one of the poorest in the country . . . Among Hartford's seventeen neighborhoods, this small area ranks highest in all kinds of preventable illnesses: obesity, heart disease, infant and neonatal mortality, preventable infections and communicable diseases.

Signifying the contradictions that Community Solutions describes, the neighborhood is characterized by the paradox of a significant level of drug abuse, and hence has been a center of HIV transmission since early in the epidemic, as well as having a set of active and dedicated community service organizations intent on building a healthier, more vibrant community. One of the latter, of course, is the Burgdorf Clinic itself.

Reflections and the Future

Reflecting on his life, Bruce remarked:

> My sadness now is that I'm 61 years old, and I know the amount of time I have left is far less than what has come before and that [there is] so much to do. And I'm a bit tired. I have to admit that it has gotten harder, and that is a sad commentary. It's gotten harder to elicit change because everything went to corporatization. And the ethical construct in the business world, and even in the not-for-profit world, is now being held to the measure of the business world. There's an acceleration in dehumanization, and the surfacing of a much more balance sheet mentality. But solving some of our very basic societal issues is going to take people just doing it because it just needs to be done, not because it pays off, not because your return on investment is within six months, a year, two years. [But our social] vision of the future has collapsed down. That's what prevents us as a society from really making changes that we need to make, for us, for our children, for our grandchildren. Change is going so slowly, that I'm just afraid that it will not come in my lifetime or certainly not in my career. And that is what drives me to do more, to push the system, to not accept the excuses.

From a clinical standpoint, to deal with complex issues that are so tied to the social and experiential lives of patients, on the one hand, and the broader, unjust social structure that deeply influences their lives on the other, Bruce emphasized the need to find ways for the healthcare system to break out of the conventional medical mold. In this effort, a good part of his time has been spent in just trying to keep the entities that own the Burgdorf Clinic from shutting it down, something they have contemplated and occasionally attempted for many years. At times, he has enlisted community support to save Burgdorf from decisions made in comfortable, well-decorated meeting rooms far removed from the neighborhoods that are home to Bruce's patients. For his untiring commitment to the poor and underserved, Bruce has earned a local reputation as a highly respected advocate for public health. No doubt, among those who have other allegiances, he has a rather different reputation. As history has shown, friends of the poor commonly have rich enemies.

In addition to his clinical work as medical director of the Burgdorf, Bruce serves as director of the Connecticut Area Health Education Center Program, which seeks to improve access to basic healthcare by linking local community groups with the resources of the University of Connecticut Health Center, and he is the medical director of Hartford's Department of Health and Human Services. Moreover, Bruce routinely participates in community health initiatives, such as building a city-wide collaboration of NGOs working on AIDS in the early years of the epidemic. It was through this participation in community initiatives that Merrill Singer, the lead author of this book, first met Bruce and was impressed to find a physician outside of the clinic working directly in the community with grassroots efforts trying to stem the AIDS epidemic. As noted, Bruce also was active in building a community garden to supply his patients with fresh vegetables that often are not available in stores near to where they live. This impressive list of commitments reflects Bruce's personal engagement with a persistent and urgent question raised for all people by Martin Luther King: "What are you doing for others?" In assessing a person's life, King asserted: "The ultimate measure of a man is not where he stands in moments of comfort and convenience, but where he stands at times of challenge and controversy" (quoted in Mintz 2015). Bruce, who was deeply impacted by the death of Reverend King, has engaged this question throughout his adult life.

Fighting a two-front war, against a dysfunctional healthcare system that is in continual retreat from serving poor and ethnic minority patients, and against the harsh health consequences of social inequality, sometimes Bruce fantasizes about getting away from the burden of the struggle for social health:

> I find that, if I leave my phone [at] home, I feel like a limb has been amputated. I'm disconnected. People can't get me 24/7. That's what I would love to do. I'm thinking of buying a sailboat because you're out in the middle of the ocean, unfortunately you still have a phone, and it may work, or it may not work, but if it works and somebody calls you, you still can't get back very quickly. You're dependent on the wind.

But, except in moments of fanciful day dreams, he has not sailed away; rather, he has stayed with his feet on the ground deep in the struggle for health and social justice, even if it often is a somewhat lonely uphill effort.

Morality Engaged

Bruce does not flee because he is bound by the moral compass he has long used to steer his life. Forged in a home experience populated by adult family members with strong ethical sensibilities and political perspectives that railed at the face of social injustice, he recognized early on that it was vital to him to do his best to remain a moral person despite living in an abidingly immoral world, a world in no small measure made immoral by greed, condescension, unfairness, and the power of social elites (Kleinman 2007). His personal mission, however ultimately unlikely to be fully achieved in the few short years of a human lifespan, has been to focus his energies on repairing the world, as he put it "to make the world a better place."

For Bruce, medicine and morality are inseparable. The issue of morality in social life has become a topic of growing interest and vibrancy in human research fields like anthropology in recent years. Anthropologists, Cheryl Mattingly (2012: 166) suggests, are particularly well situated to elicit first-person narratives in order to "illuminate the complexities of moral judgement and action in everyday life." While various paths have been trodden by different researchers concerned with morality, one line of concern involves finding a balanced approach that simultaneously focuses on the suffering caused by structural violence and political-economic inequalities, as well as on the way people attempt to construct meaningful moral lives, or what philosophers call "moral personhood." This effort entails recognizing that personal gain—in terms of material wealth, leisure hours, stature, etc.—is unacceptable if it causes harm to others, while personal sacrifice is desirable if it benefits those who are socially marginalized and structurally abused. Choosing to do the right thing in terms of this formulation is the heart and soul of moral personhood, and it is a choice that must be made by all people in and out of clinical practice. For doctors, a built-in issue in choosing to do what is right involves deciding how far to go upstream in addressing the causes of patient health problems. Is doing one's best to consciously address the immediate health disruptions of individual patients sufficient? Or do doctors have an obligation to do more than treat individual cases of disease and engage the social causes that repeatedly return patients to the clinic, fill their lives with stress and risk, subject them to injustice and exploitation, and rob them of years of life?

One of the things some anthropologists who have embarked on the assessment of morality have called for is an increase in "explicit detailed accounts of moral experience," recognizing that such experience occurs within particular historic, political, and economic contexts (Zigon and Throop 2014: 1). This goal can be achieved, they argue, by developing nuanced descriptions of social life and everyday moral experience as it is framed and conditioned by ongoing engagement with social structure. Throop (2014: 69), moreover, calls attention to the issue of moral disjunctures in which there is "a breach of expectation that reflects deeply rooted dissatisfaction with one's existential condition." Such breakdowns "provide space for moments of moral reflection . . . of our current self-experience and situation" (Throop 2014: 71). The self is "worked on" reflexively at moments of moral breakdown as well as through processes of ethical striving (Zigon 2007: 134). Moments of moral breakdown, therefore, provide windows for the anthropological assessment of the nature of morality as both an individual and social process.

The evolving anthropological discourse on morality is useful in building a nuanced understanding of Bruce's moral experience as well as his commitment to social medicine and his willingness to do battle on behalf of the well-being of the poor. Disjunctures certainly have played a role in Bruce's moral life. One of the disjunctures Bruce experienced, at the age of 9, as discussed in Chapter 3, was the assassination of his boyhood hero President Kennedy, and subsequent killings of Reverend Martin Luther King and Robert Kennedy. After the murders, Bruce's social grounding, his sense of order in a meaningful, well-arranged world was badly shaken. Camelot was shattered, and certainty and predictability became more elusive. Another disjuncture was his junior high school confrontation with choosing to be loyal to a friend over acceptance by an idolized social group that rejected that friend. This breakdown was of a very personal kind because it demanded a choice: to sacrifice popularity and stand with a friend, or to benefit from social approval by abandoning him. These experiences contributed to Bruce's ongoing focus on trying to do the right thing, the moral thing, even if it was not the easiest thing, even if it entailed sacrifice. In Bruce's view, as Martin Luther King (1964) eloquently stressed, "The time is always right to do what is right." This is not a platitude for Bruce. At his core, it is who he is.

While in high school, Bruce also experienced several disruptions while volunteering at Creedmoor State Hospital. The first was his rude introduction to how patients with mental health problems traditionally were warehoused under less than humane and healthy conditions. The second was being assigned the task of euthanizing rats for a drug experiment, an upsetting experience that brought to mind the Nazi extermination of Jews, sexual minorities, people with mentally illnesses, leftists, and others deemed to be subhuman. Both of these experiences pushed Bruce towards the embrace of a humane perspective, a moral framework in which people come first and are not subordinated to a self-aggrandizing drive for wealth, fame, or power.

While in medical school, Bruce experienced an additional disjuncture, as he watched his fellow students slowly stray from the humanist values that had first motivated them to study medicine. While many people are inspired to pursue a medical career as a way of helping people, under the influence of the cultural messages embedded in the curriculum (Hafler et al. 2011), during the long course of medical training there is a measurable decline in student idealism accompanied by a growing emphasis on the achievement of status and income. Further, for many, there comes to be a greater focus on personal lifestyle issues and family considerations (Morley et al. 2013). In other words, there tends to be a shrinking of focus from the good of humanity to the good life for self and family. As Mader and colleagues (2014) found in their study of two medical student cohorts:

> Our results provide further evidence that declines in medical student idealism may occur as early as the second year of medical education. Additionally, as students make choices in their medical careers, such as specialty choice or consideration of primary care, the influences of job security, student debt and social status increasingly outweigh idealistic motivations.

Bruce too came to be concerned about family issues and making an adequate income, but he made a fateful decision not to focus on one of the higher paying medical specialties (e.g., surgery, cardiology) and instead chose to become a primary care general internist, a field that addresses the acute and chronic healthcare needs of people from underserved communities but has only a middling ranking in the esteem hierarchy of biomedical specialties (Rosoff and Leone 1991). Drawing on his family history and values, Bruce resisted the multiple built-in messages and pressures to privilege personal advantage over doing the right thing.

The loss of idealism among medical students, it has been found, is sometimes overtly communicated by professors. Pooja Yerramilli (2014), a medical student at the Perelman School of Medicine of the University of Pennsylvania, recalls a lecture in which a professor stated: "All of you want to help people and save the world now. But, by the end of medical school, only two of you—if we're lucky—will remain idealistic." Indeed, she notes:

> Within the first three days of medical school, I had heard three different lecturers tell me that I would lose my compassion and empathy. By the end of the first three weeks, that number had grown to six. During the seventh such talk, I became frustrated. Why were my instructors telling me of "the inevitability of disillusionment" before I even hit the clinics?

As Hartzband and Groopman (2009:102) observe:

> Today's medical students are being inducted into a culture in which their profession is seen increasingly in financial terms. Add in such pressures as the need to pay off enormous debts, and it is not surprising that students' choices are dictated by the desire to maximize income and minimize work time . . . both of which press against engaging a truly social medicine approach to practice.

Yet, Bruce did not lose his compassion, his empathy, nor his idealism, in part because he had role models who did not lose theirs, and because he was on some level always engaged in a project of working on himself to assure that he stayed true to his moral obligation to the most vulnerable of patients. As a result, Bruce has become a role model for medical and other students who share his commitments. He noted:

I always tell the students and residents "don't talk with your hand on the doorknob." Take your hand off the doorknob and sit your ass down and say "tell me about it" to the patient. Because, if a patient feels that your head is not there then they may not tell you something—and that may be the last thing they tell you.

This approach impressed Connecticut State Commissioner Raul Pino who stated:

I think what best describes Bruce is this passion for . . . trying to educate his students in the same principles that he believes [in] and the idea that medicine is more than clinical practice, and having the social commitment to your patients, not only to the clinical needs but also to their social needs . . . Now we hear a lot about social determinants of health and equity, but probably without using those words he has been engaged in this practice for the longest. Probably [was] one of the pioneers if you look backwards . . . I have seen him in . . . the medical school. I have seen him teach . . . his med students. What he does is he translates to them, "This is why I have this passion and this is why you should also get engaged in this piece of work."

A fellow physician commented on Bruce's interaction with students saying:

I think he's a dynamic teacher. I haven't seen him a lot as a teacher, like directly with students. But he seems pretty dynamic as a teacher. It all depends on the subject matter, you know. He almost always would teach continuous quality improvement, which is no one's favorite topic. And so it was a little difficult to get people on board with that. However, he created a contest among the students to promote it, and having done that he actually got them involved in a way that they are enjoying it, so it wasn't necessarily the direct lecture that got them involved. He thought about a different way to get them involved in teaching—it's called stealth teaching.

Added another medical colleague:

A lot of what you're doing as a clinician is educating. And if you heard Bruce talk to his patients, he would go to great lengths to explain things to them and what this lab meant or that lab meant, really try to educate people in that sense. But he does love working with students and would always let's say . . . in his time here [at Burgdorf] he would usually be working with students or residents or a combination of the two and he was an excellent educator. He really put a lot of effort into it, was really interested in it and has very good educational skills. That translates to taking care of patients, obviously, because you're educating patients, but it also has some of the same elements of just forming personal connections with people. I would say that's probably his

> strength as an educator too is to build a strong personal bond with somebody, with a student to get them, to inspire them or get them interested and make them feel like they're engaging in something really exciting.

Physician Dr. Anton Alerte, who first met Bruce while a third-year medical student but subsequently got to know him as a colleague at the Burgdorf and at the UConn Health Center, explained:

> I've known him pretty much half my life . . . So I've seen him . . . speak on behalf of the downtrodden, you know, speak on behalf of his patients . . . work to find solutions around barriers, be the good angel, and the thorn in the side of people who may not have had the same vision or put the same priority on urban health that he did . . . All of the stuff that he kind of picks up, learns, and all of the interactions that he [has] and the connections that he makes are kind of focused back with the main topic, the theme being improving [the] health care of the underserved. So he has been very varied, you know, in his approach; he's been very varied in his way of thinking about the problem. But the central theme remains the same; the core principles remain the same. [Moreover,] he knows everybody . . . He has always been there. Whenever there's been a primary care movement, a new way of thinking, a new practice model, a new stratagem, a new way of making ends meet, a new way of enhancing services—he's always at the meeting, he's always at the table. So, I mean, there's never been one single moment; it's just kind of like the sun: it's always there . . . I participated in the Urban Service Track that he's involved with, so I've been to his house in the Berkshires [in Western Massachusetts] to do the seminars and retreats. We've been on a number of academic committees together. It's like the same people at different committee meetings all along the medical school because he is ubiquitous; he is practically ubiquitous at the medical school and heavily involved in medical education.

Dr. Keith vom Eigen, another colleague, noted:

> Well, as you probably know, Bruce is a very unique person. I would say his distinguishing characteristic is that he's a real extrovert; he's very much a people person; he is what I would call a schmoozer, that a lot of his way of interacting is very personal and very engaging and that he forms relationships very easily with people and takes interest in meeting people, you know, forming new relationships. And I think a lot of what he has been able to accomplish has come through that, for his ability to form new relationships. And I think that's sort of how he operates mostly, sort of on a personal level, on an interactive level with people. He's not really a . . . a details person, in that sort of planning something in detail and mapping it out and following through on a protocol or plan. That's not really what he does. What he does

> is, he has an idea and he talks to people and he kind of meets somebody who happens to fit his plan and then he will cultivate that relationship and kind of push things forward that way. He's always trying to move forward with his plans and ideas, and that's sort of how it happens more so than coming up with a plan that he then kind of works through systematically.

In recent years, many of the disjunctions Bruce has experienced involve the clash between his understanding of the role of medicine in society and the understandings and actions of those who head medical institutions and who privilege narrowly construed financial factors over the pressing healthcare needs of the most vulnerable patients. He stressed:

> I think that in some ways my recent battles around my clinic and everything are disheartening to me. I had not imagined that as I go into my 60s that I would be fighting the same battles I was fighting 27 years ago, as far as the existence of the clinic, the resources for the poor, and frankly the disrespect [from institutional decision-makers in local health care, their] . . . lack of moral compass. That's disturbing to me and I'm not naive . . . I would have hoped that at this point in my life and the history of the United States . . . if the *tikkun olam* era had somehow evolved . . . I do wish it were just a little easier. I wish the Burgdorf was better resourced. Again, I wish I still wasn't banging my head against everyone. Some of my students say that's the way I like it. But [he joked], enough of a good thing. It builds character, but I'm enough of a character. I say to the students, "I like what I do, but sometimes I do it more than I like."

This sentiment is reflected in a comment about Bruce by Health Commissioner Raul Pino: "His patients have his cell phone number. And sometimes it rings too much. But that says a lot. I mean, his commitment is just unparalleled, absolutely."

Disjuncture experiences pushed Bruce to find spaces, such as less overtly impacted natural settings, to reflect on his values and how to remain a moral person, as he understood it, in a world where the violation of his values is ingrained through structural violence into the hierarchies and daily processes of social life. As Bruce stated:

> The woods are . . . my special hiding place. It's a place that I go sometimes and just sit and write in my journal . . . you have to think about where do I want to be? What do I want to be doing? What type of person do I want to wind up [as] . . . Not every day, because we're all caught up in the drama of our lives, but every once in a while, to reflect a little bit about how it's going.

Watching the clock of his life, Bruce speculated on the possibility of making significant changes in Hartford over the next several years, as well as considering who would drag their feet and not let anything significant be accomplished:

> Is it possible in the next few years to pull something off? [Can we get the universities] to belly up to the bar with their resources in an open handed way to address Hartford and all of its ills? And not just to do it grant by grant [based on] what's in it for them, but to make the commitment up front and then trust that the rest will follow. I think that the [university] has enormous resources. To [allow us] to really pull together and look at the issues in Hartford and try and figure it out, sort of a Jeff Canada-type approach [with] the Harlem Children's Zone.

Canada, an educator and social activist, started the Harlem Children's Zone in a 24-block-area of Harlem, New York to increase pre-college and college graduation rates among local youth. Eventually, the zone grew to 97 blocks and has served over 13,000 students. The program is based on providing youth with a continuum of services to support their skills and knowledge development. Evaluations of the program show that it has had considerable success, including a dropout rate of less than 10 percent, which is significantly lower than the national average of 43.6 percent. Test scores on state exams also have been very high (New York Department of Education 2012). Program graduates had a 93 percent college acceptance rate in 2015 (Harlem Children's Zone 2015).

But Bruce has found it hard to push for this kind of coordinated multifaceted program for Hartford:

> Historically, organizations chase dollars and universities are no different. They identify a grant opportunity, partner with the city and others. If the grant isn't funded, as often happens, everyone walks away. UConn tries . . . a few years ago, the School of Education spearheaded a grant to create a promise zone in Hartford, part of an Obama program early in his tenure. I was involved, as were a pretty diverse collection of individuals and organizations . . . but when it didn't get funded it fell apart. What I've tried to do is get the University to the table in a more open-ended way . . . get them to work with the city and identify "Here's what needs to be done. Here are models in other cities. Now let's figure out how to get the money. Let's start doing it." Some projects don't work right away and need time, but that's the thing—I don't have many years left. So I feel pressure to stop talking and just do it. There's such a hierarchy within the system that has gotten solidified over the last several years. It used to be much more fluid. Now you have to get sign off from several layers with the likelihood that some layer will say no . . . and this stifles creativity and dissuades students and faculty from getting involved in the first place.

In the end, it is clear that Bruce's life and career choices are guided by an embrace of what has been called the struggle for bread and roses. This cultural symbolism dates to early in the twentieth century. For nine weeks in 1912, during the Lawrence Textile Strike, a labor struggle united workers of diverse immigrant communities and languages under the effective leadership of women. The strike began when workers in the cotton weaving room of the Everett Mill turned off their thunderous looms and stood silently next to their machines. When a factory official, startled by this rebellious comportment in his normally docile workers demanded to know what was going on, he was given a simple explanation: "Not enough pay." For the workers, who earned about $8.75 a week, a 32-cent cut that had been imposed on their wages meant the difference between their families surviving, if barely, in squalid tenements and starving in the streets. Even without the pay cut, workers faced horrendous conditions. They were exposed to respiratory infections such as pneumonia and tuberculosis, due to inadequate ventilation, and to diseases like chronic obstructive pulmonary disease associated with inhaling textile dust, and they were subject to routine workplace accidents that maimed their bodies or took their lives. Within a few weeks of the initial work stoppage, over 10,000 workers in Lawrence went on strike. It is said, and was written about by Upton Sinclair in his edited book, *The Cry for Justice: An Anthology of the Literature of Social Protest* (1915), that during marches, the strikers carried signs that read "We want bread, but we want roses, too!" This slogan came from a poem written by James Oppenheim, published in 1911 and republished in Oppenheim's book, that included the line "Yes, bread we fight for—but we fight for roses, too." The idea of uniting bread and roses was intended to graphically express the fundamental human need not only for sustenance but for dignity as well. The roses represented a deep-seated desire that took workers' imaginations beyond food for the body to nourishment for the human spirit. From the standpoint of the strikers, who worked 10–14-hour life- and energy-consuming labor shifts and who daily faced the brutality of social inequality, roses stood for the good life, a thing that only the rich were able to afford. The world that Bruce too seeks to achieve is a world of bread and roses, and, being a doctor, of course, a world of health, a world of well-being, and a world of meaningful and fulfilling lives for all people. For Bruce, all of this is medicine, as Virchow and all other social medicine physicians understand it. But it is not the medicine encountered by most patients in corporate America, and they are increasingly hurting, although not equally so, because of it.

Burnout

Physicians are hurting too, although certainly not in the same ways as the poor. The term that has come to label this pain is "burnout," which has been defined as feeling "emotionally exhausted, depersonalized (i.e., cynical and detached), and ineffective" (Epstein and Privitera 2016). Physicians who are burned out experience "an erosion in values, dignity, spirit, and will" (Maslach and Leiter 1997: 17). Nationally, physician burnout has reached epidemic levels (West et al. 2016). In a countrywide study of physicians across medical specialties, using an instrument called the Burnout Inventory (Shanafelt et al. 2012), 45.8 percent of physicians reported at least one symptom of burnout (e.g., loss of enthusiasm for work, feelings of cynicism, and a low sense of personal work-related accomplishment). Significant levels of differences in burnout were found by specialty, with physicians practicing family medicine, general internal medicine, and emergency medicine showing the highest rates of burnout. Compared with a probability-based sample of non-physician working adults in the US, physicians were more likely to have symptoms of burnout (37.9 percent vs. 27.8 percent) and to be dissatisfied with their work vs. non-work life balance (40.2 percent vs. 23.2 percent). Findings of other studies (e.g., Spickard, Gabbe, and Christensen 2002, Shanafelt et al. 2009) suggest that physician burnout may diminish professionalism, adversely influence quality of care, lead to a reduction in availability to patients, increase the risk for medical errors, and encourage early retirement. Burnout also appears to have negative personal consequences for physicians' personal lives, including contributing to broken relationships and divorce, the emergence of alcohol abuse, depression and suicidal ideation, and suicide (Shanafelt et al. 2011, Schernhammer 2005).

A sign of the adverse effects of physician burnout are turnover rates, although other factors impact these rates as well (e.g., the state of the economy). A survey of medical groups found an average physician turnover rate of 6.8 percent in 2012, a rise from 5.9 percent in 2009, during the recession, and from 6.4 percent in 2005 (Irving 2013). Turnover was also high (11.5 percent) among physician assistants and nurse practitioners. Turnover rates of hospital employees show they are greater than other fields of employment (Brimmer 2012).

What is driving physician burnout? One study of note examined the relationship between professionalism and burnout among medical students (Dyrbye et al. 2010). Researchers found that students suffering burnout were more likely to report engaging in one or more unprofessional actions (e.g., cheating/dishonest clinical behaviors, like reporting a physical exam finding as being normal when it was not actually assessed) than those not suffering from burnout (35.0 percent vs. 21.9 percent). Students dealing with burnout also were less likely to report having altruistic attitudes regarding their responsibility to society. Thus, they were less likely to intend to provide care for the medically underserved than those without burnout.

Another expression of this problem is the number of medical students who decide not to pursue residency training and instead are lured into corporate jobs in biotechnology, digital health, or other nonclinical positions. In California, in 2011, only 68 percent of medical school students chose to move on to a residency program, giving the schools a ranking of 117th among 123 U.S. medical schools. A national network of medically trained individuals who have dropped out of clinical practice has formed called "The Drop Out Club." It was started as a support website by six medical school classmates who left medicine for other careers. By 2015, the club had over 23,000 members, and its website is now a job-posting site. Interviews with former medical students who have left medicine have shown that they are interested in finding ways to improve doctor–patient interaction, including strengthening the patient voice in clinical encounters (e.g., through the development of patient-friendly apps, pill bottles that signal when a dose has been missed, implanted sensors, or other technologies). Dropouts also complain that those on the frontlines of healthcare, like family physicians, are poorly paid and routinely overworked (Farr 2015).

In his book *Doctored: The Disillusionment of an American Physician*, cardiologist Sandeep Jauhar (2014) provides further insight on this dilemma for medicine. He argues that being a caring and altruistic physician has become cost-prohibitive. Insurance companies do not pay doctors for spending time with patients, let alone walking out of the clinic and into the worlds patients inhabit in their communities. Insurance companies do pay for laboratory tests and high-tech scans, and as a result, these are ordered even when not fully warranted. Jauhar even reveals that his own brother, also a cardiologist, refers to patients as "commodities." To pay his medical school loans, live the comfortable lifestyle in New York City that he wants, and pay for his child's private school, Jauhar accepts speaking fees from a pharmaceutical company that makes a heart medication he prescribes to his patients. A cardiologist who Jahuar works for on weekends to make extra money told him "I tried to practice ethical medicine, but it didn't pay." He concludes, as seen in Chapter 2, that "you have to motivate doctors to do the right thing [because] nothing today influences physicians' behavior (even if unconsciously) like hard cash."

This feature of contemporary physician behavior reflects a shift that has occurred from social values to market values in biomedicine, as suggested in Chapter 2. This shift is seen by the fact that many physicians are "so alienated and angered by the relentless pricing of their day that they wind up having no desire to do more than the minimum required for the financial bottom line" (Hartzband and Groopman 2009: 102). In short, the medical industrial complex plays no small role in physician burnout and its consequences, both for physicians and patients. Corporatization processes that permeate medical schools and medical practice, turning patients and their diseases into commodities, warps biomedicine in the US, transforming a field with great potential to relieve suffering into one that all too often inflicts it, as well as one that narrowly defines its focus to billable activities and away from the upstream causes of disease.

Yet, despite growing pressures, some doctors avoid, or at least are not hampered by, this trap and provide a guiding light for others to follow. The same can be said of nurses and others working in the healthcare system. Nurses, for example, especially those employed in hospital settings, commonly complain that their work conditions are not conducive to providing their patients with the safest and highest level of care (Aiken et al. 2003). Research suggests that the work environment and staffing levels for nurses affect both nurse burnout and job satisfaction (Aiken et al. 2008), and nurses' working conditions, in turn, have been shown by the Institute of Medicine (2003) to be linked to patient satisfaction. These patterns were confirmed during Merrill Singer's recent brief hospitalization, where he was struck by the regularity of the frustration voiced in interpersonal conversations by care staff (e.g., nurses, patient care technicians) about lost staff, heavier workloads, and lost services and service units resulting from the hospital's merger several years earlier into a larger multi-hospital conglomerate. Commitment to patient care, however, remains high as many struggle for a better healthcare system (Burger, Higgins, and Ross 2015).

Modeling an Alternative

Studies on the qualities of people others look to as role models (Price-Mitchell 2015, Rakatansky 1994) have identified a number of common traits: having passion for what you do and being able to excite others to share your imagination; embracing a clear set of values and living by them; possessing a commitment to others rather than being self-focused; having a degree of selflessness and broad tolerance, and having the fortitude to overcome obstacles and roadblocks. Throughout his life, beginning in junior high school, where he was president of the Junior High Student Council, and continuing in high school where he served as the valedictorian of his graduating high school class, Bruce has comfortably fit the definition of a role model and incipient leader. In addition to being a colorful and likeable person possessed of a self-deprecating and witty sense of humor, he is highly passionate about the social responsibility he feels to address the health and social needs of disadvantaged populations. For him, to do otherwise would be to live an immoral life. His value set is firmly established and, while not inflexible, is not subject to changing whim or circumstance, or to appeals to exchange his determination to make a difference in the world for personal rewards. In his commitment to the poor, Bruce has demonstrated qualities of selflessness, although he is far from a saint or devoid of contradictions. He is a man characterized by many of the foibles and frailties common to our species and those enhanced by western cultures, but he strives to not be limited by self-doubt or other personal flaws and uncertainties. In his prolonged battle to preserve and expand the work of the Burgdorf Clinic and in other initiatives designed to challenge health inequality, Bruce has shown great stamina and the ability to get things done. It is for all of these reasons that patients, students, co-workers, and community leaders alike look to him for leadership. It is the reason the lead author, Merrill Singer, came to know Bruce, become his patient for a number of years, and decide to write this book. Some stories merit telling, and some people are exceptionally worthy of knowing. Bruce is one of them.

One place that Bruce has had a particular impact is with the medical students he teaches in his positions as Professor of Medicine and Associate Dean for Primary Care at the University of Connecticut School of Medicine. In these capacities, in 2007, he helped develop the Urban Service Track at the medical school, a special mentorship program designed to train doctors, dentists, nurses, physician assistants, social workers, and pharmacists who are committed to addressing the healthcare needs of underserved populations in Connecticut's cities. Students enrolled in this program, about fifty a year, are trained to have competencies in culture and linguistics, population health, health policy, advocacy, healthcare financing and management, leadership, community resources, working successfully in interprofessional healthcare teams, and quality improvement. Participants receive interdisciplinary in-class education about the health and social issues facing vulnerable urban populations like the poor, the homeless, children, refugees, and the elderly; attend highly interactive educational retreats with faculty and students from all of the participating disciplines; and gain enhanced service learning experience by working in homeless shelters, community health fairs, and community health centers. Commenting on his experience in the Urban Service Track, dental medicine student Marcus Moss stated:

> They put me in the very environment I wanted to be in anyway, they're the gateway, they give students the opportunity to have [their] passions reinvigorated. I just really appreciate the Urban Service Track for taking the passion that I have inside of me and showing me how to act upon that passion in a productive way. (Quoted in Urban Service Track Video 2016)

Role models are known to have a strong influence on the career choices of medical students, and students report receiving counseling and advice on their career directions from those they identify as their role models. From the perspective of medical students, a potential mentor's personality, clinical skills, competence, and teaching ability have all been found to be important (Reuler and Nardone 1994, Wright 1996). Other qualities of physician mentors that have been identified by medical students include spending time with students, stressing the importance of the doctor–patient relationship and the psychosocial aspects of patient care, and engaging in activities that build relationships with students (Wright, Wong, and Newill 1997). Again, these traits well describe Bruce's approach to teaching medical students, which is heavily influenced by his life experience:

> My own self-doubt is probably what has driven me beyond being a high school custodian, which is what I was in 11th grade. I do believe that it's the little turns along the way that sometimes are determinate of the ultimate outcome of your life. When you look at the innumerable seemingly inconsequential decisions we make every day . . . do you make that phone call, do you talk to that student, do you not answer that email of some kid? You know yours may be the moment, that little influence that changes their life.

In a study of medical student mentoring at the University of California, San Francisco, participants reported that their mentors most commonly provided them with personal support, role modeling of the physician role, and career advice. Personal support included providing motivation, moral support, and personal advice. Mentors also offered medical students assistance in selecting a medical specialty and with making decisions about the residency application process (Aagaard and Hauer 2003).

In talking about what he tries to teach medical students, Bruce recalled his time working in a nursing home and the challenges of that kind of work, which he described as "very hard work, probably the hardest thing I've ever done." But the experience, as described in Chapter 3, taught him to remain connected with

> the humanistic side of medicine because the patients that I was caring for took every ounce of compassion in me to keep caring because I was cleaning their shit and their piss and their vomit. It was exhausting, and it was also

> sad; patients asked me to kill them . . . to end their suffering. I had to find my compass at a relatively early stage. And to be honest, I've suggested to UConn that every student should do that, be a nurse's aide for a few days. It was there, in that nursing home, that I developed patient care skills that I would not have had, but I also gained insight into the health care team, and that it's not just the doctor or the nurse that make the difference in the lives of our patients. It allows you to gain respect for all those other folks and the work they do which, frankly, comes across just in your tone of voice and the way you treat coworkers and talk to people. You develop a sense of humility I guess. I'm not sure all my students or colleagues share that and that's something that I looked for when I was on [medical school] admissions for twelve years. I always tried to look for students that I sensed had that commitment and that humility . . . that someone's not so impressed with themselves and the status of the medical profession [that] they're not going to be able to interact in a very equal way with others, with colleagues from other professions, and with staff down the continuum. And that they will be able to talk to people on a humanistic level that gets them on board. There are times when you just have to tell someone to do their job. I don't have a problem with that, but for all the other interactions, my parents taught me that you catch more flies with honey. I've had students who have been very concerned about the acculturation process of medical education and that they would lose their soul [because a medical school education can produce] arrogance. But you have to work to hold onto your humanity, compassion, and empathy, and everything else. Someone who's incredibly arrogant is . . . narcissistic, and if you're narcissistic it's very hard to be empathetic, perhaps impossible to be empathetic.

One of the challenges of teaching medical students is conveying to them the realization that

> if you save people from one thing, something else is going to get them. That's cynical, but it's absolutely true. So anybody going into medicine thinking they're going to cure everybody, has a lot of frustration and disappointment in their future. But you can help every patient, absolutely. There will always be patients that you can't cure, that all you can do is be there for them. You can call it doing the social work thing, or the case manager thing, but it's doctoring. It's making sure if she's in pain she gets morphine. If she's incontinent, she gets a commode. Helping her to sit up comfortably and all those small things, those acts of caring, that maybe you think you, the doctor, shouldn't even be doing. You should have staff that can handle those things, but unfortunately [I don't] because we are caring for the underserved and the hospital has stripped us to the bone, and others have let them do it. But doing those small things have brought me ever so much closer to my patients.

Being a teacher is important to Bruce because he realizes this kind of work can have long-term impact on people's lives:

> If you can change an event now, you don't necessarily know what the ripples will be from that action. It's the metaphor of throwing a pebble into a pond, and knowing that those ripples really go on almost forever. When you are a teacher you never know when your influence stops. You don't know when you influence a kid [if] they will go on to something that they would never have done, or looking at the negative side, had you not done it, have you saved that child from some terrible fate? I have influenced a lot of people over the years, patients and families, and kids. A lot of [medical students] come here to shadow [me as I go about my clinical duties]. I find it hard to say no so I am crazy busy a good part of the time. Anyone you have hanging around shadowing requires mentoring and that takes time. And you know, that is the most precious commodity in a lot of ways now. As you get older, it becomes more precious, because there is less of it left. And I do waste a lot of my time.

In fact, for Bruce, being a teacher is a constant process, even with his patients. For example, he once treated a woman who came to the clinic with her two nieces, aged 4 and 10. Bruce showed his stethoscope to the children and taught them how to use it. They listened to his heart and to their own hearts. As they played with the stethoscope, he asked them if they wanted to be doctors when they grew up and both children replied in the affirmative. He commented:

> you never know when you are giving somebody a goal at an early age that keeps them on track . . . . There are so many ways that kids get diverted and waste their lives. If you just put out that little extra something, you may be saving someone's life. (Quoted in Meldrum 2010: 94)

Some of those Bruce has mentored over the years were not young medical students but already practicing physicians who left their home country and migrated to the US. Among those who have come to Hartford are Jews who fled discrimination in the Soviet Union:

> Burgdorf became the center of that settlement from the health care side. I was working with Jewish Family Services in doing entrance physicals and taking care of this community. Also doing counseling for a lot of Russian doctors who came here. They had to do a residency all over [again] and so the Burgdorf became the training site for a lot of these immigrant doctors. And I used to counsel them—literally—I was like a guidance counselor. And you would have these "new Americans," that's what they were called, come in and we would talk about where they were, what they had done, where

> they had worked in the Soviet Union, and what their aspirations were. We would try to get them a job in the medical field, so someone would become a phlebotomist or an EKG technician, or whatever it might be, while they were studying for their boards. And once they got those, they'd apply for medical residency. We had a whole bunch! In fact, I just got an email, you know "Season's Greetings" from Irina and David who were two residents that went through that process and came to UConn, came to the Burgdorf for the Clinic, as primary care/internal medicine residents.

New Directions, Enduring Concerns

As the interviews for this book were being conducted, Bruce made a weighty decision about his future. In April 2016, he sent a letter to all of his patients informing them that he would be leaving the Burgdorf Clinic to take the position of Medical Director of the not-for-profit Community Health Center Association of Connecticut's (CHCACT) Practice Transformation Network. CHCACT is the umbrella organization for all the federally qualified community health centers in the state. As Bruce explained:

> The Burgdorf Health Center, its staff and patients have been my medical home and my passion for nearly three decades . . . But in my new CHCACT role I can use the experience and knowledge I've gained over a lifetime of working with the underserved to assist community health centers across the state to provide more effective and efficient healthcare . . . These are exciting times of rapid transformation in healthcare delivery across the country with systems transitioning from fee-for-service, illness-based care to more global approaches to population health and prevention that promise better health, and patient healthcare experience at a more affordable cost for our nation. It is forcing clinicians to expand their focus beyond the walls of the clinic into the homes and neighborhoods where our patients live. (Quoted in Woods 2016)

In announcing Bruce's appointment, Mollie Melbourne, chief operating officer and acting CEO of the Community Health Center Association of Connecticut, Inc. stated, "For this critical new role we were searching for a leading expert who best understood the health care landscape in Connecticut and we found that in Dr. Gould and his career experience" (quoted in Woods 2016).

In assessing whether to take the position of Medical Director of the new initiative, Bruce

> decided that this as an opportunity to go out with a bang, to really do something impactful. So working with the community health centers, who treat the most challenging of our poor, and giving them the tools and resources to address those challenges, would be an absolute good. It would allow me

> to create the changes that I wanted to implement at the Burgdorf. As part of my job, I asked that even though Burgdorf is not a community health center, could I bring those resources to the Burgdorf, and they said "absolutely."

In breaking the news to his patients, in addition to the letter he sent out, he wanted to be sure to

> tell as many of my patients face to face that I'm not going to be there and would have to transition them to another doctor. This happened very, very quickly. It was an opportunity that I never expected to get at my age . . . being asked to fix the health care system. To use the sum total of your experience of 35-plus years in medicine and apply it to the reality of health care delivery to the underserved in pursuit of better outcomes, healthier populations and affordable care . . . was a challenge and an opportunity. Not a cake walk, because transforming the system to where it will need to be for a global value-based payment system, while you're still working under the same old dysfunctional fee-for-service system—is insanely difficult. Fee-for-service thrives on volume . . . the more patients you see, the more money you make . . . so the less well your patients remain, the more they need to see the doctor, the better the bottom line. That's why it's called an illness-based model. With a value-based payment, you are paid similarly whether you see the patient or not. If through effective screening and case management, patients are healthier, don't need acute care visits or urgent or emergent care, and if they are healthy enough to avoid the hospital, the most expensive and least efficient part of the system, then you get to keep more of the health care dollar. You are paid, incentivized, to keep people healthier. It's an opportunity really very much in sync with the rest of my career . . . one more and, perhaps, final opportunity. Also, it's a 3½–4 year gig, and I'll be over 65 years by the end. At that point, I might be ready to slow down. To be honest, I have two beautiful grandkids and I do want to spend time with them before they're too old to care.

One of the motivations for Bruce accepting the new job was the health problems he was starting to experience because of the building that houses the Burgdorf:

> they told me at employee health that if I kept working at the Burgdorf I would eventually get sensitized to the point that I would be symptomatic all the time and they were right . . . I've reached that point. The hospital was aware of the health issues I was having, they were informed by the occupational health docs I saw at UConn and Yale but they chose to ignore it. It was a wet building, the roof leaked from the day we walked in . . . maintenance had been deferred . . . it needed a new roof, carpets, and so on. My wife wanted me to leave, to save myself, but I couldn't do that . . . couldn't

leave my staff behind. I could get another job, many of them didn't have that option. This went on for four years . . . with UConn asking for entry into the building to inspect for mold, St. Francis refusing. I filed a Workers Comp case, not because I was going to leave, but to get them to fix the building. It was denied, and nothing was done. The hospital saved money by not doing maintenance over the last ten years and there really is no one to hold them accountable for the condition of the facility or the promises they made to the community. They believe that they are above that. That those promises don't matter. Finally, as I was leaving, the hospital finally rehabbed the building . . . new roof, ventilation system, carpets, paint . . . but why the wait?

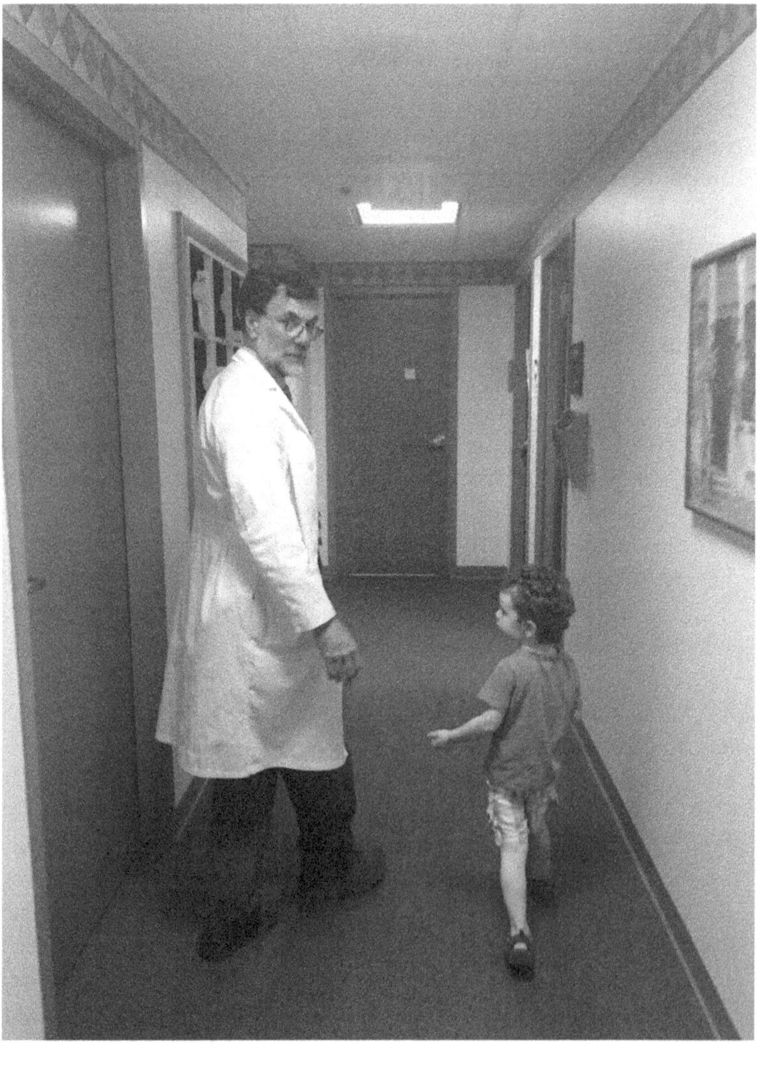

FIGURE 6.1 Bruce and his grandson

Also Bruce grew tired of recurring "discussions" with administration about staff:

> Many, if not most, of our patients are poor, old, sick and intensely complex. And I do take more time [with them]. I've been told by the committee that I take too much time; they'd prefer 15-minute visits. That I should just tell patients that we're only going to do two problems today. The rest, I'll have you come back five times in the next four weeks. But that's not the way it works. It's not the way I was taught to do good care. I don't think it's the way we want to teach our students to give care. My sense going forward, however, is that there will be a paradigm shift at some point toward value- and quality-driven care and this will reclaim health care delivery for the patients, and frankly, for the doctors, the providers. The present system is not sustainable. My hope is that as the health care system evolves toward population health and value-based payment, we will reclaim some of the dollars that have gone to Wall Street, so that you can still provide a good living, a solid wage for everyone in the health care system, perhaps less for the administrators at the top, and create a sustainable, smartly staffed health care team that creates better health for patients at an affordable cost and allows clinicians and staff to go home at night not rung out like a dishrag.

Bruce acknowledges that he has "gotten [many] letters from concierge medicine companies, that's where doctors are escaping to." Concierge or retainer medicine involves a contractual relationship between a patient and a primary care physician in which the patient pays an annual fee for private care, often in addition to other charges. In exchange for a significant fee, concierge doctors agree to limit their patient load to ensure enhanced availability of time for contracting patients. Enhanced services may include same-day access to your doctor; access to the doctor's cell phone and the ability to text message your doctor; unlimited office visits with no co-pays; limited waiting time to be seen by your doctor; a focus on preventive care; an unhurried pace during doctor–patient interactions, and appointment scheduling that is convenient for the patient. With annual fees of $5,000 or more, concierge care is not accessible to most poor and working people but, rather, is an evolving form of privileged care for the wealthy. In 2012, the American Academy of Private Physicians reported that there were 4,400 concierge doctors in the US and the number is growing. As assessed by Kathleen Stoll, deputy executive director of Families USA, a healthcare consumer advocacy organization, "It is a step towards a two-tiered healthcare system: a system where the rich get first-choice care and the not-so-rich get second-choice care" (Leonard 2012). Of course, we already have a tiered healthcare system. Under the Affordable Care Act (ACA), there are four tiers, marked by metal designations, with different levels in the percentage of healthcare costs covered by health insurance. The tiers are: platinum (90 percent coverage), gold (80 percent coverage). silver (70 percent coverage), and bronze (60 percent coverage). For example, under the ACA, almost 13,000 members of Congress and their office staffers are enrolled in gold-tier Small Business Health Option Program plans found on the Washington, DC health insurance exchange and they receive a 75 percent subsidy paid for by taxpayers. In contrast, by the end of 2015, with the ACA in effect, 28.5 million people were on the bottom even below the tier system, as they were still without health insurance coverage (Kaiser Family Foundation 2016). About 70 percent of the over 11 million people covered by the law have silver-tier plans, but 22 percent only have bronze level coverage and must pay out of pocket for 30 percent of their healthcare costs (Glover 2016).

In his new position, Bruce began providing direction and medical oversight to CHCACT's network of 15 federally qualified health centers throughout Connecticut and its new statewide federally funded CT Practice Transformation Network (CT-PTN). CT-PTN is one of 29 practice networks funded by the Centers for Medicare and Medicaid Innovation, a component of the U.S. Department of Health and Human Services, in September 2015. CT-PTN is slated to receive up to $17.25 million over four years. The mission of the PTN is to support a network of over 2,000 primary care clinicians in Connecticut to improve the quality and safety of their work by providing resources and support, enabling them to learn and draw motivation from one another, and supporting them to achieve a set of common goals, including improved patient care, better patient health, and reduced medical cost. Emphasis on quality improvement in medicine was sparked by the 1999 Institute of Medicine report entitled *To Err is Human: Building a Safer Health System* (Kohn, Corrigan, and Donaldson 1999), which acknowledged there were serious safety issues in U.S. healthcare. According to the report, at that time at least 44,000 people a year, according to one study, and as many as 98,000, according to another study, die in hospitals in the US because of medical errors that could have been prevented. The report emphasized that even based on the lower figures, medical errors in hospital exceed the toll in lives taken by motor vehicle accidents, breast cancer, or even AIDS. Other tolls exacted by medical errors include patient suffering and lost productivity, heightened medical costs, loss of trust in healthcare providers, and diminished morale among physicians. While the IOM report drew immediate professional and public attention to the need for measuring healthcare quality and outcomes in order to diminish errors, improve patient well-being, and cut costs, studies since the report show the problem remains. A meta-analysis of four more recent studies (James 2013) found that at least 210,000 and as many as 400,000 deaths per year were associated with preventable harm in hospitals. Moreover, serious patient harm appears to be 10–20 times greater than lethal harm. To reduce this significant toll in human lives and suffering, the authors of the study stress that patient harm in hospitals needed to be taken more seriously and strongly recommended fully engaging patients and their support networks during hospital stays, systematically seeking patients' perspectives on identifying harms, and implementing transparent accountability when harm occurs.

The approach implemented by the PTN to address error and improve the health benefits of primary care, called "quality improvement" (QI), is structured around a commitment to the use of quality assessment procedures. This entails training clinicians to systematically track and assess their performance as healthcare providers over time and to use this information in regularly making changes to improve their performance. Training and support provided by PTN includes furnishing information through an online portal, making available skill-building coaching and feedback, and supplying skilled intervention to help primary care practitioners to assist patients to achieve their health and quality-of-life goals (Hysong, Best, and Pugh 2006). Determination of the specific needs of individual primary care facilities like the Burgdorf Clinic begins with an outside readiness evaluation to determine preparedness for the adoption of best practices, receptivity to learning new approaches, and willingness to engage in data-driven improvements in everyday practice. The kinds of data made available to practitioners comes from two sources. First, there is information from within the medical practice itself, from registries of standardized information about patients who share a condition or experience, electronic health records, and the audit of medical charts. Second, there are data from beyond a healthcare practice, such as patients' use of emergency departments or their record of hospitalizations. Assessments suggest that without this kind of information, providers are often flying in the dark, while tending to assume their performance is better in some areas than is warranted, in part because many doctors overestimate their interpersonal skills and abilities as communicators (Fong, Anat, and Longnecker 2010, Palmieri and Stern 2009, Patel et al. 2016). A key strategy in the use of in-practice and outside patient data is known as "benchmarking." This involves comparing a practice's performance on a set of selected measures to the accepted standards in the field, such as achieving a certain level of patient adherence to specific health-maintenance behaviors (e.g., regularly measuring blood glucose levels among patients with diabetes). The PTN is specifically designed to improve health outcomes for three common conditions frequently seen at health centers like Burgdorf and similar primary care facilities: asthma, diabetes, and hypertension.

The PTN recognizes that given the existing organization of healthcare in the US, as described throughout this book, most primary care practices lack the time, resources—like new health information technologies that allow the collection of data on clinical performance—and hands-on knowledge needed to incorporate QI infrastructure into everyday healthcare routines. Instead, because of the structure of medical financing, most primary care providers require "large patient panels, leading them to focus on the daily demands of patient care rather than continuously improving the way they provide care" (Taylor et al. 2013).

A key element of the PTN is the Patient-Centered Medical Home (PCMH). The PCMH is not a place but rather a model of primary medical care that dates to the 2007 adoption by the major primary care physician associations—namely the American Academy of Family Physicians, the American Academy of Pediatrics, the American College of Physicians, and the American Osteopathic Association—of the Joint Principles of the Patient-Centered Medical Home. These principles include providing care that is patient-centered and involves including patients and their families fully in decisions about their treatment; understanding and respecting each patient's unique configuration of needs, culture, values, and preferences, treating the whole person not just their array of diseases; designation of an interprofessional team of providers as wholly accountable for prevention, wellness, acute care, and chronic care; regular communication with patients, and inclusion of QI in provider facilities. Observed Bruce:

> Cultural competence means understanding the beliefs of your patient, and reaching into those beliefs to better understand their perception of their illness or treatment, to give them comfort or to give them what they need, so that they can either make it through treatment or perhaps let go. (Quoted in Meldrum 2010: 94)

In explaining the importance of culture, he cited the case of a Puerto Rican woman he once treated:

> She was one of my patients who I had been taking care of for a whole bunch of years. I had gotten her through a marriage—an abusive marriage and divorce—now she was older. She was in her 60s. Very pleasant, nice woman and she came to me one day in the clinic, a little embarrassed, and said, "There is a spirit living in my apartment." I said, "Ok, I can deal with that." She said that a year previously she had clicked her tongue . . . discounting when some of her neighbors living in her apartment building had said that a lot of people had died in the apartment, that there were spirits running around, and she had thought [her neighbors] were crazy. And now, there was something living with her in her apartment. A presence, a spirit, that she said would lie down with her when she went to sleep and get up in the morning, and she was scared. I made sure she wasn't psychotic, you know, hearing voices, seeing ghosts or whatever. She told me that she had only told me, and her priest . . . So I called her priest and I thought, "Wow, how interesting is this—a consult with the church?" I explained what was happening. He got a little upset with me. I said, "Maybe we could do an exorcism." And he said, a bit perturbed, "We don't do that anymore!" So plan B, my social worker here [at Burgdorf] is from the island, from Puerto Rico, so we put our heads together with this patient.

The new plan was to assist the woman to visit Puerto Rico to see a traditional spiritist healer, a person experienced in identifying and removing the souls of the deceased that are stalled in their spiritual development and cling to the world of mortals. These spirits can cause illness. Although spiritist healers live and practice in the Puerto Rican community of Hartford, they are not well known to the biomedical healthcare system (Singer and Garcia 1989). Continued Bruce, in Puerto Rico his patient saw

> this woman, who basically did a ritual, you can call it an exorcism, whatever it might be, and [my patient] came back cured. And we joked that there's no way to bill [for] it. It was the interaction of mind, body and culture. People have cultural belief systems . . . We as practitioners need to be open and sensitive and value everyone's culture for a lot of reasons: (a) it's allows us to better care for our patients, (b) it allows us to really hear our patients, to listen with a different and perhaps more accepting ear so that we can effectively, within their own held belief system, try and make their lives better. I could have just clicked my tongue and gone to the backroom and said, "This lady is nuts." But instead, I listened, and I called her priest to see if he had any ideas, but I think in some ways he had clicked his tongue.

Now that he has left the Burgdorf, Bruce's attention is focused on improving the quality of care, including cultural awareness and sensitivity, at community health centers across Connecticut, including, eventually, his former clinic. This has meant a shift toward health promotion and disease prevention, and away from a concentration on one-on-one treatment of patients as diseases began to take a toll on their lives. Bruce explained:

> [While] I've been at UConn . . . I've taken on more jobs. I haven't necessarily [let go] of anything. The Burgdorf [recently] was the first thing that I stepped down from. Frankly, the Burgdorf was breaking my heart. [But now,] I'm actually rejuvenated . . . I have this whole new mission . . . improving care and assuring that the healthcare system's affordable for everyone, especially the poor . . . across the state. The job is scary. Now I'm waking up at three in the morning rather than worrying about the Burgdorf, I'm saying "what have I gotten myself into?" Because it is like herding cats more than a little bit . . . but we've got some really smart people at the community health center association so if we can pull this sucker off, incredible! Because you're talking about better outcomes of care, more intelligent care, better outreach into the community and a global and population approach to health care delivery for the underserved, for the poorest of the state, hopefully at a more affordable cost. Less emergency room use, less hospitalization, less re-hospitalization. Which you can look as "oh you're cheating them, oh my god, rationing, how terrible is that," but in fact, you have to look at it from an epidemiologic perspective. You have to look at running to the emergency room or being hospitalized as a quality indicator of system failure. If somebody needs to go to the emergency room or get admitted to the hospital, was it preventable? And preventable means they're now less healthy than they might have been had we intervened earlier. Health care advocates are very concerned, and [it is] a well-placed concern, that as you try to control cost if you do it one sided, you may disenfranchise the population from getting health care because you don't want to spend the money. That

> was the fear with managed care. Clearly that's the fear with any healthcare reform. But instead, you really have to look at hospitalization and emergency room [care]; emergency need is often a failure of primary care. There are exceptions, there are patients with cancer and other end-stage conditions. You can't cure it and so if they're in the hospital, or with heart failure, inevitably they may be in the hospital periodically. But if the health care system is well designed, and you can be preemptive, it certainly can decrease the temporal pattern of admissions, if you decrease the number needed it means the patient is probably doing better, more functional, spending more time at home with their families and enjoying better quality of life. And the care costs less. Hopefully, a win-win.

When Bruce announced to his colleagues that he was stepping down as the Medical Director of the Burgdorf, they were disheartened. Noted a pediatrician who works at the clinic:

> [Bruce is] well-liked by all his fellow physicians. Everyone loves Bruce. We all know Bruce, we all like Bruce. And we [laughs] all know Bruce is devoted and single-minded . . . I think his colleagues over in pediatrics respect him greatly, even though we have like different fields, [we] really hold Bruce in high esteem, and that goes to his staff as well. Even though Bruce isn't in pediatrics, when he announced he was leaving the Burgdorf you should have seen the looks on their faces. And these are, you know, folks in pediatrics, who really have no day-to-day interaction with him, and they were upset . . . Everyone that I've ever spoken to—and I'm Mr. Sarcastic, I find a bad thing to say about pretty much anybody—I can't find someone who dislikes Bruce. I know there are people who disagree with him and find him a burr in their saddle, but it's not the nursing staff or the people who work with him day to day.

By contrast with clinical staff, this colleague readily admitted that Bruce was not popular with the hospital administration:

> I'm not going to sugar coat it, I think they can't stand him [laughs]. Some of them really can't stand him. And I think some of them may have had the bottom line as their priority and may not have had a great understanding of the power of primary care and they have looked at it as a loss leader and something that cannot be sustained in the current financial environment. And I've heard these arguments, I've heard these pitches before at every medical staff meeting that I've ever attended, and I think that he keeps them honest, when they sometimes don't want to be particularly honest, when they have another agenda. He kind of keeps them honest, and says, "Hey, guys, you gotta look at this. It should be workable if you would just invest in this, this could [work]." And sometimes he would just go say,

> "Fine. Let me show you. I'll do it. And then we can talk about it later, since you don't really believe me," and they go from there. I think certain people just view him as the activist, loudmouth, rabble rouser, trouble maker. I do not share that view.

In fact, it was this colleague's sense that Bruce's biggest accomplishment

> was getting the Burgdorf to be a primary care medical home, with zero support from anybody else [laughs], like it was by the force of will. Okay, so to be a medical home, you need medical records, you need to have an integrated system. It would be really awesome if you had your parent hospital's support in terms of electronics and data because part of being a medical home means you have to be able to manage your population and their data. You have to know your population. We didn't get all that great support. Other clinics in the St. Francis system got that support to become primary care or medical home models, but we didn't. This was by force of [Bruce's] will. This was about Bruce saying, "We should really do this. We can do this." And of course, he did the nice thing: he asked for help, he asked for the numbers, and he got stonewalled. And he's just like, "Okay, I'm just going to do it on my own." [This was in] 2011, 2012 because St. Francis let it lapse, like we got it done, and then they let it lapse. That was pretty darned impressive because there was no infrastructure, there was no help; it was just him being able to convince a bunch of overworked, busy people to work a little harder. And he pulled it off.

Step Up, Step Out

James Orbinski, an associate professor of medicine at the University of Toronto and a founding member of the Nobel-Prize winning *Médecins Sans Frontières* (Doctors Without Borders), says that it is time for physicians to "step up and step out" on local and national levels in response to the social and environmental factors that have become the greatest threats to health in the twenty-first century (quoted in Fayerman 2016). In his book, *An Imperfect Offering: Humanitarian Action for the Twenty-First Century*, Orbinski (2008: 4) addresses a fundamental question all physicians must ask of themselves: "How am I to be, how are we to be in relation to the suffering of others?" His response is "solidarity": "In our choice to be with those who suffer, compassion leads to solidarity . . . Solidarity implies a willingness to confront the causes and conditions of suffering that persist in destroying dignity, and to demand a minimum respect for human life" (Orbinski 2008: 7–8). This choice, to step up and step out is a commitment to healthcare in the fullest sense possible. It is not just a worthy goal. In the end, in a world of widespread human-inflicted suffering, it is the only goal that if achieved could really allow physicians—in the words of the modern Hippocratic Oath (Miles 2004)—to truly "experience the joy of healing those who seek my help."

As the interviews with him were coming to an end, Bruce mused about how readers of this book would react to it, saying: "I'm a little concerned . . . this will come out as the radical manifesto . . . [laughing] and then I'll definitely have to leave Hartford or maybe the country." Needless to say, Bruce is still working to improve healthcare for the poor and has not had to leave the country, at least not yet. Without question, however, in trying times, the world of medicine needs many more physicians, nurses, dentists, and other healthcare providers with the energy, passion, and commitment to improving the health of the underserved seen in Bruce. As the U.S. health care system is now organized and in light of the forces shaping the current direction of healthcare, such commitment may indeed be seen by some as radical. The alternative, however, is amplified social and health inequality, widening disparities in access to and quality of healthcare, and increased human misery. During his whole adult life, with all of his energy and skills, Bruce has taken a laudable stand against the structural causes of much ill health and the restructuring of medicine so that it does not only serve the economic objectives of the rich at the cost in well-being to the poor, and, increasingly, to everyone who is not rich. In this, Bruce has modeled an approach to medicine and to healthcare worthy of potential broad emulation. Most importantly, Bruce has demonstrated that it is possible to practice social medicine in a country sorely in need of dramatic change in its broken healthcare system.

REFERENCES

Aagaard, E. and Hauer, M. 2003 A cross-sectional descriptive study of mentoring relationships formed by medical students. *Journal of General Internal Medicine* 18(4):298–302.

Adams, R. 2008 Socialism for the rich. *Guardian*. Retrieved from www.guardian.co.uk/commentisfree/2008/sep/17/wallstreet.useeconomy.

Advanced Medical Technology Association 2015 AdvaMed unveils innovation agenda: Policy proposals aim to renew medical technology innovation ecosystem. Retrieved from www.advamed.org/newsroom/press-releases/advamed-unveils-innovation-agenda.

Aggarwal, A., Monsivais, P., and Drewnowski, A. 2012 Nutrient intakes linked to better health outcomes are associated with higher diet costs in the US. *PLoS One* 7(5):e37533.

Aikin, K. 2003 Direct-to-consumer advertising of prescription drugs: Physician survey preliminary results. U.S. Food and Drug Administration, Division of Drug Marketing, Advertising and Communications. Retrieved from www.fda.gov/cder/ddmac/presentations.htm.

Aiken, L., Clarke, S., Sloane, D., Lake, E., and Cheney, T. 2008 Effects of hospital care environment on patient mortality and nurse outcomes. *Journal of Nursing Administration* 38(5):223–229.

Aiken, L., Clarke, S., Sloane, D., Sochalski, J., Busse, R., Clarke, H., Giovannetti, P., Hunt, J. et al. 2003 Nurses' reports on hospital care in five countries. *Health Affairs* 20(3):43–53.

Akerlof, G. and Schiller, R. 2015 The free market preys on your every weakness. *New Republic*. Retrieved from https://newrepublic.com/article/123180/free-market-preys-your-every-weakness.

Alaimo, K., Briefel, R., Frongillo, E., and Olson, C. 1998 Food insufficiency exists in the United States: Results from the third National Health and Nutrition Examination Survey (NHANES III). *American Journal of Public Health* 88:419–426.

Albert, N. 2003 A tale of two cities: The rise & fall of public housing. *Connecticut Explored*. Retrieved from http://ctexplored.org/a-tale-of-two-cities-the-rise-fall-of-public-housing/.

Alexander, J., Morlock, L., and Gifford, B. 1988 The effects of corporate restructuring on hospital policymaking. *Health Services Research* 23:311–337.

Alfirevic, Z., Devane, D., and Gyte, G. 2006 Continuous cardiotocography (CTG) as a form of electronic fetal monitoring (EFM) for fetal assessment during labour. *Cochrane Database of Systematic Reviews* (3):CD006066.

Alonso-Magdalena, P., Quesada, I., and Nadal, A. 2011 Endocrine disruptors in the etiology of type 2 diabetes mellitus. *Nature Reviews of Endocrinology* 7(6):346–353.

Altman, L. 1982 Prescription drugs are advertised to patients, breaking with tradition. *New York Times*. Retrieved from www.nytimes.com/1982/02/23/science/prescription-drugs-are-advertised-to-patients-breaking-with-tradition.html?pagewanted=all.

American Academy of Pediatrics 2012 Policy statement. Breastfeeding and the use of human milk. *Pediatrics* 129(3):e827–e841.

American Diabetes Association 2016 Diabetes symptoms. Retrieved from www.diabetes.org/diabetes-basics/symptoms/.

American Medical Association 2016 Creating the medical school of the future. Retrieved from https://www.ama-assn.org/ama/pub/about-ama/strategic-focus/accelerating-change-in-medical-education/innovations.page.

Anderson, J. 2014 Health care equity causes a paradigm shift in medicine. Association of American Medical Colleges. Retrieved from https://www.aamc.org/newsroom/reporter/june2014/384704/health-care-equity.html.

Anderson, M. 2012 Howard Waitzkin's *Medicine and Public Health at the End of Empire*: *Social Medicine* 7(1):1–3.

Anderson, S. and Cavanagh, J. 2007 The rise of corporate global power. Retrieved from www.ips-dc.org/reports/top200.htm.

Andrews, M., Nord, M., Bickel, G., and Carlson, S. 1999. Measuring food security in the United States: household food security in the United States. Washington, DC: U.S. Department of Agriculture, Economic Research Service, Food Assistance and Nutrition Research report no. 8.

Andreyeva, T., Blumenthal, D., Schwartz M., Long, M., and Brownell, K. 2008 Availability and prices of foods across stores and neighborhoods: The case of New Haven, Connecticut. *Health Affairs* 27(5):1381–1388.

Angell, M. 2004 *The Truth about the Drug Companies: How They Deceive Us and What to Do about It*. New York: Random House.

Armbruster, B. 2009 GOP rep. admits that health insurance companies control the market and dictate medical decisions. Retrieved from https://thinkprogress.org/gop-rep-admits-that-health-insurance-companies-control-the-market-and-dictate-medical-decisions-a0d91f87225f#.juegaim7a.

Asante-Muhammed, D., Collins, C., Hoxie, J., and Nieves, E. 2016 *The Ever-Growing Gap: Without Change, African-American and Latino Families Won't Match White Wealth for Centuries*. Washington, DC: Institute for Policy Studies and CFED.

Association of American Medical Colleges 2009 Scientific foundations for future physicians. Report of the AAMC-HHMI Committee. Retrieved from https://www.aamc.org/download/271072/data/scientificfoundationsforfuturephysicians.pdf.

Association of American Medical Colleges 2015 *AAMC Annual Report*. Retrieved from https://www.aamc.org/about/451624/annual-report-2015.html.

Austad, K., Avorn, J., Franklin, J., Kowal, M., Campbell, E. and Kesselheim, A. 2013 Physician trainees and the pharmaceutical industry: A national survey. *Journal of General Internal Medicine* 28(8):1064–1071.

Austin, P. 2009 *Something for the Pain: Compassion and Burnout in the ER*. New York: W. W. Norton & Company.

Avorn, J. 2005 *Powerful Medicine: The Benefits, Risks and Costs of Prescription Drugs*. New York: Vintage Books.

Bailey, M. 2016 Looming question for medical students: Will they be shut out of advanced training? *Stat*. Retrieved from https://www.statnews.com/2016/03/17/medical-students-match-day/.

Bailin, D., Goldman, G., and Phartiyal, P. 2014 *Sugar-Coating Science: How the Food Industry Misleads Consumers on Sugar*. Washington, DC: Union of Concerned Scientists.

Baker, D. 2017 Trump is proving the rich aren't necessarily insightful. *TruthOut*. Retrieved from www.truth-out.org/opinion/item/39363-donald-trump-and-the-unhinged-rich.

Barbaccia, J. 1976 Introducing quality assurance and medical audit into the UCSF Medical Center curriculum. *Journal of Medical Education* 51:386–491.

Barker, D. and Osmond, C. 1986 Infant mortality, childhood nutrition, and ischaemic heart disease in England and Wales. *Lancet* 1:1077–1081.

Bass, T. 2012 The double game of the U.S. health insurance companies. *Huffington Post*. Retrieved from www.huffingtonpost.com/thomas-a-bass/the-double-game-of-the-us_b_1558794.html.

Baxandall, P. and Smith, D. 2013 *Picking Up the Tab 2013: Average Citizens and Small Businesses Pay the Price for Offshore Tax Havens*. Washington, DC: U.S. Public Interest Research Group.

Bean, W. 1961 Physicians for a growing America: Report of the Surgeon General's Consultant Group on Medical Education. *Public Health Service Publication No. 709*. Retrieved from http://jamanetwork.com/journals/jamainternalmedicine/article-abstract/566494.

Beck, A. 2004 The Flexner Report and the standardization of American medical education. *Journal of the American Medical Association* 291(17):2139–2140.

Beck, M. 2015 Innovation is sweeping through U.S. medical schools. *Wall Street Journal*. Retrieved from www.wsj.com/articles/innovation-is-sweeping-through-u-s-medical-schools-1424145650.

Becker, A. 2010 Free: 1 day Of care. *Hartford Courant*. Retrieved from http://articles.courant.com/2010-01-25/news/10012512585943_1_free-clinics-one-day-clinics-dr-bruce-gould.

Bell, R., Kravatz, R., and Wilkes, M. 1999 Direct-to-consumer prescription drug advertising and the public. *Journal of General Internal Medicine* 14(11):651–657.

Bendix, J., Verdon, D., Ritchie, A., Marbury, D., and Mazzolini, C. 2014 Top 10 challenges facing physicians in 2013. *Medical Economics*. Retrieved from http://medicaleconomics.modernmedicine.com/medical-economics/content/tags/affordable-care-act/top-10-challenges-facing-physicians-2014?page=0,3.

Ben-Shalom, Y., Moffitt, R., and Scholz, J. 2011 An assessment of the effectiveness of anti-poverty programs in the United States. The National Bureau of Economic Research. Retrieved from www.nber.org/papers/w17042.

Beverly, E., Hultgren, B., Brooks, K., Ritholz, M., Abrahamson, M., and Weinger, K. 2011 Understanding physicians' challenges when treating Type 2 diabetic patients' social and emotional difficulties. *Diabetes Care* 34(5): 1086–1088.

Biehl, J. 2007 *Will to Live: AIDS Therapies and the Politics of Survival*. Princeton, NJ: Princeton University Press.

Boggess, B. and Bogue, H. 2016 The health of U.S. agricultural worker families: A descriptive study of over 790,000 migratory and seasonal agricultural workers and dependents. *Journal of Health Care for the Poor and Underserved* 27(2):778–792.

Bourgois, P. 2003 *In Search of Respect: Selling Crack in El Barrio*, 2nd ed. Berkeley: University of California Press.

Boynton, C. 2007 The secret life of shade tobacco. *New York Times*. Retrieved from www.nytimes.com/2007/09/23/nyregion/nyregionspecial2/23mainct.html?_r=0.

Bradley, I. 2010 Talk to your doctor: Direct-to-consumer advertising of prescription drugs (Part 1). *Clinical Correlations*. Retrieved from www.clinicalcorrelations.org/?p=2867.

Bragg, M., Miller, A., Elizee, J., Dighe, S., and Elbel, B. 2016 Popular music celebrity endorsements in food and nonalcoholic beverage marketing. *Pediatrics* (June). doi:10.1542/peds.2015-3977.

Bragg. M., Yanamadala, S., Roberto, C., Harris, J., and Brownell, K. 2013 Athlete endorsements in food marketing. *Pediatrics* 132(5):1–6.

Braveman, P., Egerter, S. and Mockenhaupt, R. 2011a Broadening the focus: The need to address the social determinants of health. *American Journal of Preventive Medicine* 40(Suppl. 1):S4–S18.

Braveman, P., Egerter, S., and Williams, D. 2011b The social determinants of health: Coming of age. *Annual Review of Public Health* 32(1):381–398.

Breslow, L. 1999 From disease prevention to health promotion. *Journal of American Medical Association* 281:1030–1033.

Brimmer, K. 2012 PwC report shows hospitals saw increased employee turnover. *HealthCare Finance*. Retrieved from www.healthcarefinancenews.com/news/pwc-report-shows-hospitals-saw-increased-employee-turnover.

Buchanan, M. and Abraham, M. 2015 Connecticut has more concentrated poverty (and wealth) than most metros: The story in numbers. *TrendCT.Org*. Retrieved from http://trendct.org/2015/05/27/connecticut-has-more-concentrated-poverty-and-wealth-than-most-metros/.

Burger, D., Higgins, K., and Ross, J. 2015 Letter from the Council of Presidents, Nurses United. Retrieved from http://nnumagazine.uberflip.com/i/489502-national-nurse-magazine-march-2015.

Bushnell Park Foundation 2016 Park history. Retrieved from www.bushnellpark.org/about-2/history-2.

Caldwell, P. 2016 Elizabeth Warren rips into Paul Ryan's anti-poverty plan. *Mother Jones*. Retrieved from www.motherjones.com/politics/2016/06/elizabeth-warren-rips-paul-ryans-poverty-plan.

California Newsreel 2008 *Unnatural Causes: Is Inequality Making Us Sick?* Television documentary series. San Francisco, CA.

Candia, J., Banavar, J., and Losert, W. 2013 Understanding health and disease with multidimensional single-cell methods. *Journal of Physics: Condensed Matter* 26(7). Retrieved from http://iopscience.iop.org/article/10.1088/0953-8984/26/7/073102/meta.

Carlson, S., Andrews, M., and Bickel, G. 1999 Measuring food insecurity and hunger in the United States: Development of a national benchmark measure and prevalence estimates. *Journal of Nutrition* 129:510–516.

Carrion, I., Castaneda, H., Martinez Tyson, D., and Kline, N. 2011 Barriers impeding access to primary oral health care among farmworker families in central Florida. *Social Work in Health Care* 50(10):828–844.

Carroll, D., Georges, A. and Saltz, R. 2011 Changing characteristics of U.S. farm workers: 21 years of findings from the National Agricultural Workers Survey. Washington, DC: U.S. Department of Labor.

Casselman, B. 2016 Americans don't miss manufacturing—they miss unions. *FiveThirtyEight*. Retrieved from http://fivethirtyeight.com/features/americans-dont-miss-manufacturing-they-miss-unions/.

Castaneda, H., Carrion, I., Kline, N., and Martinez Tyson, D. 2010 False hope: Effects of social class and health policy on oral health inequalities for migrant farmworker families. *Social Science and Medicine* 71(1):2028–2037.

Cato Institute 2013 Four reasons not to raise the minimum wage. Retrieved from https://object.cato.org/sites/cato.org/files/four_reasons_not_to_raise_the_minimum_wage.pdf.

CDC (Centers for Disease Control and Prevention) 2007 National diabetes fact sheet: United States, 2007. Atlanta, GA: Centers for Disease Control and Prevention.

CDC (Centers for Disease Control and Prevention) 2014 National diabetes statistics report: Estimates of diabetes and its burden in the United States, 2014. Atlanta, GA: U.S. Department of Health and Human Services.

Center for Food Safety 2016 State labeling initiatives. Retrieved from www.centerforfoodsafety.org/issues/976/ge-food-labeling/state-labeling-initiatives.

Centers for Medicare & Medicaid Services 2010 Shining a light on health insurance rate increases. Retrieved from https://www.cms.gov/CCIIO/Resources/Fact-Sheets-and-FAQs/ratereview.html#_ftn1.

Charles, B. 2014 Teen pregnancy in Connecticut: City birth rates twice state average. *New Haven Register*. www.nhregister.com/general-news/20140322/teen-pregnancy-in-connecticut-city-birth-rates-twice-state-average.

Chesanow, N. 2014 Doctors are talking: EHRs destroy the patient encounter. *MedScape*. Retrieved from http://ontariorheum.ca/images/uploads/content_documents/EMR_erode_Pt_Experience.pdf.

Chomsky, N. 2014 Chomsky: How America's great university system is being destroyed. *Alternet*. Retrieved from www.alternet.org/corporate-accountability-and-workplace/chomsky-how-americas-great-university-system-getting.

Chren, M. 1999 Interactions between physicians and drug company representatives. *American Journal of Medicine* 107:182–183.

Chui, M., Manyika, J., and Miremadi, M. 2015 Four fundamentals of workplace automation. *McKinsey Quarterly*. Retrieved from www.mckinsey.com/business-functions/digital-mckinsey/our-insights/four-fundamentals-of-workplace-automation.

Clark, K. and Esch, C. 2016 SO1-5 "Pregnant? We can help. *MarketPlace.com*. Retrieve from www.marketplace.org/topics/uncertain-hour.

Clay, R. 2008 The corporatization of higher education. *Monitor on Psychology* 39(11):50.

Cogswell, M., Gunn, J., Kennedy, Y., Park, S., and Merritt, R. 2015 Sodium and sugar in complementary infant and toddler foods sold in the United States. *Pediatrics* 135(4):416–423.

Cohn, J. 2009 The new republic: Health care lobbyist playing nice. *NPR*. Retrieved from www.npr.org/templates/story/story.php?storyId=105648205.

Colins, M. 2006 *Hot Lights, Cold Steel: Life, Death and Sleepless Nights in a Surgeon's First Years*. New York: St. Martin's Press.

Commission on Social Determinants of Health 2008 Closing the gap in a generation: Health equity through action on the social determinants of health. Final Report of the Commission on Social Determinants of Health. Geneva: World Health Organization.

Community Solutions 2016 Healthy communities: Northeast Hartford. Retrieved from https://cmtysolutions.org/blog/healthy-communities-northeast-hartford.

Condon, T. 2016 Will Hartford's crisis force a CT property tax overhaul? *Connecticut Mirror*. Retrieved from http://ctmirror.org/2016/08/31/will-hartfords-crisis-force-a-ct-property-tax-overhaul/.

Connecticut by the Numbers 2014 Hartford ranked #35, New Haven #39 in income inequality among US cities; Bridgeport-Stamford-Norwalk is nation's most disparate region. Retrieved from http://ctbythenumbers.info/2014/04/22/hartford-ranked-35-new-haven-39-income-inequality-among-us-cities/.

Connecticut Department of Community Development 2013 Connecticut income data. Retrieved from www.ct.gov/ecd/cwp/view.asp?a=1106&q=250652.

Connecticut Department of Public Health 2002 *Epidemiologic Profile of HIV and AIDS*. Hartford: Connecticut Department of Public Health.

Consumer Reports 2009 Consumer Reports adwatch. Retrieved from www.consumerreports.org/health/prescription-drugs/adwatch/overview/adwatch-hub.htm.

Consumer Reports 2011 Consumer Reports adwatch. Retrieved from www.consumerreports.org/health/prescription-drugs/adwatch/overview/adwatch-hub.htm.

Consumer Reports 2012 Sluggish economy forces Americans to cut corners to pay for medications. Retrieved from www.consumerreports.org/cro/2012/09/sluggish-economy-forces-americans-to-cut-corners-to-pay-for-medications/index.htm.

Consumer Reports 2015 Is there a cure for high drug prices? Retrieved from www.consumerreports.org/drugs/cure-for-high-drug-prices/.

Contopoulos-Ioannidis, D., Ntzani, E., and Ioannidis, J. 2003 Translation of highly promising basic science research into clinical applications. *American Journal of Medicine* 114(6):477–484.

Cooke, M., Irby, D., Sullivan, W., and Ludmerer, K. 2006 American medical education 100 years after the Flexner Report. *New England Journal of Medicine* 355:1339–1344.

Corn, D. 2012 SECRET VIDEO: Romney tells millionaire donors what he REALLY thinks of Obama voters. *Mother Jones*. Retrieved from www.motherjones.com/politics/2012/09/secret-video-romney-private-fundraiser.

Cramer, R. 2016 Improving the state of our welfare state. *New America Weekly*, edition 128. Retrieved from https://www.newamerica.org/weekly/edition-128/improving-state-our-welfare-state/.

Currie, J. 2007 Poverty among inner-city children. Retrieved from https://www.princeton.edu/~jcurrie/publications/inman_june07.pdf.

CVS Health 2016 Cost is the biggest barrier to medication adherence. Retrieved from https://cvshealth.com/thought-leadership/cvs-health-research-institute/cost-biggest-barrier-medication-adherence.

Daemmrich, A. 2011 U.S. healthcare reform and the pharmaceutical industry. Working Paper 12-015. Harvard Business School. Retrieved from www.hbs.edu/faculty/Publication%20Files/12-015.pdf.

DataHaven 2016 Living in a poor neighborhood changes everything about your life. Retrieved from http://ctdatahaven.org/blog/living-poor-neighborhood-changes-everything-about-your-life.

Davis, K., Stremikis, K., Squires, D., and Schoen, C. 2014 *Mirror, Mirror on the Wall, 2014 Update: How the U.S. Health Care System Compares Internationally*. New York: The Commonwealth Fund.

Declercq, E., Sakala, C., Corry, M., and Applebam, S. 2007 Listening to mothers II: Report of the Second National U.S. Survey of Women's Childbearing Experiences. *Journal of Perinatal Education* 16(4):15–17.

DeFrancesco, C. 2014 Hartford's Burgdorf Clinic is rooted in the community. *UCONN Today*. Retrieved from http://today.uconn.edu/2014/08/hartfords-burgdorf-clinic-is-rooted-in-the-community/.

Delaney, A. 2012 Paul Ryan wants "Welfare reform round 2." *Huffington Post*. Retrieved from www.huffingtonpost.com/2012/03/20/paul-ryan-welfare-reform_n_1368277.html.

Department of Justice 2010 Two Johnson & Johnson subsidiaries to pay over $81 million to resolve allegations of off-label promotion of Topamax. Retrieved from https://www.justice.gov/opa/pr/two-johnson-johnson-subsidiaries-pay-over-81-million-resolve-allegations-label-promotion.

Derber, C. 1998 *Corporation Nation: How Corporations are Taking Over Our Lives and What We Can Do about It*. NY: St Martin's Press.

Desilver, D. 2015 5 facts about the minimum wage. *Pew Research Center*. Retrieved from www.pewresearch.org/fact-tank/2015/07/23/5-facts-about-the-minimum-wage/.

Desjarlais, R. and Throop, C. 2007 Phenomenological approaches in anthropology. *Annual Review of Anthropology* 40:87–102.

Deyo, R. 2002 Cascade effects of medical technology. *Annual Review of Public Health* 23:23–44.

Doland, K. and Kroll, L. 2015 Inside the 2015 Forbes 400: Facts and figures about America's wealthiest. *Forbes*. Retrieved from www.forbes.com/sites/luisakroll/2015/09/29/inside-the-2015-forbes-400-facts-and-figures-about-americas-wealthiest/#7b18febd28f8.

Donohue, J., Cevasco, M., and Rosenthal, M. 2007 A decade of direct-to-consumer advertising of prescription drugs. *New England Journal of Medicine* 357:673–681.

Dorio, G. 2015 The corporate practice of medicine is overwhelming American health care. Retrieved from www.kevinmd.com/blog/2015/12/corporate-practice-medicine-overwhelming-american-health-care.html.

Doty, M., Edwards J., and Holmgren, A. 2005 Seeing red: Americans driven into debt by medical bills. Issue brief. The Commonwealth Fund. Retrieved from www.commonwealthfund.org/usr_doc/837_Doty_seeing_red_medical_debt.pdf?section=4039.

Douglas, S. and Michaels, M. 2005 *Go To "The Mommy Myth": The Idealization of Motherhood and How It Has Undermined All Women*. New York: Free Press.

Dressler, W and Bindon, J. 2000 The health consequences of cultural consonance: Cultural dimensions of lifestyle, social support, and arterial blood pressure in an African American community. *American Anthropologist* 102:244–260.

Drewnowski, A. and Specter, S. 2004 Poverty and obesity: The role of energy density and energy costs. *American Journal of Clinical Nutrition* 79(1):6–16.

Dwan, K., Altman, D., Arnaiz, J., Bloom, J., Chan, A.-W., Cronin, E., Decullier, E. et al. 2008 Systematic review of the empirical evidence of study publication bias and outcome reporting bias. *PLoS One* 3(8):e3081.

Dyrbye, L., Massie, M., Eacker, A., Harper, W., Power, D., Durning, S., Thomas, M., Moutier, C., Satele, D., Sloan, J., and Shanafelt, T. 2010 Relationship between burnout and professional conduct and attitudes among US medical students. *Journal of the American Medical Association* 304(11):1173–1180.

Ehrenreich, B. and Ehrenreich, J. 1971 *The American Health Empire: Power, Profits, and Politics*. New York: Random House.

Ehrenreich, J. 2016 *Third Wave Capitalism: How Money, Power, and the Pursuit of Self-Interest Have Imperilled the American Dream*. Ithaca, NY: Cornell University Press.

Eichenwald, K. 2016 Trump's many business failures, explained. *Newsweek*. Retrieved from www.newsweek.com/2016/08/12/donald-trumps-business-failures-election-2016-486091.html.

Eisenmann, J., Bartree, R., and Wang, M. 2002 Physical activity, TV viewing, and weight in U.S. youth: 1999 Youth Risk Behavior Survey. *Obesity Research* 10(5):379–385.

Elliot, C. and Conlon, M. 2014 Packaged baby and toddler foods: Questions of sugar and sodium. *Pediatric Obesity* 10:149–155.

Epstein, R. and Privitera, M. 2016 Doing something about physician burnout. *Lancet* 388(10057):2216–2217.

Esch, C. 2016 The legacy of welfare reform, 20 years later. *MarketPlace.com*. Retrieved from www.marketplace.org/2016/08/17/world/legacy-welfare-reform-20-years-later.

Faerber, A. and Kreling, D. 2013 Content analysis of false and misleading claims in television advertising for prescription and nonprescription drugs. *Journal of General Internal Medicine* 29(1):110–118.

Falbe, J., Thompson, H., Becker, C., Rojas, N., McCulloch, C., and Madsen, K. 2016 Impact of the Berkeley excise tax on sugar-sweetened beverage consumption. *American Journal of Public Health* 106(10):1865–1871.

Families USA 2012 Dying for coverage: The deadly consequences of being uninsured. Retrieved from http://familiesusa.org/sites/default/files/product_documents/Dying-for-Coverage.pdf.

Farmer, P., Nizeye, B., Stulac, S., and Keshavjee, S. 2006 Structural violence and clinical medicine. *PLoS Med* 3(10):e449.

Farr, C. 2015 Siren song of tech lures new doctors away from medicine. *NPR*. Retrieved from www.npr.org/sections/health-shots/2015/07/19/423882899/siren-song-of-tech-lures-new-doctors-away-from-medicine.

Fayerman, P. 2016 Doctors at Vancouver conference called to action over health effects of climate change. *Vancouver Sun*. Retrieved from http://vancouversun.com/news/local-news/doctors-at-vancouver-conference-called-to-action-over-health-effects-of-climate-change.

Ferdman, R. 2016 Why the sugar industry hates the FDA's new Nutrition Facts label. *Washington Post*. Retrieved from https://www.washingtonpost.com/news/wonk/wp/2016/05/20/why-the-sugar-industry-hates-the-fdas-new-nutrition-facts-label/.

Ferguson, C., Munoz, M., and Medrano, M. 2012 Advertising influences on young children and parental influences. *Journal of Pediatrics* 160(3):452–455.

Ferguson, R., Rhim, E., Belizaire, W., Egede, L., Cartern K., and Lansdale, T. 1999 Encounters with pharmaceutical sales representatives among practicing internists. *American Journal of Medicine* 107:149–151.

Ferguson, T. 1995 *Golden Rule: The Investment Theory of Party Competition and the Logic of Money-Driven Political Systems*. Chicago, IL: University of Chicago Press.

Fitzgerald, S. 2016 Ryan: Minimum wage hikes "do more harm than good." *Newsmax.com*. Retrieved from www.newsmax.com/Politics/US-ryan-minimum-wage-hikes/2016/06/07/id/732700/.

Fitzgibbon, M., Blackman, L., and Avellone, M. 2000 The relationship between body image discrepancy and Body Mass Index across ethnic groups. *Obesity* 8(8):582–589.

Flexner, A. 1910 *Medical Education in the United States and Canada: A Report to the Carnegie Foundation for the Advancement of Teaching*. New York: The Carnegie Foundation.

Flexner. A. 1925 *Medical Education: A Comparative Study*. New York: MacMillan.

Fong, J., Anat, D., and Longnecker, N. 2010 Doctor-patient communication: A review. *Ochsner Journal* 10(1):38–43.

Foucault, M. 1972 *The Archaeology of Knowledge*. New York: Pantheon Books.

Foucault, M. 1975 *The Birth of the Clinic: An Archaeology of Medical Perception*. New York: Vintage Books.

Frank, J. 2015 Nook Farm. *Connecticut History.Org*. Retrieved from http://connecticuthistory.org/hartfords-nook-farm/.

Frase, P. 2017 Will automation benefit humanity and the planet, or a tiny elite? *TruthOut*. Retrieved from www.truth-out.org/opinion/item/39320-four-futures-including-options-to-greed.

Freakonomics 2015 How many doctors does it take to start a healthcare revolution? Retrieved from http://freakonomics.com/2015/04/09/how-many-doctors-does-it-take-to-start-a-healthcare-revolution-full-transcript/.

Freel, A. 1998 Achievement in urban schools: What makes the difference? A conversation with Kati Haycock. *Education Digest* 64(1):17–22.

Freeman, J. 2012 Health is not a commodity: Let us get the language right. *Physicians for a National Health Program*. Retrieved from www.pnhp.org/news/2012/november/health-is-not-a-commodity-let-us-get-the-language-right.

Friedberg, M., Chen, P.G., Busum, K.R., Aunon, V., Chau Pham, F., Caloyeras, J. et al. 2013 *Factors Affecting Physician Professional Satisfaction and Their Implications for Patient Care, Health Systems, and Health Policy*. Santa Monica, CA: RAND Corporation.

Friedman, L. and Jennings, K. 2013 The US has a staggering gap between black and white life expectancy. *US News and World Report*. Retrieved from www.businessinsider.com/huge-black-white-gap-in-life-expectancy-in-us-2014-8.

Frohlich, T. 2015 The cities where no one wants to drive. *USA Today*. Retrieved from www.usatoday.com/story/money/cars/2015/02/14/247-wall-st-cities-no-one-wants-drive/23363835/.

Frosch, D., Krueger, P., Hornik, R., Cronholm, P., and Barg, F. 2007 Creating demand for prescription drugs: A content analysis of television direct-to-consumer advertising. *Annals of Family Medicine* 5(1):6–13.

Fry, R. and Kochhar, R. 2014 America's wealth gap between middle-income and upper-income families is widest on record. Pew Research Center. Retrieved from www.pewresearch.org/fact-tank/2014/12/17/wealth-gap-upper-middle-income/.

Furberg, C., Furberg, B., and Sasich, L. 2016 *Knowing Your Medications*. St. Louis, MO: Express Scripts.

Gabriel, T. 2016 Donald Trump fields questions on jobs in Iowa. *New York Times*. Retrieved from www.nytimes.com/politics/first-draft/2015/11/20/donald-trump-fields-questions-on-jobs-in-iowa/.

Gagnon, M. and Lexchin, J. 2008 The cost of pushing pills: A new estimate of pharmaceutical promotion expenditures in the United States. *PLoS Med* 2008(5):e1.

Gammell, B. 2014 Cash crop: L.B. Haas & Co. and the history of tobacco in Connecticut. *ConnecticutHistory.Org*. Retrieved from http://connecticuthistory.org/cash-crop-l-b-haas-co-and-the-history-of-tobacco-in-connecticut/.

Garfield, R. and Damico, A. 2016 The coverage gap: Uninsured poor Adults in states that do not expand Medicaid—an update. The Henry J. Kaiser Family Foundation. Retrieved from http://kff.org/health-reform/issue-brief/the-coverage-gap-uninsured-poor-adults-in-states-that-do-not-expand-medicaid-an-update/.

Gewertz, D. and Errington, F. 2010 *Cheap Meat: Flap Food Nations in the Pacific Islands*. Berkeley: University of California Press.

Geyman, J. 2015 *How Obamacare Is Unsustainable: Why We Need a Single-Payer Solution For All*. Friday Harbor, WA: Copernicus Healthcare.

Giancoli, A. and Soto, R. 2011 *Sugary Drinks: A Big Problem for Kids*. Davis, CA: California Center for Public Health Advocacy.

Gibson, G. and Smith, G. 2016 Clinton outpaces rivals in drug company donations. *Reuters*. Retrieved from www.reuters.com/article/us-usa election-pharmaceuticals-idUSKCN 0Z22F1.

Giovannucci, E., Harlan, D., Archer, M., Bergenstal, R., Gapstur, S., Habel, L. et al. 2010 Diabetes and cancer: A consensus report. *Diabetes Care* 33(7):1675–1685.

Giris, L. 2015 Will corporate greed destroy the American healthcare system? *Dr. Linda*. Retrieved from http://drlinda-md.com/2015/01/corporate-greedhealthcare-system/.

Gladwell, M. 2008 *Outliers: The Story of Success*. New York: Little Brown & Company.

Glasmeier, A. 2016 Living wage calculation for Hartford County, Connecticut. Retrieved from http://livingwage.mit.edu/counties/09003.

Glover, L. 2016 Bronze, silver, gold: Which health insurance tier best buy for you? *USA Today*. Retrieved from www.usatoday.com/story/money/personalfinance/2016/10/30/bronze-silver-gold-health-insurance-tier/92666622/.

Good B. 1994 *Medicine, Rationality and Experience*. Cambridge: Cambridge University Press.

Gordon D. 1988 Tenacious assumptions in Western medicine. In: Lock, M. and Gordon, D., eds. *Biomedicine Examined*. Dordrecht: Kluwer Academic Publishers, pp. 19–56

Gould, B. 2004 Adding continuous quality improvement to a medical school curriculum: Problems and possibilities. *The AMA Journal of Ethics* 6(6), PMID:23260637.

Gould, B., Grey, M., Huntington, C., Gruman, C., Rosen, J., Storey, E., Abrahamson, L., Conaty, A., Curry, L., Ferreira, M., Harrington, K., Paturzo, D., and Van Hoof, T. 2002

Improving patient care outcomes by teaching quality improvement to medical students in community-based practices. *Academic Medicine* 77(10):1011–1018.

Gould, B., O'Connell, M., Russell, M., Pipas, C., and McCurdy, F. 2004 Teaching quality measurement and improvement, cost-effectiveness, and patient satisfaction in undergraduate medical education: The UME-21 experience. *Family Medicine* 36(Supplement):S57–S62.

Gould, E. 2005 Prognosis worsens for workers' health care: Fourth consecutive year of decline in employer-provided insurance coverage. Washington, DC: Economic Policy Institute. Retrieved from www.epi.org/publication/bp167/.

Gravlee, C. and Dressler, W. 2005 Skin pigmentation, self-perceived color, and arterial blood pressure in Puerto Rico. *American Journal of Human Biology* 2005(17):195–206.

Greene, J. and Herzberg, D. 2010 Hidden in plain sight: Marketing prescription drugs to consumers in the twentieth century. *American Journal of Public Health* 100(5):793–803.

Greene, R. 2012 Farmworkers plagued by pesticides, red tape. The Center for Public Integrity. Retrieved from https://www.publicintegrity.org/2012/06/25/9159/farm workers-plagued-pesticides-red-tape.

Greenstone, M., Looney, A., Patashnik, J., and Yu, M. 2013 Thirteen economic facts about social mobility and the role of education. The Hamilton Project. Retrieved from www.brookings.edu/research/reports/2013/06/13-facts-higher-education.

Greenwald, G. 2012 Obamacare architect leaves White House for pharmaceutical industry job. *Guardian*. Retrieved from https://www.theguardian.com/commentisfree/2012/dec/05/obamacare-fowler-lobbyist-industry1.

Haar, D. 2016 Why Hartford is headed for bankruptcy. *Hartford Courant*. Retrieved from http://www.courant.com/community/hartford/hc-haar-hartford-bankruptcy-bronin-20160826-column.html.

Hafferty, F. and Hafler, J. 2011 The hidden curriculum, structural disconnects, and the socialization of new professionals. In: Hafler, J., ed. *Extraordinary Learning in the Workplace*. Berlin: Springer Science, pp. 17–35.

Hafler, J., Ownby, A., Thompson, B., Fasser, C., Grigsby, K., Haidet, P., Kahn, M., and Hafferty, F. 2011 Decoding the learning environment of medical education: A hidden curriculum perspective for faculty development. *Academic Medicine* 86:440–444.

Hall, R. and Deardorf, A. 2006 Lobbying as legislative subsidy. *American Political Science Review* 100(1):69–84.

Hamill, S. 2016 In reporting on effects of hospital closures, granular tales tell the real story. *Center for Health Journalism*. Retrieved from www.centerforhealthjournalism.org/resources/lessons/reporting-effects-hospital-closures-granular-tales-tell-real-story.

Harkinson, J. 2013 Walmart ads target "low income" consumers with junk food. *Mother Jones*. Retrieved from www.motherjones.com/mojo/2013/11/walmart-targets-low-income-consumers-junk-food.

Harlem Children's Zone 2015 Our results. Retrieved from http://hcz.org/results/.

Harris, J., Fleming-Milici, F., Frazier, W., Haraghey, K., Romo-Palafox, M., Seymour, N. et al. 2016 *Baby Food Facts 2016: Nutrition and Marketing of Baby and Toddler Food and Drinks*. Storrs, CT: UConn Rudd Center for Food Policy and Obesity.

Hartford Department of Health and Human Services 2010 Critical health indicators: Working for a healthy Hartford, 2010. Retrieved from www.hartfordinfo.org/issues/wsd/Health/2010_Critical_Health_Indicators_Final.pdf.

Hartzband, P. and Groopman, J. 2009 Money and the changing culture of medicine. *New England Journal of Medicine* 350:101–103.

Health Care for America Now 2012 Health insurance industry. Retrieved from http://healthcareforamericanow.org/ourissues/health-insurance-industry/.

Henderson, J. 2012 Is medicine science? *KevinMD*. Retrieved from www.kevinmd.com/blog/2012/04/medicine-science.html.

Henderson, V. and Kelly, B. 2005 Food advertising in the age of obesity: Content analysis of food advertising on general market and African American television. *Journal of Nutrition Education and Behavior* 37:191–196.

Hightower, J. and DeMarco, S. 2009 *Swim against the Current: Even a Dead Fish Can Go with the Flow*. Hoboken, NJ: John Wiley & Sons.

Hill, J. 2013 Understanding the social factors that contribute to diabetes: A means to informing health care and social policies for the chronically ill. *The Permanente Journal* 17(2):67–72.

Hillman, B., Joseph, C., Mabry, M, Sunshine, J., Kennedy, S., and Noether, M. 1990 Frequency and costs of diagnostic imaging in office practice: Comparison of self-referring and radiologist-referring physicians. *New England Journal of Medicine* 323(23):1604–1608.

Himmelstein, D., Jun, M., Busse, R., Chevreul, K., Geissler, A., Jeurissen, P., Thomson, S., Vinet, M.-A., and Woolhandler, S. 2014 A comparison of hospital administrative costs in eight nations: US costs exceed all others by far. *Health Affairs* 33(9):1586–1594.

Himmelstein, D., Thorne, D., Warren, E., and Woolhandler, S. 2009 Medical bankruptcy in the United States, 2007: Results of a national study. *American Journal of Medicine* 122(8):741–746.

Himmelstein, D., Warren, T., and Woolhandler, S. 2005 Illness and injury as contributors to bankruptcy. *Health Affairs*. Retrieved from http://content.healthaffairs.org/cgi/reprint/hlhaff.w5.63v1.

Hiss, T. 1991 *The Experience of Place: A New Way of Looking at and Dealing with Our Radically Changing Cities and Countryside*. New York: Vintage Books.

Ho, J. and Preston, S. 2011 International comparisons of U.S. mortality. Unpublished data analyses for the NAS/IOM Panel on Understanding Cross-National Health Differences Among High-Income Countries. Population Studies Center, University of Pennsylvania.

Holland, B. 1999 *Wasn't the Grass Greener? Thirty-Three Reasons Why Life Isn't as Good as It Used to Be*. New York: Harcourt, Inc.

Holocaust Museum 2016 Martin Niemöller: "First they came for the Socialists ...." Retrieved from https://www.ushmm.org/.

Horowitz, J. 2005 Does corporate ownership matter? Service provision in the hospital industry. National Bureau of Economic Research. Retrieved at www.nber.org/papers/w11376.pdf.

Horton, S. 2016 *They Leave Their Kidneys in the Field: Illness, Injury and Illegality among U.S. Farmworkers*. Oakland, CA: University of California Press.

Horton, S. and Barker, J. 2010 Stigmatized biologies: Examining the cumulative effects of oral health disparities for Mexican American farmworker children. *Medical Anthropology Quarterly* 34(2):199–219.

Housing Assistance Council. 2001 No refuge from the fields: Findings from a survey of farmworker housing conditions in the United States. Retrieved from www.ruralhome.org/storage/documents/norefuge.pdf.

Howard, D., Bach, P., Berndt, E., and Conti, R. 2015 Pricing in the market for anticancer drugs. *Journal of Economic Perspectives* 29(1):139–162.

Hoynes, H., Page, M., and Stevens, A. 2006 Poverty in America: Trends and explanations. *Journal of Economic Perspectives* 20(1):47–68.

Hucklenbroich, P. 2014 "Disease entity" as the key theoretical concept of medicine. *Journal of Medicine and Philosophy* 39:609–633.

Hudson, J. and Bruckman, A. 2004 The bystander effect: A lens for understanding patterns of participation. *Journal of the Learning Sciences* 13(2):165–195.

Hyman, P. 2009 Eastern European immigrants in the United States. *Jewish Women: A Comprehensive Historical Encyclopedia*. Jewish Women's Archive. Retrieved from http://jwa.org/encyclopedia/article/eastern-european-immigrants-in-united-states.

Hysong, S., Best, R., and Pugh, J. 2006 Audit and feedback and clinical practice guideline adherence: Making feedback actionable. *Implementation Science* 1(9). doi:10.1186/1748-5908-1-9.

Ingraham, C. 2015 As the rich become super-rich, they pay lower taxes. For real. *Washington Post*. Retrieved from https://www.washingtonpost.com/news/wonk/wp/2015/06/04/as-the-rich-become-super-rich-they-pay-lower-taxes-for-real/.

Institute of Medicine 2000 *Crossing the Quality Chasm: A New Health System for the 21st Century*. Washington, DC: National Academies Press.

Institute of Medicine 2002 *Unequal Treatment: Confronting Racial and Ethnic Disparities in Health Care*. Washington, DC: National Academies Press.

Institute of Medicine. 2003 *Keeping Patients Safe: Transforming the Work Environment of Nurses*. Washington, DC: National Academies Press.

Institute of Medicine 2005 *Food Marketing to Children and Youth: Threat or Opportunity?* Washington, DC: National Academies Press.

Ioannididis· J. 2008 Why most discovered true associations are inflated. *Epidemiology* 19(5):640–648.

Ioannidis, J. 2005 Contradicted and initially stronger effects in highly cited clinical research. *Journal of the American Medical Association* 294(2):218–228.

Irving, F. 2013 Physician turnover rate hits all-time high. *HealthCare Finance News*. Retrieved from www.healthcarefinancenews.com/news/physician-turnover-rate-hits-all-time-high.

Jacobs, D., Wilson, J., Dixon, S., Smith, J., and Evens, A. 2009 The relationship of housing and population health: A 30-year retrospective analysis. *Environmental Health Perspectives* 117(4):597–604.

Jacobs, K., Perla, Z., Perry, I., and Graham-Squire, D. 2016 Producing poverty: The public cost of low-wage production jobs in manufacturing. University of California, Berkeley Labor Center. Retrieved from http://laborcenter.berkeley.edu/producing-poverty-the-public-cost-of-low-wage-production-jobs-in-manufacturing/.

James, J. 2013 A new, evidence-based estimate of patient harms associated with hospital care. *Journal of Patient Safety* 9(3):122–128.

Jargowsky, P. 2003 *Stunning Progress, Hidden Problems: The Dramatic Decline of Concentrated Poverty in the 1990s*. Dallas: University of Texas.

Jauhar, S. 2014 *Doctored: The Disillusionment of an American Physician*. New York: Farrar, Straus and Giroux.

Johnson, K. 1991 Take our poor, angry Hartford tells suburbs. *New York Times*. Retrieved from www.nytimes.com/1991/02/12/nyregion/take-our-poor-angry-hartford-tells-suburbs.html?pagewanted=all.

Joint Center for Political and Economic Studies 2012 *Place Matters for Health in Baltimore*. Washington, DC: Joint Center for Political and Economic Studies.

Jorgensen, P. 2013 Pharmaceuticals, political money, and public policy: A theoretical agenda. *Journal of Law, Medicine and Ethics* 41(3):561–570.

Kaiser Family Foundation 2015 Employer health benefits survey. Retrieved from http://kff.org/health-costs/report/2015-employer-health-benefits-survey/.

Kaiser Family Foundation 2016 Key facts about the uninsured population. Retrieved from http://kff.org/uninsured/fact-sheet/key-facts-about-the-uninsured-population/.

Kamins M. 1989 Celebrity and non-celebrity advertising in a two-sided context. *Journal of Advertising Research* 29(3):34–42.

Karnik, A., Tschannel, A., and Anderson, M. 2015 What is a social medicine doctor? *Social Medicine* 9(2):56–62.

Katz, P. 1999 *The Scalpel's Edge: The Culture of Surgeons*. Boston, MA: Allyn and Bacon.

Kearns, C., Schmidt, L., and Glantz, S. 2016 Sugar industry and coronary heart disease research: A historical analysis of internal industry documents. *Journal of the American Medical Association*. Retrieved from doi:10.1001/jamainternmed.2016.5394.

Keating, C. 2010 Juan Figueroa drops out of Governor's race; cites raising money as a major problem; no deal for Lt. Governor. *Hartford Courant Capitol Watch Blog*. Retrieved from https://blogs.courant.com/capitol_watch/juan-figueroa-drops-out-of-gov.html.

Keehan, S., Poisal, J. Cuckler, G., Sisko, A., Smith, S., Madison, A. et al. 2016 National health expenditure projections, 2015–25: Economy, prices, and aging expected to shape spending and enrollment. *Health Affairs* (online before print). Retrieved from doi:10.1377/hlthaff.2016.0459.

Kelly Report 2015 Health disparities in America. Retrieved from https://robinkelly.house.gov/sites/robinkelly.house.gov/files/2015%20Kelly%20Report.pdf.

Keppel, K., Pearcy, J., and Wagener, D. 2002 Trends in racial and ethnic-specific rates for the health status indicators: United States, 1990–1998. *Healthy People 2000 Statistical Notes* 23:1–6.

Kidder, T. 2003 An interview with Tracy Kidder. *Bookbrowse.Com*. Retrieved from https://www.bookbrowse.com/author_interviews/full/index.cfm/author_number/940/tracy-kidder?

Kidder, T. 2004 *Mountains beyond Mountains: The Quest of Dr. Paul Farmer, a Man Who Would Cure the World*. New York: Random House Trade Paperbacks.

Kimbrell, A. 2016 Why the GMO "labeling" bill that Obama just signed into law is a sham—and a national embarrassment. *NPR*. Retrieved from www.huffingtonpost.com/andrew-kimbrell/why-the-gmo-labeling-bill_b_11335918.html.

King, M. 1977. *Strength to Love*. Cleveland, OH: Collins and World.

King, M. 1964 The future of integration. Speech to Oberlin College. Retrieved from www.oberlin.edu/external/EOG/BlackHistoryMonth/MLK/MLKmainpage.html.

Kirk, N. 2011 Health center history: There's more to explore. *UConn Today*. Retrieved from http://today.uconn.edu/2011/07/health-center-history-there%E2%80%99s-more-to-explore/#/.

Kirsch, A. 2007 This hospital serves any and everybody. *Poor Magazine*. Retrieved from http://img.alternet.org/story/64343/will_your_community_lose_its_hospital.

Kleinman, A. 2007 *What Really Matters: Living a Moral Life Amidst Uncertainty and Danger*. Oxford: Oxford University Press.

Kluegel, J. and Bobo, L. 1993 Dimensions of whites' belief about black-white socio-economic status, 1977–1989. *American Sociological Review* 55:512–525.

Kluger, J. 2009 Is drug-company money tainting medical education? *Time*. Retrieved from http://content.time.com/time/health/article/0,8599,1883449,00.html.

Kohn, L., Corrigan, J., and Donaldson, M. (Eds.) 1999 *To Err Is Human: Building a Safer Health System*. Washington, DC: The National Academies Press.

Kohn, N., Cash, D., and Brown, K. 2005 *Heartache in the heartland: Kansans speak about the burden of medical debt*. Boston, MA: The Access Project.

Konczal, M. 2009 GI Bill and suburbanization. Retrieved from https://rortybomb.wordpress.com/2009/09/11/gi-bill-and-suburbanization/.

Kornbluh, P. 2003 *The Pinochet File: A Declassified Dossier on Atrocity and Accountability*. New York: The New Press.

Kovner, J. 2015 Fewer pediatric services for residents of Hartford's North End. *Hartford Courant*. Retrieved from www.courant.com/news/connecticut/hc-saint-francis-clinics-1008-20151008-story.html.

Krieger, J. and Higgins, D. 2002 Housing and health: Time again for public health action. *American Journal of Public Health* 92(5):758–768.

Krieger, N. 2005 *Health Disparities and the Body*. Boston, MA: Harvard School of Public Health.

Krieger, N. 2007 Ecosocial theory. In: Anderson, N., ed. *Encyclopedia of Health and Behavior*. Thousand Oaks, CA: Sage Publications.

Kumanyika, S. 2005 Obesity, health disparities, and prevention paradigms: Hard questions and hard choices. *Preventing Chronic Disease* 2(4). Retrieved from https://www.cdc.gov/pcd/issues/2005/oct/05_0025.htm.

Kuzawa, C. and Sweet, E. 2009 Epigenetics and the embodiment of race: Developmental origins of US racial disparities in cardiovascular health. *American Journal of Human Biology* 21:2–15.

Kwallek, N., Woodson, H., Lewis, C., and Sales, C. 1996 Impact of three interior color schemes on worker mood and performance relative to individual environmental sensibility. *Color Research and Application* 22(2):121–132.

Lagu, T., Hannon, N., Rothberg, M., Wells, A., Green, L., Windom, M., Dempsey, K., Pekow, P., Avrunin, J., Chen, A., and Lindenauer, P. 2013 Access to subspecialty care for patients with mobility impairment: A survey. *Annals of Internal Medicine* 158(6):441–446.

Lancet Editorial 2016 WHO's war on sugar. *Lancet* 388(10055):1956.

Langreth, R. 2014 Big pharma's favorite prescription: Higher prices. *Bloomberg.com*. Retrieved from www.bloomberg.com/news/articles/2014-05-08/why-prescription-drug-prices-keep-rising-higher.

Laugesen, M. and Glied, S. 2011 Higher fees paid to US physicians drive higher spending for physician services compared to other countries. *Health Affairs* 30(9):1647–1656.

Leonard, D. 2012 Is concierge medicine the future of health care? *Bloomberg.com*. Retrieved from www.bloomberg.com/news/articles/2012-11-29/is-concierge-medicine-the-future-of-health-care.

Leontief, W. 1986 *Input-Output Economics*. Oxford: Oxford University Press.

Lerner, B. 2006 A case that shook medicine. *Washington Post*. Retrieved from www.washingtonpost.com/wp-dyn/content/article/2006/11/24/AR2006112400985.html.

Levins, R. 2000 Is capitalism a disease? The crisis in U.S. public health. *Monthly Review* 52(4):8–33.

Levy, B. 2013 Poverty, social injustice, and health. *Social Medicine* 7(3):169–171.

Lewis, J., Beavers, W., Gossett, J., and Phillips, V. 1976 *No Single Thread: Psychological Health in Family Systems*. Oxford: Brunner/Mazel.

Lichter, D., Parisi, D., and Taquinob, M. 2015 Segregation within and between metropolitan cities and suburbs. *American Sociological Review* 80(4):843–873.

Lichter, P. 2008 Debunking myths in physician–industry conflicts of interest. *American Journal of Ophthalmology* 146(2):159–171.

Lindert, P. and Williams, J. 2016 *Unequal Gains: American Growth and Inequality since 1700*. Princeton, NJ: Princeton University Press.

Liu, J. 2007 Health professional shortage and health status and health access. *Journal of Health Care for the Poor and Underserved* 18(3):590–598.

Lo, B. and Field, M., eds. 2009 *Conflict of Interest in Medical Research, Education, and Practice*. Washington, DC: Institute of Medicine.

Lock, M. and Nguyen, V-K. 2010 *An Anthropology of Biomedicine*. Malden, MA: John Wiley and Sons.

Loder, N. 2013 Let them eat nothing. *Economist*. Retrieved from www.economist.com/blogs/democracyinamerica/2013/08/food-stamps.

Long, D., Hunter, C., and van der Geest, S. 2008 When the field is a ward or a clinic: Hospital ethnography. *Anthropology and Medicine* 15(2):71–78.

Longo, D., Jameson, J., Loscalzo, J., Fauci, A., Kasper, D., Hauser, S. 2015 *Harrison's Principles of Internal Medicine.* New York: McGraw-Hill Education.

Los Angeles County Department of Public Health 2007 *Los Angeles County Health Survey.* Los Angeles, CA: Office of Health Assessment and Epidemiology.

Ludwig, M. 2015 How much of Big Pharma's massive profits are used to influence politicians? *TruthOut.* Retrieved from www.truth-out.org/news/item/33010-how-much-of-big-pharma-s-massive-profits-are-used-to-influence-politicians.

Lumeng, J., Appuglese, C., Cabral, H., Bradley, R., and Zuckerman, B. 2006 Neighborhood safety and overweight status in children. *Archives of Pediatric and Adolescent Medicine* 160(1):25–31.

Lynch, H. 2013 Discrimination at the doctor's office. *New England Journal of Medicine* 368:1668–1670.

Macintyre, S. and Ellaway, A. 2000 Ecological approaches: Rediscovering the role of the physical and social environment. In Berkman, L. and Kawachi, I., eds. *Social Epidemiology.* New York: Oxford University Press, pp. 332–348.

Mack, J. 2016 Annual spending on direct-to-consumer drug advertising ties an all-time high. *Pharma Marketing Blog.* Retrieved from http://pharmamkting.blogspot.com/2016/03/annual-spending-on-direct-to-consumer.html.

Mackenbach, J., Stirbu, L., Roskam, A., Schaap, M., Menvielle, G., Leinsalu, M., Kunsa, A., and the European Union Working Group on Socioeconomic Inequalities in Health. 2008 Socioeconomic inequalities in health in 22 European countries. *New England Journal of Medicine* 358(23):2468–2481.

Mader, E., Roseamelia, C., and Morely, C. 2014 The temporal decline of idealism in two cohorts of medical students at one institution. *BMC Medical Education* 14:58.

Majerol, M., Newkirk, V., and Garfield, R. 2015 Key facts about health insurance and the uninsured in an era of health reform. Kaiser Family Foundation. Retrieved from http://files.kff.org/attachment/primer-the-uninsured-a-primer-key-facts-about-health-insurance-and-the-uninsured-in-the-era-of-health-reform.

Makary, M. 2012 *Unaccountable: What Hospitals Won't Tell You and How Transparency Can Revolutionize Health Care.* New York: Bloomsbury Press.

Malani, P. 2012 Research paper insight: *Harrison's Principles of Internal Medicine. Journal of the American Medical Association* 308(17):1813. Retrieved from doi:10.1001/jama.308.17.1813.

Malik, V., Schulze, M., and Hu, F. 2006 Intake of sugar-sweetened beverages and weight gain: a systematic review. *American Journal of Clinical Nutrition* 4(2):274–288.

Mangan, D. 2016 Most want drug ads off TV, oppose faster approvals. *CNBC.* Retrieved from www.cnbc.com/2016/05/11/.

Manning, R., Levine, M. and Collins, A. 2007 The Kitty Genovese murder and the social psychology of helping: The parable of the 38 witnesses. *American Psychologist* 62(6):555–562.

Markel, H. 2008 The House of God: 30 years later. *Journal of the American Medical Association* 299(2):227–229.

Marmot, M. 2005 Social determinants of health inequalities. *Lancet* 365:1099–1004.

Marmot, M. 2015 *The Health Gap: The Challenge of an Unequal World.* London: Bloomsbury Press.

Marmot, M. and Wilkinson, R. 2005 *The Social Determinants of Health.* Oxford: Oxford University Press.

Marmot, M., Rose, G., Shipley, R., and Hamilton, P. 1978 Employment grade and coronary heart disease in British civil servants. *Journal of Epidemiology and Community Health* 32:244–249.

Marmot, M., Shipley, M. and Rose, G. 1991a Health inequalities among British civil servants: The Whitehall II study. *Lancet* 337:1387–1393.

Marmot, M., Shipley, M., and Rose, G. 1991b Inequalities in death: Specific explanations of a general pattern. *Lancet* 1(8284):1003–1006.

Maslach, C. and Leiter, M. 1997 *The Truth about Burnout*. San Francisco, CA: Jossey-Bass.

Massey, D. 1996 The age of extremes: Concentrated affluence and poverty in the twenty-first century 33(4):395–412.

Massey, D. and Denton, N. 1993. *American Apartheid: Segregation and the Making of the Underclass*. Cambridge, MA: Harvard University Press.

Mattingly, C. 2012 Two virtue ethics and the anthropology of morality. *Anthropological Theory* 12(2):161–184.

Mayo Clinic 2016 Diabetes. Retrieved from www.mayoclinic.org/diseases-conditions/diabetes/basics/complications/con-20033091.

Mayoral, J., Alonso, J., Garin, O., Herrador, Z., Astray, J., Baricot, M., Castilla, J., Canton, R., Castro, A. et al. 2012 Social factors related to the clinical severity of influenza cases in Spain during the A (H1N1) 2009 virus pandemic. *BMC Public Health* 13:118. Retrieved from doi:10.1186/1471-2458-13-118.

McGandy, R., Hegsted, D., and Stare, F. 1967a Dietary fats, carbohydrates and atherosclerotic vascular disease [Part 1]. *New England Journal of Medicine* 277(4):186–192.

McGandy, R., Hegsted, D., and Stare, F. 1967b Dietary fats, carbohydrates and atherosclerotic vascular disease [Part 2]. *New England Journal of Medicine* 277(5):245–247.

McGaphie, W. 2002 Assessing readiness for medical education: Evolution of the Medical College Admission Test. *Journal of the American Medical School Association* 388(9):1085–1090.

McKenna, B. 2010 Take back medical education: The "primary care" shuffle. *Medical Anthropology* 29(1):6–14.

McWilliams, J., Meara, E., Zaslavsky, A., and Ayanian, J. 2007 Use of health services by previously uninsured Medicare beneficiaries. *New England Journal of Medicine* 357(2):143–153.

Meehan, E. 2013 The debate over who could occupy World War II public housing in West Hartford. *ConnecticutHistory.Org*. Retrieved from http://connecticuthistory.org/the-debate-over-who-could-occupy-world-war-ii-public-housing-in-west-hartford/.

Meldrum, H. 2010 *Characteristics of compassion: Portraits of exemplary physicians*. Burlington, MA: Jones & Bartlett.

Mensah, G., Mokdad, A., Ford, E., Greenlund, K., and Croft, J. 2005 State of disparities in cardiovascular health in the United States. *Circulation* 111:1233–1241.

Migrant Farm Worker Clinics Video 2016 About the clinics. Retrieved from www.publichealth.uconn.edu/migrant-farm-worker-clinics.html.

Miles, S. 2004 *The Hippocratic Oath and the Ethics of Medicine*. Oxford: Oxford University Press.

Miller, T. 2016 Closure of Colusa's only hospital "disaster for the community." *KCRA*. Retrieved from www.kcra.com/news/only-hospital-in-colusa-county-to-close/38831148.

Minkel, J. 2007 Complications: The toll of diabetes. *Scientific American*. Retrieved from www.scientificamerican.com/article/complications-the-toll-of-diabetes/.

Mintz, Z. 2015. MLK Day quotes: 15 sayings to honor Martin Luther King Jr. in 2015. *IBTimes.com*. Retrieved from www.ibtimes.com/mlk-day-quotes-15-sayings-honor-martin-luther-king-jr-2015-1785998.

Mises Institute 2016 What is the Mises Institute? Retrieved from https://mises.org/about-mises/what-is-the-mises-Institute.

Mishel, L., Bernstein, J., and Allegretto, S. 2005 *The State of Working America 2004–2005*. Ithaca, NY: Cornell University Press.

Mokdad, A., Ford, E., Bowman, B., Diez, W., Vinicor, F., Bales, V., and Marks, J. 2003 Prevalence of obesity, diabetes, and obesity-related health risk factors, 2001. *Journal of the American Medical Association* 289:76–79.

Moore, P. 2014 Poll results: Punishment. Retrieved from https://today.yougov.com/news/2014/09/17/poll-results-punishment/.

Moreno, G., Morales, L., Nuñez de Jaimes, F., Tseng, C., Isiordia, M., Noguera, C., and Mangione, C. 2014 Neighborhood perceptions and health-related outcomes among Latinos with diabetes from a rural agricultural community. *Journal of Community Health* 39(6):1077–1084.

Morley, C., Roseamelia, C., Smith, J., and Villarreal, A. 2013 Decline of medical student idealism in the first and second year of medical school: A survey of pre-clinical medical students at one institution. *Medical Education Online* 18:21194.

Morone, J. 1990 *The Democratic Wish: Popular Participation and the Limits of American Government*. New York: Basic Books.

Morrison, R., Busby, J., and Wells, H. 2010 Guess who's turning 100? Tracking a century of American eating. United States Department of Agriculture, Economic Research Service. Retrieved from www.ers.usda.gov/amber-waves/2010-march/guess-who%E2%80%99s-turning-100tracking-a-century-of-american-eating.aspx#.V5XrCthTFjo.

Moyers, B. 2016 We, the plutocrats vs. we, the people: Saving the soul of democracy. *TomDispatch*. Retrieved from www.tomdispatch.com/blog/176184/.

Mustain, P. 2014 The point-by-point response to beverage industry script that was removed from a news station website. *Scientific American*. Retrieved from http://blogs.scientificamerican.com/food-matters/the-point-by-point-response-to-beverage-industry-script-that-was-removed-from-a-news-station-website/.

National Center for Children in Poverty 2016 Child poverty. Retrieved from www.nccp.org/topics/childpoverty.html.

National Center for Farmworker Health 2014 *Regional Migrant Health Profile*. Buda, TX: NCFH.

National Center for Health Statistics 2012 Health, United States, 2011: With special feature on socioeconomic status and health. Hyattsville, MD: National Center for Health Statistics. *Health Affairs* 31(8):1803–1813.

National Public Radio 2015 Ebola doctor to grads: Enter the suffering of others. *NPR*. Retrieved from www.npr.org/2015/05/17/407447354/ebola-doctor-to-grads-enter-the-suffering-of-others.

New York City Department of Education 2012 Progress report 2011–12: Harlem Children's Zone/Promise Academy Charter School. Retrieved from http://schools.nyc.gov/OA/SchoolReports/2011-12/Progress_Report_2012_HS_M284.pdf.

Newport, F. 2016 Majority in U.S. support idea of Fed-funded healthcare system. *Gallup*. Retrieved from www.gallup.com/poll/191504/majority-support-idea-fed-funded-health care-system.aspx.

NHS Health Scotland 2004 Public Health Institute for Scotland. Available online at: www.phis.org.uk.

Nolte, E. and McKee, M. 2011 Variations in amenable mortality: Trends in 16 high income nations. *Health Policy* 103(1):47–52.

Nuland, S. 1988 *Doctors: The Biography of Medicine*. New York: Alfred A. Knopf.

O'Hare, W. and Mather, M. 2003 *The Growing Number of Kids in Severely Distressed Neighborhoods: Evidence from the 2000 Census*. Baltimore, MD: Annie E. Casey Foundation.

O'Rourke, M. 2014 Doctors tell all—and it's bad. *The Atlantic*. Retrieved from www.theatlantic.com/magazine/archive/2014/11/doctors-tell-all-and-its-bad/380785/.

Oberlander, J. 2006 The political economy of unfairness in U.S. health policy. *Law and Contemporary Problems* 60:244–264.

Ockene, J., Quick, M., Goldberg, R., Kristeller, J., Donnelly, G., Kalan, K., Gould, B. et al. 1988 A residents' training program for the development of smoking intervention skills. *Archives of Internal Medicine* 148(5):1039–1045.

Olshansky, S., Antonucci, T., Berkman, L., Binstock, R., Boersch-Supan, A., Cacioppo, J., Carnes, B. et al. 2012 Differences in life expectancy due to race and educational differences are widening, and many may not catch up. *Health Affairs* 31(8): 1803–1813.

Olshansky, S., Passaro, D., Hershow, R., Layden, J., Carnes, B., Brody, J., Hayflick, L. et al. 2005 A potential decline in life expectancy in the United States in the 21st century. *New England Journal of Medicine* 352(11):1138–1145.

Orbinski, J. 2008 *An Imperfect Offering: Humanitarian Action for the Twenty-First Century*. New York: Walker.

Ornstein, C. 2010 Lawsuits say pharma illegally paid doctors to push their drugs. *ProPublica.org*. Retrieved from https://www.propublica.org/article/lawsuits-say-pharma-illegally-paid-doctors-to-push-their-drugs.

Ornstein, C. 2014 Our first dive into the new open payments system. *ProPublica.org*. Retrieved from https://www.propublica.org/article/our-first-dive-into-the-new-open-payments-system.

Ornstein, C. and Jones, R. 2015 A pharma payment a day keeps docs' finances okay. *ProPublica.org*. Retrieved from https://www.propublica.org/article/a-pharma-payment-a-day-keeps-docs-finances-ok.

Ornstein, C. and Jones, R. 2016 Doctors at Southern hospitals take the most payments from drug, device companies. *NPR*. Retrieved from www.npr.org/sections/health-shots/2016/06/29/483895152/industry-finds-receptive-doctors-at-for-profit-southern-hospitals.

Ornstein, C., Jones, R., and Tigas, M. 2016 Now there's proof: Docs who get company cash tend to prescribe more brand-name meds. *ProPublica.org*. Retrieved from https://www.propublica.org/article/doctors-who-take-company-cash-tend-to-prescribe-more-brand-name-drugs.

Palmieri, J. and Stern, T. 2009 Lies in the doctor-patient relationship. *Primary Care Companion Journal of Clinical Psychiatry* 11(4):163–168.

Park, J. and Grow, J. 2008 The social reality of depression: DTC advertising of antidepressants and perceptions of the prevalence and lifetime risk of depression. *Journal of Business Ethics* 79(4):379–393.

Parrott, S. 2014 Commentary: Ryan report distorts safety net's picture. *Center on Budget and Policy Priorities. CBPP.Org*. Retrieved from www.cbpp.org/commentary-ryan-report-distorts-safety-nets-picture.

Patel, V., Ashrafian, H., Uzoho, C., Nikiteas, N., Panzarasa, P., Sevdalis, N. et al. 2016 Leadership behaviours and healthcare research performance: Prospective correlational study. *Postgraduate Medical Journal*. Retrieved from doi:10.1136/postgradmedj-2016-134088.

Patternson, R. and Katz, H. 1983 Investor-owned and not-for-profit hospitals: A comparison based on California data. *New England Journal of Medicine* 309:347–353.

Pease, B. 2011 Theorizing normalization as hidden privilege. In Fahlgren, S., Johansson, A. and Mulinari, D., eds. *Normalization and "Outsiderhood": Feminist Readings of a Neoliberal Welfare State*. Dubai: Bentham Science Publishers, pp. 69–79.

Petryna, A. and Kleinman, A. 2006 The pharmaceutical nexus. In Petryna, A., Lakoff, A. and Kleinman, A., eds. *Global Pharmaceuticals: Ethics, Market, Practices*. Durham, NC: Duke University Press, pp. 1–32.

Pew Research Center 2016 America's shrinking middle class: A close look at changes within metropolitan areas. Retrieved from www.pewsocialtrends.org/2016/05/11/americas-shrinking-middle-class-a-close-look-at-changes-within-metropolitan-areas/.

Philibert, I. and Amis, S. 2011 *The ACGME 2011 Duty Hour Standards: Enhancing Quality of Care, Supervision, and Resident Professional Development*. Chicago, IL: Accreditation Council for Graduate Medical Education.

Piketty, T. 2014 *Capital in the Twenty-First Century*. Cambridge, MA: Belknap Press.

Pipes, S. 2015 Letting patients buy Canadian drugs will only import trouble. *The Hill*. Retrieved from http://thehill.com/blogs/congress-blog/healthcare/231320-letting-patients-buy-canadian-drugs-will-only-import-trouble.

Piven, F. 2007 The neoliberal challenge. *Contexts* 6(3):13–15.

Pofeldt, E. 2016 How anger is fraying the doctor-patient relationship. *Medical Economics* 93(10):30–33.

Polk, J. 2008 *The Triumph of Ignorance and Bliss: Pathologies of Public America*. Montreal: Black Rose Books.

Porter, D. 2011 Direct-to-consumer (DTC) pharmaceutical marketing: Impacts and policy implications. *SPNHA Review* 1(5). Retrieved from http://scholarworks.gvsu.edu/spnhareview/vol7/iss1/5.

Prevention Institute 2002 Eliminating health disparities: the role of primary prevention. Briefing paper for the California Endowment Board of Directors. San Francisco.

Price-Mitchell, M. 2010 Civic learning at the edge: Transformative stories of highly engaged youth. Doctoral Dissertation, Fielding Graduate University, Santa Barbara, CA.

Price-Mitchell, M. 2015 *Tomorrow's Change Makers: Reclaiming the Power of Citizenship for a New Generation*. Bainbridge Island, WA: Eagle Harbor Publishing.

Proctor, B., Semenga, J., and Kollar, M. 2016 Income and Poverty in the United States: 2015. United States Census Bureau. Retrieved from https://www.census.gov/library/publications/2016/demo/p60-256.html.

Quiley, F. 2016 Disgusted with sky-high drug prices, California voters take on Big Pharma. *TruthOut*. Retrieved from www.truth-out.org/news/item/37260-disgusted-with-sky-high-drug-prices-california-voters-take-on-big-pharma.

Radcliffe, D. 1998 *Charter Oak Terrace: Life, Death and Rebirth of a Public Housing Project*. Hartford, CT: Southside Media.

Rakatansky, H. 1994 The role of the role model. *Rhode Island Medicine* 77:339–340.

Rao, P. 2007 *Heat Related Illnesses*. Washington, DC: Farmworker Justice and Migrant Clinicians Network.

Rappeport, A. 2015 Making it rain: Members of Congress are mostly millionaires. *New York Times*. Retrieved from www.nytimes.com/politics/first-draft/2015/01/12/making-it-rain-members-of-congress-are-mostly-millionaires/.

Ratner, C. 2013 False consciousness. In: T. Teo, ed. *The Encyclopedia of Critical Psychology*. New York: Springer Publishing Co, pp. 673–685.

Reese, D. 1998 Fundamentals: Rudolf Virchow and modern medicine. *Western Journal of Medicine* 169(2):105–108.

Reich, R. 2016 Why a single-payer health care system is inevitable. *Arca Max*. Retrieved from www.arcamax.com/politics/fromtheleft/robertbreich/s-1865349-p2.

Relman, A. 1980 The new medical-industrial complex. *New England Journal of Medicine* 303:963–970.

Reuler, J. and Nardone, D. 1994 Role modeling in medical education. *Western Journal of Medicine* 160:335–337.

Rhodes, L. 1996 Studying biomedicine as a cultural system. In: Sargent, C. and Johnson, T., eds. *Medical Anthropology: Contemporary Theory and Practice*, pp. 165–180. Westport, CT: Praeger.

Richardson, B., Hulka, B., Peck, J., Hughes, C., van den Berg, B., Christianson, R., and Calvin, J. 1998. Levels of maternal serum alpha-fetoprotein (AFP) in pregnant women and subsequent breast cancer risk. *American Journal of Epidemiology* 148(8):719–727.

Richardson, E. and Hemenway, D. 2011 Homicide, suicide, and unintentional firearm fatality: Comparing the United States with other high-income countries, 2003. *Journal of Trauma and Acute Care Surgery* 70(1):238–243.

Roach, R. 2002 Unequal treatment: Confronting racial and ethnic disparities in health care. *Black Issues in Higher Education* 19(7):26.

Rose, G., Merchant, A., and Bakir, A. 2012 Fantasy in food advertising targeted to children. *Journal of Advertising* 41(3):75–90.

Rose, N. 2007 *The Politics of Life Itself: Biomedicine, Power, and Subjectivity in the Twenty-First Century*. Princeton, NJ: Princeton University Press.

Roseblum, K. and Travis, T. 1996 Experiencing difference: Framework essay. In: Rosenblum, K. and Travis, T., eds. *The Meaning of Difference: American Construction of Race, Sex, and Gender, Social Class and Sexual Orientation*. New York: McGraw-Hill.

Rosenthal, A. 1999 *Thirty-Eight Witnesses: The Kitty Genovese Case*. Berkeley, CA: University of California Press.

Rosoff, S. and Leone, M. 1991 The public prestige of medical specialties: Overviews and undercurrents. *Social Science and Medicine* 32(3):321–326.

Sahadi, J. 2012 Romney paid 14% effective tax rate in 2011. *CNN Money*. Retrieved from http://money.cnn.com/2012/09/21/pf/taxes/romney-tax-return/index.html.

Saluja, S., Woolhandler, S., Himmelstein, D., and McCormick, M. 2016a Unsafe drugs were prescribed more than one hundred million times in the United States before being recalled. *International Journal of Health Services* 46(3):523–530.

Saluja, S., Zallman, L., Nardin, R., Bor, D., Woolhandler, S., Himmelstein, D., and McCormick, D. 2016b Support for National Health Insurance seven years into Massachusetts Healthcare Reform. *International Journal of Health Services* 46:185–200.

Sawyer, B., Williams, M. DeLapp, R., and Davis, D. 2016 Posttraumatic stress disorder. In Breland-Noble, A., Al-Mateen, C. and Singh, N., eds. *Handbook of Mental Health in African American Youth*. New York: Springer, pp. 237–247.

Saydah, S. and Lochner. K. 2010 Socioeconomic status and risk of diabetes-related mortality in the U.S. *Public Health Reports* 125(3):377–388.

Scheiber, N. 2016 Doctors unionize to resist the medical machine. *New York Times*. Retrieved from www.nytimes.com/2016/01/10/business/doctors-unionize-to-resist-the-medical-machine.html.

Schernhammer, E. 2005 Taking their own lives: The high rate of physician suicide. *New England Journal of Medicine* 352:2473–2376.

Schofferman, J. 2011 The medical–industrial complex, professional medical associations, and continuing medical education. *Pain Medicine*. Retrieved from doi:http://dx.doi.org/10.1111/j.1526-4637.2011.01282.

Seifert, R. 2005 *Home Sick: How Medical Debt Undermines Housing Security*. Boston, MA: The Access Project: Boston.

Shalof, T. 2010 *A Nurse's Story*. Toronto: McClelland and Stewart.

Shanafelt, T., Balch, C., Bechamps, G., Russell. T., Dyrbye, L., Satele, D., Collicott, P., Novotny, P., Sloan. J., and Freischlag, J. 2009 Burnout and career satisfaction among American surgeons. *Annals of Surgery* 250(3):463–471.

Shanafelt, T., Balch, C., Dyrbye, L., Bechamps, G., Russell, T., Satele, D., Rummans, T., Swartz, K., Novotny, P., Sloan, J., and Oreskovich, M. 2011 Special report: Suicidal ideation among American surgeons. *Archives of Surgery* 146(1):54–62.

Shanafelt, T., Boone, S., Tan, L., Dyrbye, L., Sotile, W., Satele, D., West, D., Sloan, J., and Oreskovich, M. 2012 Burnout and satisfaction with work-life balance among US physicians relative to the general US population. *Archives of Internal Medicine* 172(18):1377–1386.

Shapiro. D. 2004 Drug companies get too close for med school's comfort. *New York Times.* January 20:F5.

Shea, J., Bridge, P. Gould, B., and Harris, I. 2004 UME-21 local evaluation initiatives: Contributions and challenges. *Family Medicine* 36(supplement):S133–S137.

Shem, S. 1978 *The House of God.* New York: Dell.

Shem, S. 2002 Fiction as resistance. *Annals of Internal Medicine* 137(11):934–937.

Shem, S. 2012 Samuel Shem, 34 years after "The House of God," *The Atlantic.* Retrieved from www.theatlantic.com/health/archive/2012/11/samuel-shem-34-years-after-the-house-of-god/265675/.

Shrank, W. and Avorn, J. 2007 Educating patients about their medications: The potential and limitations of written drug information. *Health Affairs* 26(3):731–740.

Shy, K., Larson, E., and Luthy, D. 1987 Evaluating a new technology: The effectiveness of electronic fetal monitoring. *Annual Review of Public Health* 8:165–90.

Silverman, S. 2015 In an era of healthcare delivery reforms, the corporate practice of medicine is a matter that requires vigilance. *Health Law and Policy Brief* 9(1):1–23.

Simonsen, L., Clarke, M., Williamson, G., Stroup, D. Arden, N., and Schonberger, L. 1997 The impact of influenza epidemics on mortality: Introducing a severity index. *American Journal of Public Health* 87(12):1944–1950.

Sinclair, U. 1915 *The Cry for Justice: An Anthology of the Literature of Social Protest.* Philadelphia, PA: The John C. Winston Co.

Singer, M. 1994 AIDS and the health crisis of the U.S. urban poor: The perspective of critical medical anthropology. *Social Science and Medicine* 39(7):931–948.

Singer, M. 2006 *Something Dangerous: Emergent and Changing Illicit Drug Use and Community Health.* Prospect Heights, IL: Waveland Press.

Singer, M. 2009 Desperate measures: A syndemic approach to the anthropology of health in a violent city. In: Rylko-Bauer, B., Whiteford, L., and Farmer, P., eds. *Global Health in Times of Violence.* Santé Fe, NM: School for Advanced Research Press, pp. 137–156.

Singer, M. (Ed.) 2016 *A Companion to the Anthropology of Environmental Health.* San Francisco, CA: Wiley-Blackwell.

Singer, M. and Baer, H. 2009 Introduction: Hidden harm: The complex world of killer commodities. In: Singer, M. and Baer, H., eds. *Killer Commodities: Public Health and the Corporate Production of Harm.* Lanham, MD: Altamira, pp. 1–32.

Singer, M. and Garcia, R. 1989 Becoming a Puerto Rican espiritista: Life history of a female healer. In: McClain, C., ed. *Women as Healers.* New Brunswick, NJ: Rutgers University Press, pp. 157–185.

Singer, M., Ostrach, B., and Evans, J. 2013 "Pharmacopatienthood": The patient constructed in direct-to-consumer drug advertising. *Anthropology* 1:1.

Sinsky, C., Colligan, L., Li, M., Prgomet, M., Reynolds, S., Goeders, L., Westbrook, J. Tutty, M., and Blike, G. 2016 Allocation of physician time in ambulatory practice: A time and motion study in 4 specialties. *Annals of Internal Medicine* 165(11):753–760.

Skrepnek, G., Mills, J., and Armstrong, D. 2015 A diabetic emergency one million feet long: Disparities and burdens of illness among diabetic foot ulcer cases within emergency departments in the United States, 2006–2010. *PLoS One* 10(8):e0134914.

Smarsh, S. 2014 Poor teeth. *Aeon.* Retrieved from https://aeon.co/essays/there-is-no-shame-worse-than-poor-teeth-in-a-rich-world.

Smedley, B., Stith, A., and Nelsen, A. 2002 *Unequal Treatment: Understanding Racial and Ethnic Disparities in Health Care*. Washington, DC: National Academies Press.

Smedley, T. 2006 Poor people in rich nations: The United States in comparative perspective. *Journal of Economic Perspectives* 20(1):69–90.

Sommeiller, E., Price, M., and Wazeter, E. 2016 *Income Inequality in the U.S. by State, Metropolitan Area, and County*. Washington, DC: Economic Policy Institute.

Sondheimer, H., Xierali, I., Young, G., and Nivet, A. 2015 Placement of US medical school graduates into graduate medical education, 2005 through 2015. *Journal of the American Medical Association* 314(22):2409–2410.

Spencer, L. 2015 Coltsville, USA: Inside America's gun-funded utopia. *Atlas Obscura*. Retrieved from www.atlasobscura.com/articles/coltsville_abandoned_utopian_guns_village.

Spickard, A., Gabbe, S., and Christensen, J. 2002 Mid-career burnout in generalist and specialist physicians. *Journal of the American Medical Association* 288(12):1447–1450.

Squires, D. 2012 Explaining high health care spending in the United States: An international comparison of supply, utilization, prices, and quality. The Commonwealth Fund. Retrieved from www.commonwealthfund.org/publications/issue-briefs/2012/may/high-health-care-spending.

Squires, G. and Kubrin, C. 2006 Privileged places: Race, opportunity and uneven development in urban America. *National Housing Institute Shelterforce Online* 147. Retrieved from http://nhi.org/online/issues/147/privilegedplaces.html.

Starfield, B., Shi, L., and Macinko, J. 2005 Contribution of primary care to health systems and health. *Milbank Quarterly* 83(3):457–502.

Starr, P. 1982 *The Social Transformation of American Medicine*. New York: Basic Books.

Steinwald, B. and Neuhauser, D. 1970 The role of the proprietary hospital. *Law and Contemporary Problems* 35(4):817–838.

Sterner, D. 2012 *A Guide to Historic Hartford, Connecticut*. Charleston, SC: The History Press.

Stiglitz, J. 2013 *The Price of Inequality*. New York: W.W. Norton.

Stoeckle, J. and Reiser, S. 1992 The corporate organization of hospital work: Balancing professional and administrative responsibilities. *Annals of Internal Medicine* 116(5):407–413.

Strauss, M. and Paschall, M. 2009 Corporal punishment by mothers and development of children's cognitive ability: A longitudinal study of two nationally representative age cohorts. *Journal of Aggression, Maltreatment & Trauma* 18:159–183.

Stringhini, S., Sabia, S., Shipley, M., Brunner, E., Nabi, H., Kivimaki, M., and Singh-Manoux, A. 2010 Association of socioeconomic position with health behaviors and mortality. *Journal of the American Medical Association* 303(12):1159–1166.

Stringhini, S., Carmeli, C., Jokela, M., Avendaño, M., Muennig, P., Guida, F., Ricceri, F., d'Errico, A., Barros, H., Bochud, M., Chadeau-Hyam, M., Clavel-Chapelon, F., Costa, G., Delpierre, C., Fraga, S., Goldberg, M., Giles, G., Krogh, V., Kelly-Irving, M., Layte, R., Lasserre, A., Marmot, M., Preisig, M., Shipley, M., Vollenweider, P., Zins, M., Kawachi, I., Steptoe, A., Mackenbach, J., Vineis, P., and Kivimäki, M. 2017 Socioeconomic status and the 25×25 risk factors as determinants of premature mortality: A multicohort study and meta-analysis of 1.7 million men and women. *Lancet* 380(10068): 477–572.

Student Doctor Network 2004 Your most frustrating illness to treat? Retrieved from http://forums.studentdoctor.net/threads/your-most-frustrating-illness-to-treat.1144772/.

Sustain 2014 A children's future fund: How food duties could provide the money to protect children's health and the world they grow up in. Retrieved from https://www.sustainweb.org/publications/a_childrens_future_fund/.

Swartz, M. 1995 Not what the doctor ordered. Texas Monthly. Retrieved from www.texasmonthly.com/articles/not-what-the-doctor-ordered-2/.

Swift, M. 2001 City loses blacks to suburbs. *Hartford Courant*. Retrieved from www.courant.com/hc-census-0321-story.html.

Taibbi, M. 2013 Everything is rigged: The biggest price-fixing scandal ever. *Rolling Stone*. Retrieved from www.rollingstone.com/politics/news/everything-is-rigged-the-biggest-financial-scandal-yet-20130425.

Tan, L. and Ong, K. 2002 The impact of medical technology on healthcare today. *Hong Kong Journal of Emergency Medicine* 9(4):231–236.

Taylor, C., Manganello, J., Lee, S., and Rice, J. 2010 Mothers' spanking of 3-year-old children and subsequent risk of children's aggressive behavior. *Pediatrics* 125(5):e1057– e1065.

Taylor, E., Genevro, J., Peikes, D., Geonnotti, K., Wang, W., and Meyers, D. 2013 Building quality improvement capacity in primary care: Supports and resources. Agency for Healthcare Research and Quality. Retrieved from www.ahrq.gov/professionals/prevention-chronic-care/improve/capacity-building/pcmhqi2.html.

Taylor, R. 1985 Medicine as social science: Rudolf Virchow on the typhus epidemic in Upper Silesia. *International Journal of Health Services* 15(4):547–559.

Temkin, O. 1963. The scientific approach to disease: Specific entity and individual sickness. In: Crombie, A.C., ed. *Scientific Change*. New York and London: Heinemann, pp. 629–647.

The AHEC Bulletin 1983 Center news. Retrieved from https://www.nationalahec.org/publications/documents/BulletinMay1983VolumeI.pdf.

The Segal Group 2015 Segal health plan cost trend survey. Retrieved from https://www.segalco.com/media/2138/ps-trend-survey-2016.pdf.

Thomas, L. 2014 Hospitals, doctors moving out of poor city neighborhoods to more affluent areas. *Journal Sentinel*. Retrieved from www.jsonline.com/news/health/hospitals-doctors-moving-out-of-poor-city-neighborhoods-to-more-affluent-areas-b99284882z1-262899701.html.

Throop, C. 2014 Moral moods. *Ethos* 42(1):65–83.

Tirado, L. 2013 This is why poor people's bad decisions make perfect sense. *Huffington Post*. Retrieved from www.huffingtonpost.com/linda-tirado/why-poor-peoples-bad-decisions-make-perfect-sense_b_4326233.html.

Tirodkar, M. and Jain, A. 2003 Food messages on African American television shows. *American Journal of Public Health* 93(3):439–441.

Tomoda, A., Suzuki, H., Rabi, K., Sheu, Y-S., Polcari, A., and Teicher, M. 2009 Reduced prefrontal cortical gray matter volume in young adults exposed to harsh corporal punishment. *Neuroimage* 47(Supplement 2):T66–T71.

Trinity College 2001 *A Hartford Primer and Field Guide*. Hartford, CT: Cities Data Center, Trinity College.

Trinity College 2014 Hispanic Hartford. Hispanic Studies Program. Retrieved from www.hispanichartford.org/community/history/.

Trump, D. 2011 *Time to Get Tough*. Washington, DC: Regnery Publishing.

Tumulty, K. 2009 Interview with Max Baucus, Health Care Reform Newsmaker Series. Kaiser Family Foundation. Retrieved from http://khn.org/news/newsmaker-baucus-2/.

Twedt, S. 2009 UPMC to close Braddock hospital. *Pittsburgh Post-Gazette*. Retrieved from www.post-gazette.com/local/east/2009/10/17/UPMC-to-close-Braddock-hospital/stories/200910170164.

Tylee, J. 2016 Should the Olympics allow fast-food sponsors? *Campaign*. Retrieved from www.campaignlive.co.uk/article/olympics-allow-fast-food-sponsors/1404057#.

Ubel, P. 2014 Is the profit motive ruining American healthcare? *Forbes*. Retrieved from www.forbes.com/sites/peterubel/2014/02/12/is-the-profit-motive-ruining-american-healthcare/#31ffc808a0ce.

UConn Health 2009 Primary care champion honored by health center board. Retrieved from http://today.uchc.edu/newsreleases/2009/may09/gould.html.

UConn Migrant Farm Worker Clinics 2016 Clinic brochure. Retrieved from www.publichealth.uconn.edu/assets/mfwclinicbrochure2016.pdf.

Ulrich, R. 1983 Aesthetic and affective response to natural environment. In: Altman, I and Wohlwill, J., eds. *Human Behavior and Environment*, Vol. 6 New York: Plenum, pp. 85–125.

Union of Concerned Scientists 2012 Industry influence on drug and medical device safety at FDA. Retrieved from www.ucsusa.org/sites/default/files/legacy/assets/documents/scientific_integrity/industry-influence-drug-medical-device-safety-FDA.pdf.

Union of Concerned Scientists 2016 Sugar industry paid Harvard scientists to shift blame to fat. *EcoWatch*. Retrieved from www.ecowatch.com/sugar-industry-2004899240.html.

Urban Service Track Video 2016 About Urban Service Track. Retrieved from www.publichealth.uconn.edu/urban-service-track.html.

U.S. Census Bureau 2008 Income, poverty, and health insurance coverage in the United States: 2007. Retrieved from www.census.gov/prod/2008pubs/p60-235.pdf.

U.S. Census Bureau 2015 QuickFacts: Hartford City, Connecticut. Retrieved from www.census.gov/quickfacts/table/PST045215/0937000.

US Department of Health and Human Services. 2000 *Healthy People 2010*, 2nd ed. Washington, DC: U.S. Government Printing Office.

U.S. Department of Labor 2005 The National Agricultural Workers Survey. Retrieved from https://www.doleta.gov/agworker/naws.cfm.

U.S. Department of Labor 2016 Minimum wage mythbusters. Retrieved from https://www.dol.gov/featured/minimum-wage/mythbuster.

U.S. Food and Drug Administration 2011 The impact of direct-to-consumer advertising. Retrieved from www.fda.gov/Drugs/ResourcesForYou/Consumers/ucm143562.htm.

U.S. Preventative Services Task Force 2016 Published recommendations. Retrieved from https://www.uspreventiveservicestaskforce.org/BrowseRec/Index.

UT Southwestern Medical Center 2016 Curriculum: Year One, Retrieved from www.utsouthwestern.edu/education/medical-school/academics/curriculum/first-year.html.

Vallejos, Q., Quandt, S., Grywacz, J., Isom, S., Chen, H., Galvan, L., Whalley, L. et al. 2011 Migrant farmworkers' housing conditions across an agricultural season in North Carolina. *American Journal of Internal Medicine* 54(7):533–544.

Vasquez, D. 2003 Latinos in Hartford, Connecticut. Boston, MA: Gastón Institute Publications, University of Massachusetts, Paper 64.

Verghese, A. 1994 *My Own Country: A Doctor's Story*. New York: Simon Schuster.

Volpentesta, E. 2015 The doctor is out: Insurers controlling health care. *Hartford Courant*. Retrieved from www.courant.com/opinion/op-ed/hc-op-volpintesta-doctor-patient-insurance-0208-20150206-story.html.

Wacquant, L. 2002 Deadly symbiosis: Rethinking race and imprisonment in twenty-first-century America. *Boston Review* April/May. Retrieved from http://bostonreview.net/BR27.2/wacquant.html.

Waitzkin, H. 2006 One and a half centuries of forgetting and rediscovering: Virchow's lasting contributions to social medicine. *Social Medicine* 1(1):5–10.

Waitzkin, H. 2011 *Medicine and Public Health at the End of Empire*. Boulder, CO: Paradigm Publishers.

Wall, L. and Brown, D. 2002 Pharmaceutical sales representatives and the doctor/patient relationship. *Obstetrics and Gynecology* 100(3):594–599.

Wall, T. and Nasseh, K. 2013 Dental-related emergency department visits on the increase in the United States. The American Dental Association's Health Policy Institute. Retrieved from www.ada.org/~/media/ADA/Science%20and%20Research/HPI/Files/HPIBrief_0513_1.pdf.

Wang, Y., Bleich, S., and Gortmaker, S. 2008 Increasing caloric contribution from sugar-sweetened beverages and 100% fruit juices among US children and adolescents, 1988–2004. *Pediatrics* 121(6):1604–1616.

Wardle, J. 2002 Sex differences in association with SES and obesity. *American Journal of Public Health* 92:1299–1304.

Wattles, J. 2015 Paul Ryan gets a sweet pay raise. *CNN*. Retrieved from http://money.cnn.com/2015/10/29/pf/jobs/paul-ryan-pay-hike/.

Webster, B. and Bishaw, SA. 2006 In*come, Earnings, and Poverty Data From the 2005 American Community Survey*. Washington, DC: U.S. Department of Commerce.

Weeks, W., Robinson, M., Brooks, W., and Batalden, P. 2000 Using early clinical experiences to integrate quality-improvement learning into medical education. *Academic Medicine* 75:81–84.

Weiner, L. 2014 What to do about physician unions. *Health Leaders*. Retrieved by www.healthleadersmedia.com/hr/what-do-about-physician-unions.

Weiss, R. 1988 *The American Myth of Success: From Horatio Alger to Norman Vincent Peale*. Chicago, IL: University of Chicago Press.

Weissman, J. 2016 Why I can't stop laughing at Paul Ryan's anti-poverty plan. *Slate*. Retrieved from www.slate.com/blogs/moneybox/2016/06/07/i_can_t_stop_laughing_at_paul_ryan_s_anti_poverty_plan.html.

Weissman, R. 2011 The GOP's deregulation obsession. *The Nation*. Retrieved from http://eds.a.ebscohost.com.ezproxy.lib.uconn.edu/ehost/pdfviewer/pdfviewer?sid=3f5d1210-08cd-4bbd-8e84-4055ca468dd3%40sessionmgr4008&vid=1&hid=4205.

Welch, J. 2003 Ritual in western medicine and its role in placebo healing. *Journal of Religion and Health* 42(1):21–33.

Wen, M., Hawkley, L., and Cacioppo, J. 2007 Objective and perceived neighborhood environment, individual SES and psychosocial factors, and self-rated health: An analysis of older adults in Cook County, Illinois. *Social Science and Medicine* 63(10):2575–2590.

Wenner, D. 2016 Penn State-Hershey teaches docs to be "change agents" for patients. *Pennlive*. Retrieved from www.pennlive.com/news/2016/03/ama_medical_school_reform_penn.html.

Wessel, D. 2012 Big U.S. firms shift hiring abroad. *Wall Street Journal*. Retrieved from https://www.wsj.com/articles/SB10001424052748704821704576270783611823972.

West, C., Dyrbye, L., Erwin, P., and Shanafelt, T. 2016 Interventions to prevent and reduce physician burnout: A systematic review and meta-analysis. *Lancet* 399(10052). Retrieved from doi:http://dx.doi.org/10.1016/S0140-6736(16)31279-X.

Wexner, L. 1954 The degree to which color (hues) are associated with mood tones. *Journal of Applied Psychology* 38:432–435.

Whitehead M. 1990 *The Concepts and Principles of Equity and Health*. Copenhagen: World Health Organization.

Wiesel, E. 1993 Elie Wiesel's remarks at the dedication ceremonies for the United States Holocaust Memorial Museum. Retrieved from https://www.ushmm.org/research/ask-a-research-question/frequently-asked-questions/wiesel.

Wilkinson, R. and Marmot, M., eds. 1998 *Social Determinants of Health: The Solid Facts*. Copenhagen: World Health Organization.

Wilkinson, R. and Marmot, M., eds. 2003 *The Solid Facts*, 2nd ed. Geneva: World Health Organization.

Wilkinson, R. and Pickett, K. 2011 *The Spirit Level: Why Greater Equality Makes Societies Stronger*. New York: Bloomfield Press.

Williams, J. 2005 Advertising of food and beverage products to children, teen, and adult multicultural markets. Working paper. Austin: University of Texas.

Williams, J. 2013 What happens when a town's only hospital shuts down? *U.S. News*. Retrieved from http://health.usnews.com/health-news/hospital-of-tomorrow/articles/2013/11/08/what-happens-when-the-only-hospital-closes.

Wilper, A., Woolhandler, S., Lasser, K., McCormick, D., Bor, D., and Himmelstein, D. 2009 Health insurance and mortality in US adults. *American Journal of Public Health* 99:2289–2295.

Wimer, C., Fox, L., Garfunkel, I., Kaushal, N., and Waldfogel, J. 2013 Trends in poverty with anchored supplemental poverty measures. Columbia Population Research Center. Retrieved from https://courseworks.columbia.edu/access/content/group/c5a1ef92-c03c-4d88-0018-ea43dd3cc5db/Working%20Papers%20for%20website/Anchored%20SPM.December7.pdf.

Winship, M. 2016 The Democrats ignore the 500-pound lobbyist in the room. *TruthOut*. Retrieved from www.truth-out.org/news/item/36745-the-democrats-ignore-the-500-pound-lobbyist-in-the-room.

Winter, D. and Leighton, D. 2001 Introduction to structural violence. In: Christie, D., Wagner, R. and Winter, D., eds. *Peace, Conflict, and Violence: Peace Psychology for the 21st Century*. Englewood Cliffs, NJ: Prentice-Hall, p. 203.

Wirt, J., Rooney, P., Choy, S., Provasnik, S., Sen, A., and Tobin, R. 2004 *The Condition of Education 2004* (NCES 2004-077). Washington, DC: National Center for Educational Statistics, Institute of Education Sciences.

Woods, L. 2016 Dr. Bruce Gould named medical director at Community Health Center Association of Connecticut. *UConn Today*. Retrieved from http://today.uconn.edu/school-stories/dr-bruce-gould-named-medical-director-at-community-health-center-association-of-connecticut/.

Woolhandler, S. and Himmelstein, D. 1991 The deteriorating administrative efficiency of the U.S. health care system. *New England Journal of Medicine* 324:1253–1258.

Working America 2010 Sending jobs overseas: The cost to America's economy and working families. Cornell University Digital Commons. Retrieved from http://digitalcommons.ilr.cornell.edu/cgi/viewcontent.cgi?article=1023&context=laborunions.

World Health Organization 2001 *The Optimal Duration of Exclusive Breastfeeding: A Systematic Review*. Geneva: World Health Organization.

World Health Organization 2011 Homicide, suicide, and unintentional firearm fatality: Comparing the United States with other high-income countries, 2003. *Journal of Trauma and Acute Care Surgery* 70(1):238–243.

World Health Organization 2015 *Guidelines: Sugar Intake for Adults and Children*. Geneva: WHO.

World Health Organization 2016 *International Classification of Diseases (ICD)*. Retrieved from www.who.int/classifications/icd/en/.

World Health Organization and Pan American Health Organization 2001 *Guiding Principles for Complementary Feeding of the Breastfed Child*. Washington, DC: WHO.

Wright, S. 1996 Examining what residents look for in their role models. *Academic Medicine* 71:290–292.

Wright, S., Wong, A., and Newill, C. 1997 The impact of role models on medical students. *Journal of General Internal Medicine* 12:53–56.

Yerramilli, P. 2014 How medical students can change the culture of medicine. *Kevinmd.com*. Retrieved by www.kevinmd.com/blog/2014/12/medical-students-can-change-culture-medicine.html.

Yildirim, K., Akalin-Baskaya, A., and Hidayetoglu, M. 2007 Effects of indoor color on mood and cognitive performance. *Building and Environment* 42(9):3233–3240.

Zajonc, R. 2000 Feeling and thinking: Closing the debate over the independence of affect. In: Forgas J. (Ed.) *Feeling and Thinking: The Role of Affect in Social Cognition. Studies in Emotion and Social Interaction*, pp. 31–58. New York: Cambridge University Press.

Zeldin, C. and Rukavina, M. 2007 *Borrowing to Stay Healthy: How Credit Card Debt Is Related to Medical Expenses*. Boston, MA: The Access Project.

Zigon, J. 2007 Moral breakdown and the ethical demand: A theoretical framework for an anthropology of moralities. *Anthropological Theory* 7(2):131–150.

Zigon, J. and Throop, C. 2014 Moral experience: Introduction. *Ethos* 42(1):1–15.

Zipkin, D. and Steinman, M. 2005 Interactions between pharmaceutical representatives and doctors in training: A thematic review. *Journal of General Internal Medicine* 20(8): 777–780.

INDEX

www.ingramcontent.com/pod-product-compliance
Lightning Source LLC
LaVergne TN
LVHW021125300926
849160LV00010B/861
* 9 7 8 1 6 2 9 5 8 4 2 6 3 *